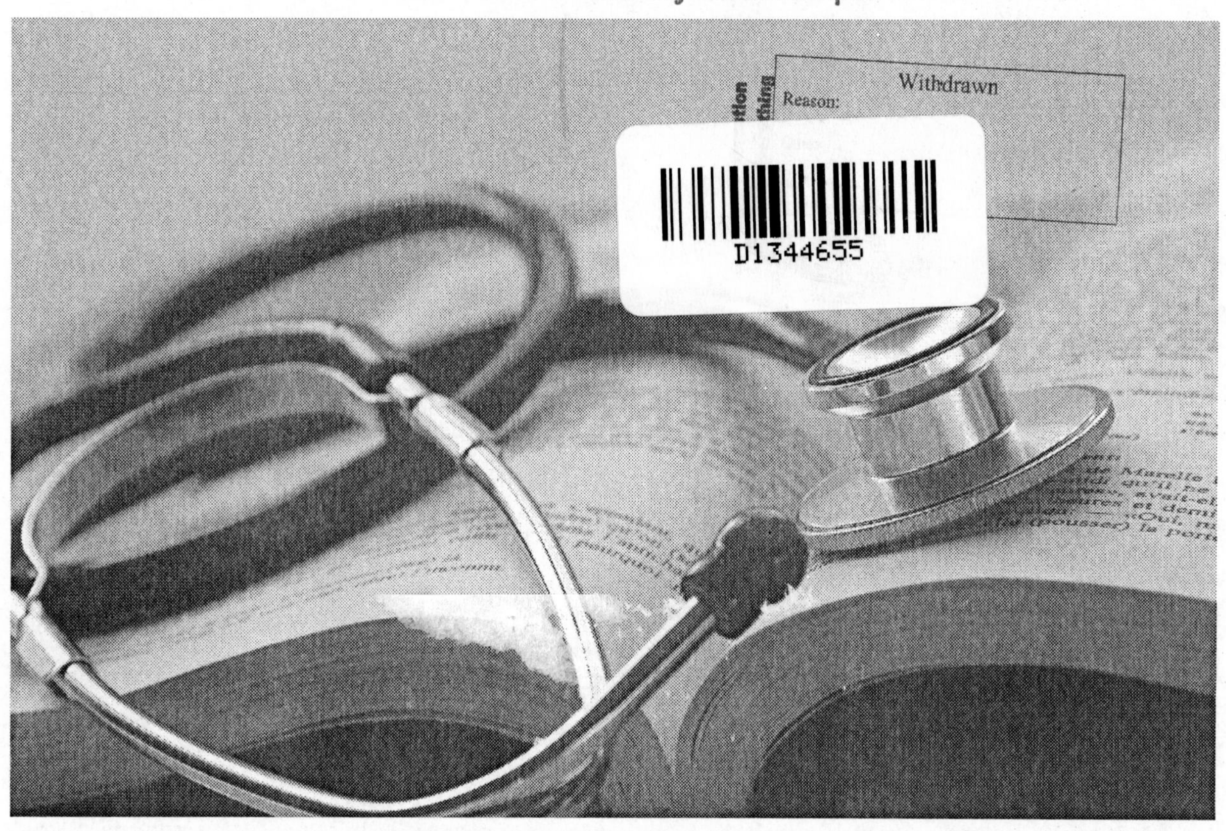

Succeeding in your Medical School Finals: Instant Revision Notes

Edited by
Alexander Young & William Dougal

BPP
LEARNING MEDIA

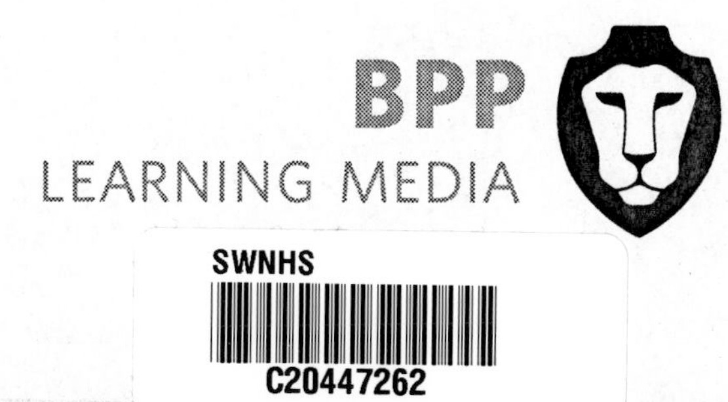

First edition December 2012

ISBN 9781 4453 8168 8
e-ISBN 9781 4453 9392 6

British Library Cataloguing-in-Publication Data
A catalogue record for this book is available from the British Library

Published by
BPP Learning Media Ltd
BPP House, Aldine Place
London W12 8AA

www.bpp.com/health

Printed in the United Kingdom by
Ricoh
Ricoh House
Ullswater Crescent
Coulsdon
CR5 2HR

Your learning materials, published by BPP Learning Media Ltd, are printed on paper sourced from sustainable, managed forests.

A note about copyright

Dear Customer

What does the little © mean and why does it matter?

Your market-leading BPP books, course materials and e-learning materials do not write and update themselves. People write them on their own behalf or as employees of an organisation that invests in this activity. Copyright law protects their livelihoods. It does so by creating rights over the use of the content.

Breach of copyright is a form of theft – as well as being a criminal offence in some jurisdictions, it is potentially a serious beach of professional ethics.

With current technology, things might seem a bit hazy but, basically, without the express permission of BPP Learning Media:

- Photocopying our materials is a breach of copyright
- Scanning, ripcasting or conversion of our digital materials into different file formats, uploading them to facebook or e-mailing them to your friends is a breach of copyright

You can, of course, sell your books, in the form in which you have bought them – once you have finished with them. (Is this fair to your fellow students? We update for a reason.) But the e-products are sold on a single user license basis: we do not supply 'unlock' codes to people who have bought them secondhand.

And what about outside the UK? BPP Learning Media strives to make our materials available at prices students can afford by local printing arrangements, pricing policies and partnerships which are clearly listed on our website. A tiny minority ignore this and indulge in criminal activity by illegally photocopying our material or supporting organisations that do. If they act illegally and unethically in one area, can you really trust them?

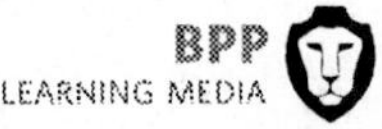

Contents

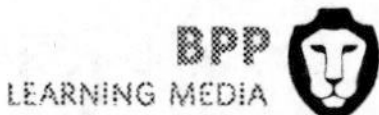

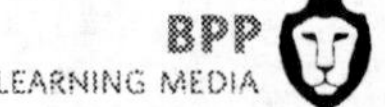
BPP
LEARNING MEDIA

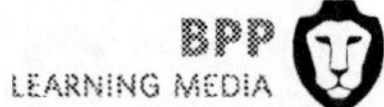

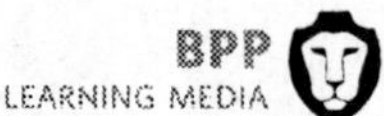
BPP
LEARNING MEDIA

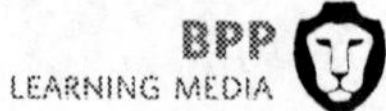
BPP
LEARNING MEDIA

About the Publisher

BPP Learning Media is dedicated to supporting aspiring professionals with top quality learning material. BPP Learning Media's commitment to success is shown by our record of quality, innovation and market leadership in paper-based and e-learning materials. BPP Learning Media's study materials are written by professionally-qualified specialists who know from personal experience the importance of top quality materials for success.

Every effort has been made to ensure the accuracy of the material contained within this guide. However it must be noted that medical treatments, drug dosages/formulations, equipment, procedures and best practice are currently evolving within the field of medicine.

Readers are therefore advised always to check the most up-to-date information relating to:

- The applicable drug manufacturer's product information and data sheets relating to recommended dose/formulation, administration and contraindications.
- The latest applicable local and national guidelines.
- The latest applicable local and national codes of conduct and safety protocols.

It is the responsibility of the practitioner, based on their own knowledge and expertise, to diagnose, treat and ensure the safety and best interests of the patient are maintained.

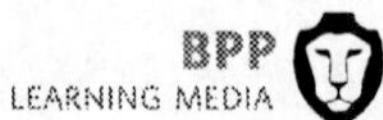

About the Editors

Alexander Young MBChB MSc MRCS

Alexander is a Core Surgical Trainee in Trauma and Orthopaedic Surgery in Bristol. He has over ten publications in various medical journals together with a certificate in medical education. Outside of medicine he plays football for a non-league side five divisions below the Football Conference and is a keen marathon runner. He is the founder of Future Orthopaedic Surgeons and a member of the Royal Society of Medicine.

William Dougal MBChB (Hons)

William is a Foundation Year 1 doctor with an Honours degree in Medicine from the University of Bristol. He is keen on a career in General Practice or Emergency Medicine. He plays football for a local Bristol team and writes for the University of Bristol Student Newspaper, *The Epigram*.

List of Contributors

Dr Richard Bond MBBS MRCP
Specialist Registrar Cardiology, Severn Deanery, UK

Dr Dan Bromage MBChB MRCP
Specialist Registrar Cardiology, Severn Deanery, UK

Dr Krishnaraj Sinhji Rathod MRCP
Specialist Registrar, Cardiology, Severn Deanery, UK

Dr Raveen Kandan MRCP
Specialist Registrar Cardiology, Royal United Hospital, Bath, UK

Dr Philip Mitchelmore MBChB MRCP
Specialist Registrar Respiratory, Musgrove Park Hospital Taunton, UK

Dr Rahul Shrimanker MBChb MRCP
Specialist Registrar Respiratory, Musgrove Park Hospital Taunton, UK

Dr Utti Chelvaratnam MBChB MRCP
Specialist Registrar Gastroenterology, Severn Deanery, UK

Dr Barnaby Hole MBChB BSc (Hons) MRCP
Clinical Teaching Fellow, North Bristol NHS Trust, UK

Dr Duncan Whitehead MBBS FRCP
Consultant Physician Renal Medicine & Acute Care, Musgrove Park Hospital Taunton, UK

Dr Rajeev Raghavan MBChB MRCP
Specialist Registrar Endocrinology, Severn Deanery, UK

Dr Madhu Ramamoorthi MBChB MRCP
Specialist Registrar Neurology, Severn Deanery, UK

Dr Winifred French MBChB MRCP
Specialist Registrar Haematology, Musgrove Park Hospital, Taunton, UK

Dr David Veale MBChB MRCP
Specialist Registrar Haematology, Musgrove Park Hospital, Taunton, UK

Dr Mahdi Abusalameh MBChB MRCP
Specialist Registrar Rheumatology, Musgrove Park Hospital Taunton, UK

Dr Begoña Bovill MSc, FRCP
Consultant Physician Infectious Disease, Southmead Hospital, UK

Dr Daniel Newton MBChB
Core Medical Trainee, Gloucester Royal Hospital, UK

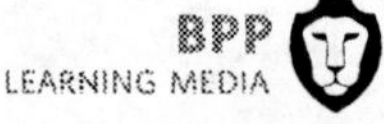

Mr John Loy MBChB MSc MRCS
Specialist Registrar General Surgery, Severn Deanery, UK

Miss Jane Carter, MB ChB, MRCS
Clinical Teaching Fellow, Gloucestershire Royal Hospital, UK

Miss Sarah Vestey, MD, FRCS
Consultant Breast & Oncoplastic Surgeon, Gloucestershire Royal Hopsital, UK

Mr Dermot Mallon MBChB BSc MSc MRCS DOHNS
Core Surgical Trainee, Oxford Deanery, UK

Mr John M Henderson BMBS BMedsci (Hons) MRCS (Eng)
Specialist Registrar Urology, Oxford Deanery, UK

Mr Joseph G Manjaly BSc (Hons) MBChB MRCS DOHNS
Core Surgical ENT Trainee, Wessex Deanery, UK

Mr Peter J Kullar MA MBChir MRCS DOHNS
Academic ENT Trainee, Northern Deanery, UK

Dr Jonathan A Dunne BSc (Hons) MBChB
Core Surgical Trainee (Plastic Surgery), Yorkshire Deanery, UK

Mr Jeremy M Rawlins MBChB (Hons) MPhil FRCS (Plast)
Consultant Plastic, Reconstructive and Burns Surgeon, Wakefield, UK

Mr Samuel Carter Jonas MBChB BSc MRCS
Core Surgical Trainee (Orthopaedic Surgery), Gloucester Royal Hospital, UK

Dr Tom Teare MBChB MRCP
Specialist Trainee ACCS, Severn Deanery, UK

Dr Tara Bader MBChB (Hons) BSc (Hons)
Core Trainee (Ophthalmology), Severn Deanery, UK

Dr Sarah Blackstock MBChB
Core Trainee Paediatrics, London, UK

Dr Sarah Bird MBChB
Core Trainee Paediatrics, London, UK

Dr Philip Brooks MBChB
Specialist Registrar Psychiatry, London, UK

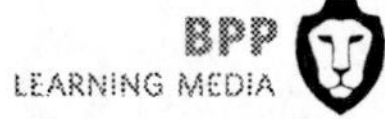

Acknowledgements

The authors would like to thank everyone at BPP for their help with the text, in particular Matt Green and Jennifer Brookbanks. The authors would also like to thanks their families and the contributors for their help and support with the text.

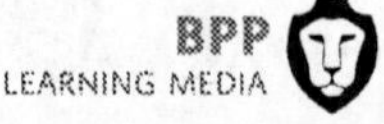

Abbreviations

AAA	Abdominal aortic aneurysm
Ab	Antibody
ABC	Airway, breathing, circulation
ABG	Arterial blood gas
ABPI	Ankle brachial pressure index
ACE	Angiotensin-converting enzyme
ACh	Acetylcholine
AChE	Acetylcholinesterase
ACTH	Adrenocorticotrophic hormone
ADH	Antidiuretic hormone
ADLs	Activities of daily living
ADP	Adenosine diphosphate
AIDS	Acquired immunodeficiency syndrome
ALT	Alanine aminotransferase
ANP	Atrial natriuretic peptide
ANS	Autonomic nervous system
APTT	Activated partial thromboplastin time
ARDS	Adult respiratory distress syndrome
ASD	Atrioseptal defect
AST	Aspartate aminotransferase
ATLS	Advanced trauma and life support
ATP	Adenosine triphosphate
AV	Atrioventricular
AVP	Arginine vasopressin
BCG	Bacille Calmette-Guérin
BMR	Basal metabolic rate
BP	Blood pressure
CABG	Coronary artery bypass grafting
cAMP	Cyclic adenosine monophosphate
CCF	Congestive cardiac failure
CCK	Cholecystokinin
CNS	Central nervous system
CO	Cardiac output
COPD	Chronic obstructive pulmonary disease

CPAP	Continuous positive airway pressure
CRP	C-reactive protein
CSF	Cerebrospinal fluid
CVA/E	Cerebrovascular accident /event
CVP	Central venous pressure
DCT	Distal convoluted tubule
DHEA	Dehydroepiandrosterone
DVT	Deep vein thrombosis
ECF	Extracellular fluid
ECG/EKG	Electrocardiogram
ERV	Expiratory reserve volume
ESR	Erythrocyte sedimentation rate
FBC	Full blood count
FiO_2	Fraction of inspired oxygen
FEV	Forced expiratory volume
FFA	Free fatty acid
FOB	Faecal occult blood
FRC	Functional residual capacity
FVC	Force vital capacity
GCS	Glasgow coma scale
GFR	Glomerular filtration rate
HCT	Haematocrit
ICF	Intracellular fluid
ICU	Intensive care unit
IDDM	Insulin dependent diabetes mellitus
IPSP	Inhibitory postsynaptic potential
IRV	Inspiratory reserve volume
IVC	Inferior vena cava
IVDU	Intravenous drug user
JVP	Jugular venous pressure
KUB	Kidney, ureter, bladder
LFT	Liver function test
LVF	Left ventricular failure
MAP	Mean arterial pressure

MEN	Multiple endocrine neoplasia
MI	Myocardial infarction
NIDDM	Non-insulin dependent diabetes mellitus
NO	Nitric oxide
PCT	Proximal convoluted tubule
PDGF	Platelet-derived growth factor
PND	Paroxysmal nocturnal dyspnoea
PNS	Parasympathetic nervous system
PT	Prothrombin time
PVR	Pulmonary vascular resistance
R-A-A	Renin-angiotensin-aldosterone
RV	Residual volume
RVF	Right ventricular failure
SA	Sinoatrial
SIADH	Syndrome of inappropriate ADH
SLE	Systemic lupus erythematosus
SNS	Sympathetic nervous system
SVC	Superior vena cava
TLC	Total lung capacity
TLV	Total lung volume
TSH	Thyroid-stimulating hormone
TV	Tidal volume
U&Es	Urea & electrolytes
VC	Vital capacity
V/Q	Ventilation/perfusion ratio
VSD	Ventriculoseptal defect
WCC	White cell count

How to Use this Book

Medical school finals can be an extremely daunting time with students expected to revise the entire medical curriculum prior to sitting both written and OSCE examinations.

This book is designed as a quick reference guide and is best used in conjunction with online question banks and self-test questions provided to consolidate learning. The mnemonics, boxes, tables and figures have all been handpicked based on learning principles and topics are given appropriate weighting in the book as they appear in finals examination.

The single best answer and extended matching questions are all based on questions previously seen in finals examinations.

Readers are encouraged to annotate the text with information collected from course notes, online questions and other resourses to personalise the test for examinations at your medical school.

Instant Revision Notes for Medical Finals utilises the mnemonic PASSIT CP as a succinct aide memoire to facilitate learning and recall of the salient points for each topic examined in medical school finals.

This framework is used throughout the book with some minor alterations when topics do not fit directly into each sub-heading.

List of Icons: PASSIT CP

P	Pathology
A	Aetiology
S	Signs
Sx	Symptoms
I	Investigations
T	Treatment
C	Complications
Pr	Prognosis

We hope that the book serves you well for both your final examinations and beyond.

Good Luck.

Normal Reference Values

Hb	Male 13.5–18.0 g/dl
	Female 11.5–16.0 g/dl
MCV	76–96 fL
PLTs	150–400 × 10^9 / uL
WCC	4.5–11.0 × 10^9/uL
Neutrophils	2.0–7.5 × 10^9/L
Lymphocytes	1.3–3.5 × 10^9/L
Eosinophils	0.04–0.44 × 10^9/L
Basophils	0.0–0.10 × 10^9/L
Na	135–145 mmol/L
K	3.5–5.1 mmol/L
Urea	2.5–6.7 mmol/L
Creat	70–150 μmol/L
eGFR	>90
Billirubin	3–17 μmol/L
ALT	5–35 iU/L
ALP	30–150 iU/L
AST	5–35 iU/L
Albumin	35–50 g/L

Chapter 1

Cardiology

Dr Richard Bond, Dr Raveen Kandan, Dr Krishnaraj Sinhji Rathod and Dr Dan Bromage

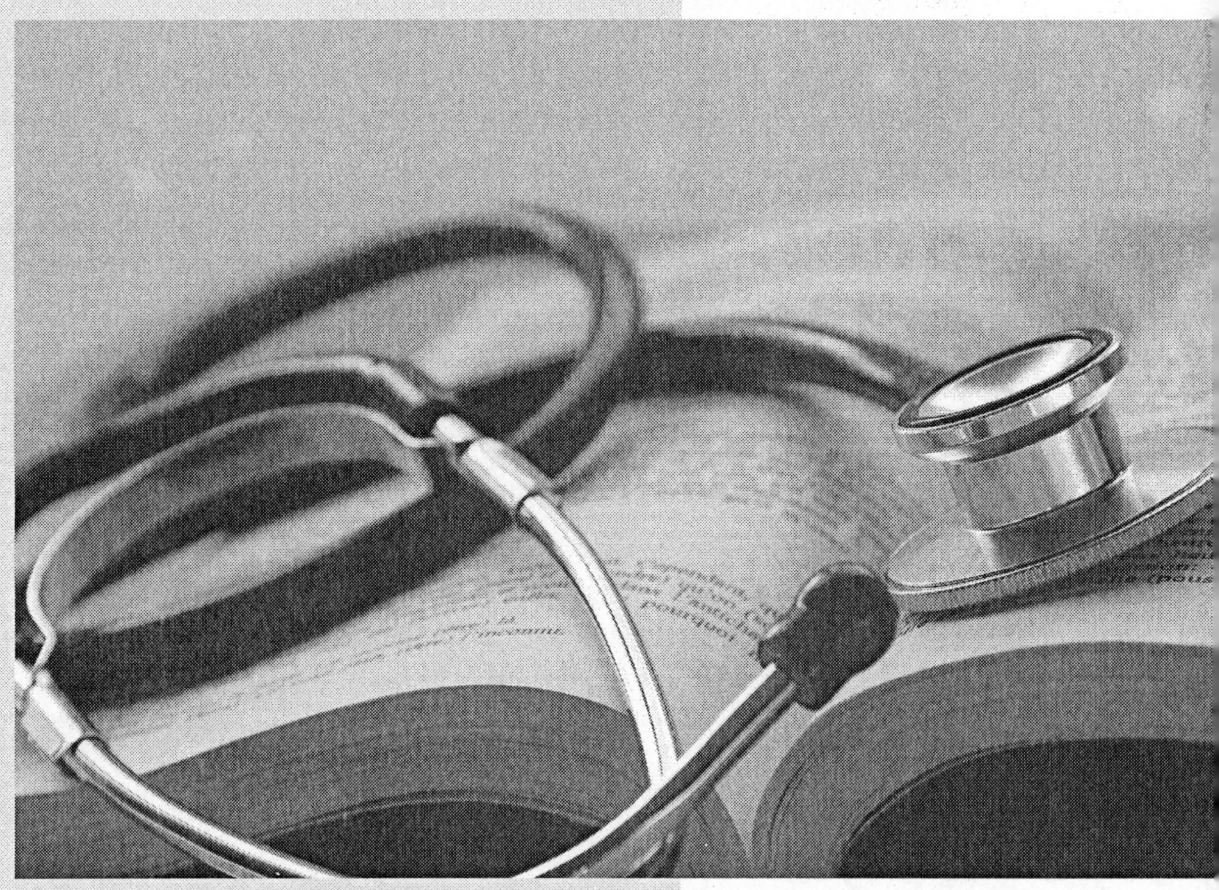

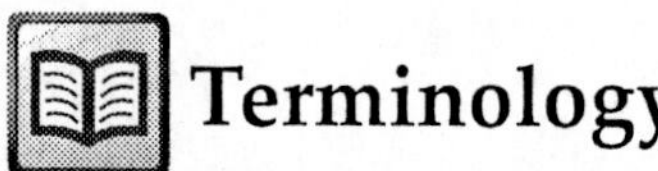

Terminology

- **ECG**: electrocardiogram, electrical tracing of the heart
- **ECHO**: trans oesophageal (TTO) or trans thoracic (TTE) sonogram of the heart
- **Holter monitor**: 24-hour ECG recorder
- **ICD**: implantable cardioverter defibrillator
- **LAE**: left atrial enlargement
- **LVH**: left ventricular hypertrophy
- **PPM**: permanent pacemaker
- **RAE**: right atrial enlargement
- **RVH**: right ventricular hypertrophy
- **TPW**: temporary pacing wire

Angina and Acute Coronary Syndromes (ACS)

Stable angina

P Pain caused by myocardial ischaemia when myocardial oxygen demand exceeds supply.

A Usually coronary stenosis due to atheroma, but can result from anything that causes demand-supply mismatch including tachycardia, anaemia, left ventricular hypertrophy, aortic stenosis, and hypotension.

S Patients usually identify ischaemic pain with an open palm or fist over the centre of the chest (Levine's sign), rather than by pointing.

Sx Central chest heaviness or tightness precipitated by exertion or emotional stress and relieved by rest.

Heavy arms, nausea, fatigue, breathlessness.

I FBC, U&E, lipid profile, blood glucose, 12-lead ECG, exercise tolerance test, stress echocardiogram, myocardial perfusion scan, cardiac magnetic resonance imaging, coronary CT, coronary angiography.

T Lifestyle adjustment, reverse precipitants, aspirin, anti-anginals (nitrates, nicorandil, β-receptor antagonists, calcium antagonists), aggressive risk factor control, including tight control of hypertension, hyperlipidaemia and diabetes.

C Acute coronary syndromes, arrhythmias, heart failure.

Pr Clinical trial data estimate an annual risk of non-fatal MI and mortality of 9–14% and 5–26% respectively.

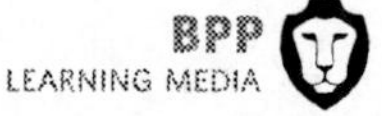

Acute coronary syndromes

Unstable angina / Non-ST elevation MI (NSTEMI)

P Part of the acute coronary syndrome spectrum of conditions that result from acute myocardial ischaemia.

A Atheromatous plaque rupture and partial luminal obstruction by thrombus.

S Levine's sign, diaphoresis, dyspnoea.

Sx Central chest heaviness or tightness, leaden arms, nausea, and breathlessness, although beware 'atypical' presentations. Symptoms may occur with increasing frequency or severity, at rest or at a lower threshold, escape the control of anti-anginals, or be new onset and severe.

I FBC, U&E, lipid profile, blood glucose, serial biochemical markers of myocardial injury (their presence indicates NSTEMI while their absence indicates unstable angina), ECG monitoring, 12-lead ECG within ten minutes (transient or permanent ST depression or T wave inversion (see Figure 1.1), (however normal ECG does not exclude the diagnosis), portable CXR, echocardiogram, risk stratification (see Box 1.1), early coronary angiography.

T Bed rest, analgesia and oxygen as required, nitrates, β-receptor antagonists (± cautious diltiazem), aspirin, thienopyridine (clopidogrel or prasugrel), (low molecular weight) heparin, glycoprotein IIb/IIIa receptor antagonists (tirofiban), coronary angioplasty or surgery, secondary prevention (including a statin and ACE inhibitor).

C Progression to Q wave (transmural) infarct, arrhythmias, LV failure, sudden death, RV failure, pericarditis, systemic embolism of mural thrombus, pulmonary embolism, mitral regurgitation, Dressler's syndrome, depression and anxiety.

Pr Hospital mortality in NSTEMI is 3–5%, and 13% at six months. Unstable angina/ NSTEMI associated with high incidence of late events (30% rate of death, MI and refractory angina at six months in PRAIS-UK study).

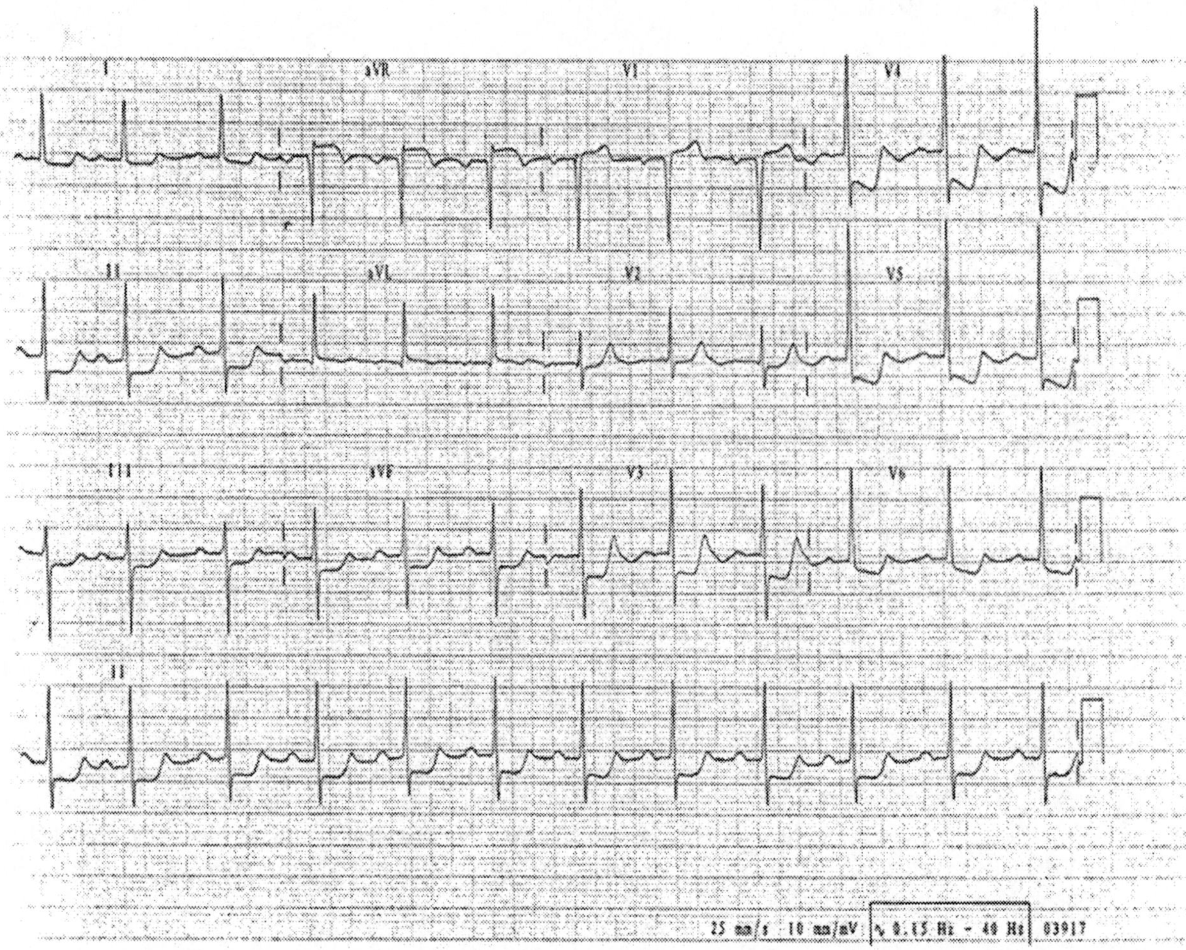

Figure 1.1: Acute myocardial ischaemia. (Reproduced with permission from SW Deanery.)

TIMI risk score	GRACE score
• Age ≥65 years	• Age
• ≥3 risk factors for CAD	• Heart rate
• Known CAD (≥50% stenosis)	• Systolic BP
• ST deviation ≥05 mm	• Serum creatinine
• ≥2 episodes of angina in last 24 hours	• Killip class
• Aspirin use in last 7 days	• Cardiac arrest at admission
• Raised cardiac markers	• Elevated cardiac markers
	• ST-segment deviation

Box 1.1: Examples of risk stratification scores

ST-segment elevation MI (STEMI)

P Part of the acute coronary syndrome spectrum of conditions that result from acute myocardial ischaemia.

A Atheromatous plaque rupture and total luminal obstruction by thrombus, results in transmural (Q wave) infarction.

S Levine's sign, diaphoresis, and dyspnoea.

Sx Central chest heaviness or tightness, leaden arms, nausea, and breathlessness, although beware 'atypical' presentations (including back pain, syncope, shock, acute pulmonary oedema, and many more, especially in the elderly and diabetics (so-called 'silent' infarcts)).

Pain may be more severe, more persistent and cause more distress than angina. Not relieved by GTN.

I Diagnosis is made on the basis of history and 12-lead ECG (ST-segment elevation (see Figure 1.2) or new LBBB).

Do not delay reperfusion therapy to wait for investigations: FBC, U&E, lipid profile, blood glucose, serial biochemical markers of myocardial injury, ECG monitoring, portable CXR ECHO.

T Stabilise in a high-dependency area, IV access, diamorphine, antiemetic, oxygen, nitrates, aspirin and a thienopyridine (follow local protocols).

The priority of management is early reperfusion.

The gold standard is primary percutaneous coronary intervention.

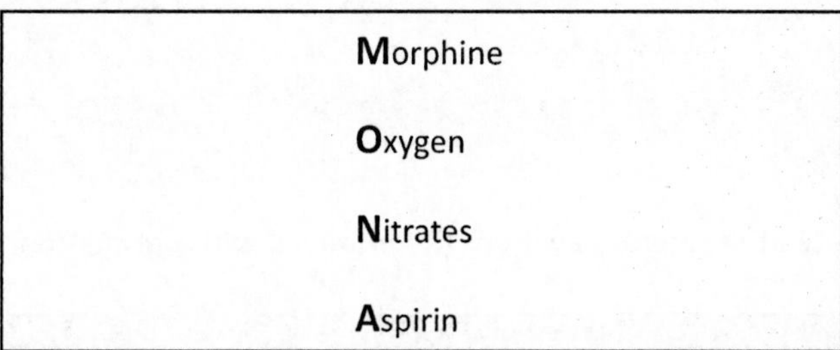

Box 1.2: Mnemonic for the initial management of acute myocardial infarction

C Arrhythmias, LV failure, sudden death, fever, RV failure, pericarditis, systemic embolism of mural thrombus, pulmonary embolism, tamponade, mitral regurgitation, ventricular septal defect, LV aneurysm, Dressler's syndrome, depression and anxiety.

Pr Prognosis with STEMI is better than NSTEMI and continues to fall, 50% of patients who die from acute MI do so in the first two hours (highlighting the importance of early reperfusion).

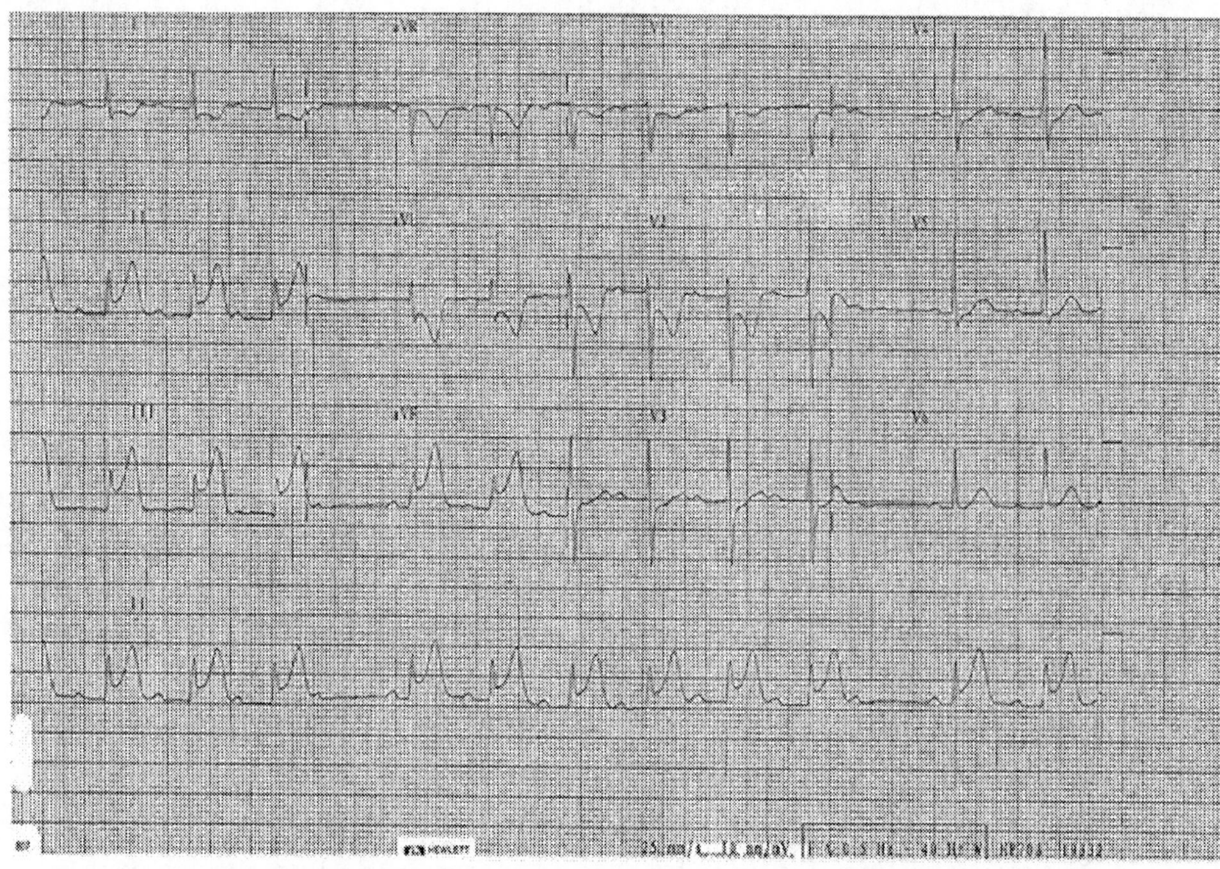

Figure 1.2: Acute ST-segment elevation. (Reproduced with permission from SW Deanery.)

Indications	Absolute contraindications
• Typical-sounding chest pain within 12 hours and ST-elevation within 2 contiguous leads (>2 mm V1-6 or >1 mm in limb leads) • Typical-sounding chest pain with new or presumed new LBBB	• Active uncontrollable bleeding, bleeding diathesis or warfarin therapy • Suspected aortic dissection • Previous haemorrhagic stroke • Recent head trauma or intracranial malignancy • Ischaemic stroke within past six months • Known allergy to thrombolytic • Trauma or surgery, including liver biopsy, dental extraction and lumbar puncture, within past month • Pregnancy or post-partum

Box 1.3: Thrombolysis

Arrhythmias

Tachycardias

Sinus tachycardia

P Tachycardia (rate >100) originating from sino-atrial node.

A Can be normal as a result of increased sympathetic drive ie exercise or anxiety.

Pathological conditions include infection/sepsis, hyperthyroidism, pulmonary embolism and phaeochromocytoma.

S Regular fast pulse.

Sx Usually asymptomatic, fast, regular palpitations.

I FBC, TFTs, ECG, 24-hour ECG/Holter monitor and 24-hour urinary collection for catecholamines.

T Treat underlying cause appropriately – reassurance.

C Complications are related to aetiology.

Pr Depends on aetiology, usually good.

Atrial fibrillation (AF)

P AF is the most common sustained cardiac arrhythmia.

During AF the atria contract at 400–600bpm, ventricular rate is determined by conduction through the atrio-ventricular node. It is classified as

- **Paroxysmal**: terminates spontaneously and lasts less than seven days
- **Persistent**: lasts more than seven days and is terminated by drug treatment or cardioversion
- **Permanent**: cannot restore sinus rhythm

AF is a major risk factor for stroke, low flow within the atria and atrial appendage leads to thrombus formation.

A See Box 1.4.

- AF is common in patients with structural heart disease
- Rheumatic valvular disease (remains a major aetiological factor in developing countries)
- Hypertension
- Ischaemic heart disease
- Congestive heart failure
- Valvular heart disease (mainly mitral stenosis)
- Diabetes mellitus
- Cigarette smoking
- Excessive alcohol consumption (>3drinks/day)
- Pulmonary diseases (COPD/PE)
- Cardiothoracic surgery
- Hyperthyroidism
- Lone AF

Box 1.4: Risk factors for AF

S Irregularly, irregular pulse which can be slow, fast or normal.

BP may be elevated, may present with signs of heart failure or stroke.

Sx Can be asymptomatic and picked up on routine screening.

Irregular fast palpitations, SOB, dizziness and decreased exercise tolerance.

I FBC, TFTs, BP, ECG (no visible P waves and irregularly irregular QRS complexes), Holter monitor, ECHO.

T Rate/rhythm control and anticoagulation.

Rate control: beta blockers, calcium blockers, digoxin or a combination.

Rhythm control: pharmacological (IV or PO) or electrical (DCCV) IV flecainide or amiodarone can be used to cardiovert AF of acute onset.

Antithrombotic: an individual patient's risk for embolisation must be considered and scores are available to calculate this (see Table 1.1). Warfarin, aspirin.

$CHADS_2$
CCF – 1pt
HYPERTENSION – 1pt
AGE (>75) – 1pt
DIABETES – 1pt
STROKE/TIA – 2pts
Stroke risk
0 = 1.9%
1 = 2.8%
2 = 4.0%
3 = 5.9%
4 = 8.5%
5 = 12.5%
6 = 18.2%
Score of 2+ indicates warfarin as anticoagulant of choice
Score of 1 – discuss risks and benefits of anticoagulation with patient

Table 1.1: Scores to calculate thromboembolic risk and bleeding risk in AF

Ablation: pulmonary vein isolation (PVI) or PPM in patients with severe symptoms and drug refractory AF.

C Stroke, TIA, impaired exercise capacity, heart failure and dementia.

Pr AF is associated with an increase in mortality.

Atrial flutter (AFL)

P The atria contract at approx 240–300bpm. The atrial impulses are usually conducted to the ventricles in a 2:1 manner resulting in a ventricular rate of approximately 150bpm.

A Similar to AF. AFL also develops around scar so is more common in patients who have had surgery involving the atria eg ASD closure/repair.

S Similar to AF however pulse is regular.

Sx Similar to AF, patients may complain of regular palpitations.

I ECG: typically has a saw-tooth pattern (see Figure 1.3).

T Rhythm control: DCCV, anti-arrhythmic drugs can terminate AFL however are less successful than in AF, pacing wire, AFL ablation, anticoagulation.

C Similar to AF.

Pr AFL leads to an increased mortality.

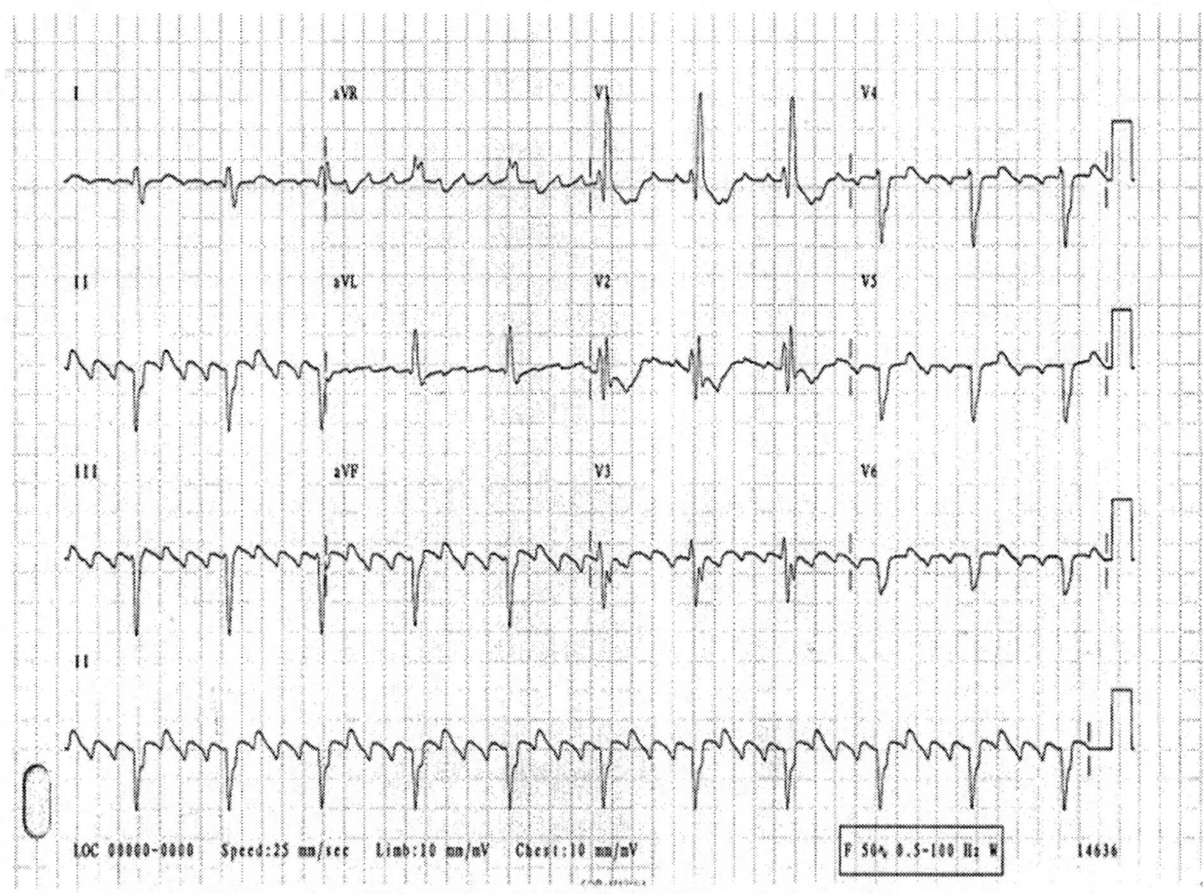

Figure 1.3: Atrial flutter: Note saw-tooth baseline.
Rate is approximately 75bpm so conduction through AV node is 4:1.
(Reproduced with permission from SW Deanery.)

Narrow complex tachycardia

P Narrow complex tachycardias or supraventricular tachycardias (SVTs) are divided into two main groups.

- Atrioventricular nodal re-entrant tachycardia (AVNRT): re-entrant circuits within the AV node (AVNRT)
- Atrioventricular re-entrant tachycardia (AVRT): dependent on an accessory pathway between the atria and ventricles (AVRT or Wolff-Parkinson-White syndrome/WPW).

A In AVNRT there is an extra pathway within or close to the AV node, usually presents in the late teens or early twenties, can be precipitated by stress, emotion, exertion, caffeine, alcohol, hyperthyroidism and electrolyte abnormalities.

In AVRT there is an accessory pathway between the atria and ventricles.

S Rapid regular pulse, BP may be low.

Sx Patients describe fast regular palpitations sometimes radiating into neck and ears, dizziness, pre-syncope or syncope.

I ECG: narrow complex tachycardia at approximately 200bpm (see Figure 1.4). ECG at rest is also important to assess for pre-excitation.

ECHO, Holter monitor.

T Vagal manoeuvres eg Valsalva, carotid sinus massage, ice cold drink IV adenosine (transiently blocks the AV node). DCCV, accessory pathway ablation.

C Sudden death in WPW occurs in approximately 0.4% of patients however if patients are symptomatic the risk is increased therefore ablation of the accessory pathway is the treatment of choice.

Pr Excellent when treated.

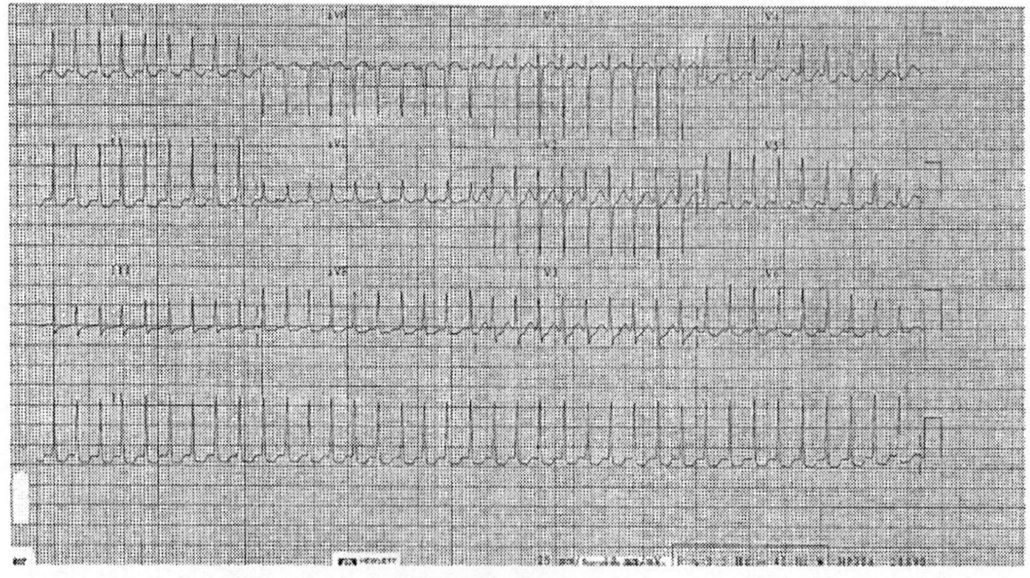

Figure 1.4: Narrow complex tachycardia. (Reproduced with permission from SW Deanery.)

Ventricular tachycardia (VT)

P Broad complex tachycardias are VT until proven otherwise.

Non sustained VT is defined as three continuous beats of ventricular ectopics for less than 30-seconds.

A Most VT is the result of damage to the myocardium (scar) and structural heart disease eg MI or cardiomyopathies.

Other causes of VT include the inherited channelopathies eg Brugada syndrome, arrythymogenic right ventricular cardiomyopathy (ARVC) and long QT syndrome.

S If the patient makes it to hospital – some can be minimally symptomatic whereas others will present with cardiogenic shock.

Sx Pre-syncope, syncope, SOB, chest pain, palpitations.

I ECG: see Figure 1.5.

ECHO.

Diagnostic coronary angiography +/- PCI.

Cardiac MRI can be useful when the cause is unclear.

- Regular rhythm
- Broad complexes
- Capture or fusion beats
- Concordance across chest leads
- AV dissociation

Box 1.5: ECG characteristics of monomorphic VT. (Reproduced with permission from SW Deanery.)

T Acute: this is a medical emergency.

Pulseless VT is a cardiac arrest and should be treated with DCCV as per ALS guidelines.

Long term: amiodarone.

Beta blockers, sotalol and mexilitine can also be tried.

ICD implantation.

C Death, injuries from syncope, side effects of drug treatment especially amiodarone, inappropriate shock therapy from ICD.

Pr Prognosis without treatment is poor, treatment with an ICD improves prognosis but the mortality rate is still significant when compared to a normal population.

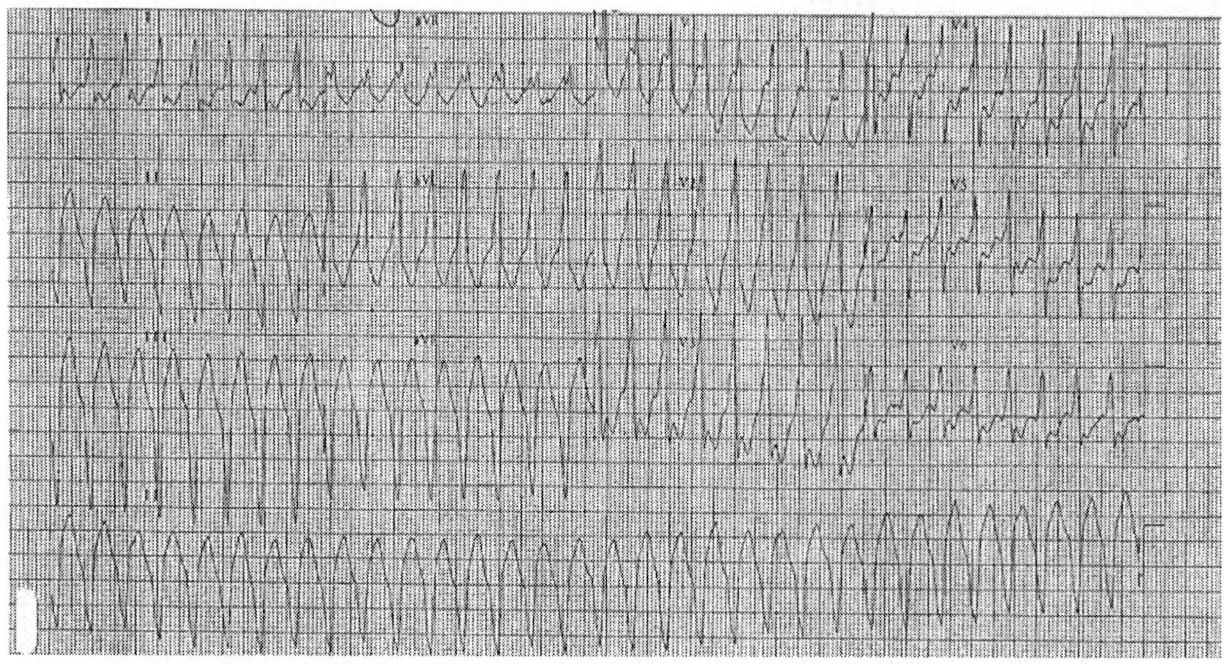

Figure 1.5: Monomorphic VT. Note broad complexes at 192bpm. Extreme left axis deviation. Concordance across chest leads. No clear P waves. (Reproduced with permission from SW Deanery.)

Bradycardias

Sinus bradycardia

P Sinus rhythm at a rate <60bpm.

A Can be normal, as in athletes or during sleep, or secondary to drug therapy (eg beta blockers, digoxin, calcium channel blockers and anti-arrhythmics), MI, sick sinus syndrome, hypothyroidism and hypothermia.

S Slow regular pulse.

Sx In non-pathological conditions patients are asymptomatic.

Symptomatic patients complain of SOB, pre-syncope, syncope, chest pain.

I Full drug history, FBC, TFTs, digoxin levels, ECG, Holter monitor.

T IV atropine, temporary pacing wire, permanent pacemaker.

Beta blocker overdose: Glucagon.

Digoxin toxicity: Digibind.

C Usually none.

Pr Usually good.

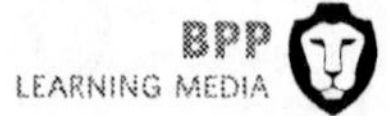

Heart block

1st degree

P Decrease in conduction of impulse from atria to ventricles through AV node.

Manifested as a prolonged PR interval (>0.2s) on ECG.

A Drug therapy eg beta blockade, fibrosis of conductive tissue, lyme disease, acute rheumatic fever, aortic valve disease sarcoidosis, myocarditis, MI, idiopathic.

S None.

Sx Usually none.

I ECG: see Figure 1.6.

T None required.

C None.

Pr Good

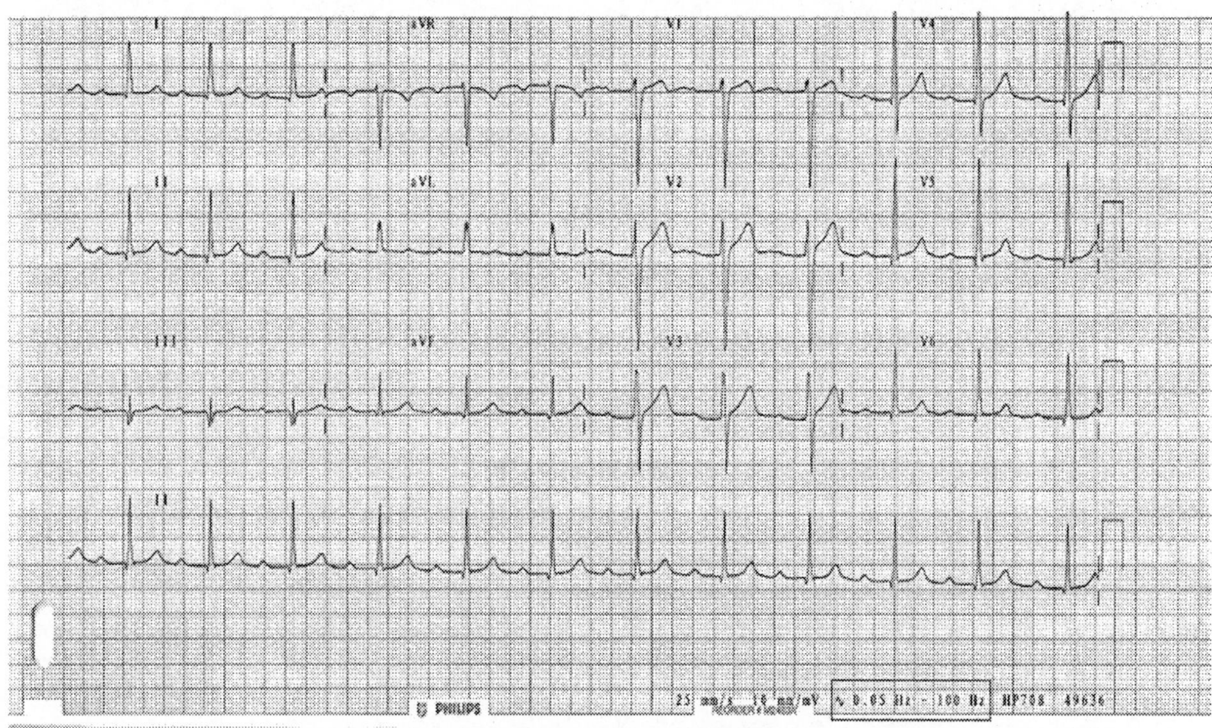

Figure 1.6: 1st degree heart block with PR interval of 292ms. (Reproduced with permission from SW Deanery.)

2nd degree

P Intermittent failure of atrial impulse to be conducted to ventricles through AV node and His bundle, subdivided into Mobitz type 1 (Wenckebach) or Mobitz type 2.

- *Mobitz type 1*: delay in AV conduction progressively increases until an impulse is not conducted, on the ECG the PR interval gets longer and longer until there is a dropped beat
- *Mobitz type 2*: intermittent failure of conduction of the atrial impulse to the ventricles usually in a 2:1 ratio, the PR interval does not lengthen

A Mobitz type 1 can be due to increased vagal tone and often occurs during sleep. Mobitz type 2 is always pathological and has a similar aetiology to 1st degree AV block.

S Bradycardia, hypotension.

Sx Can be asymptomatic, SOB, chest pain, pre-syncope/syncope.

I Full drug history.

ECG: see Figures 1.7 and 1.8, Holter monitor.

ECHO: if LV function is also impaired then the patient may benefit from CRT rather than a normal PPM.

T Stop offending medications. A TPW may be required, Mobitz type 2 always requires a permanent pacemaker.

C Death, injuries from syncope.

Pr Both Mobitz type 1 and 2 can progress to complete heart block and mortality is increased.

Prognosis is good following PPM implantation.

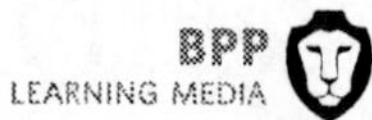

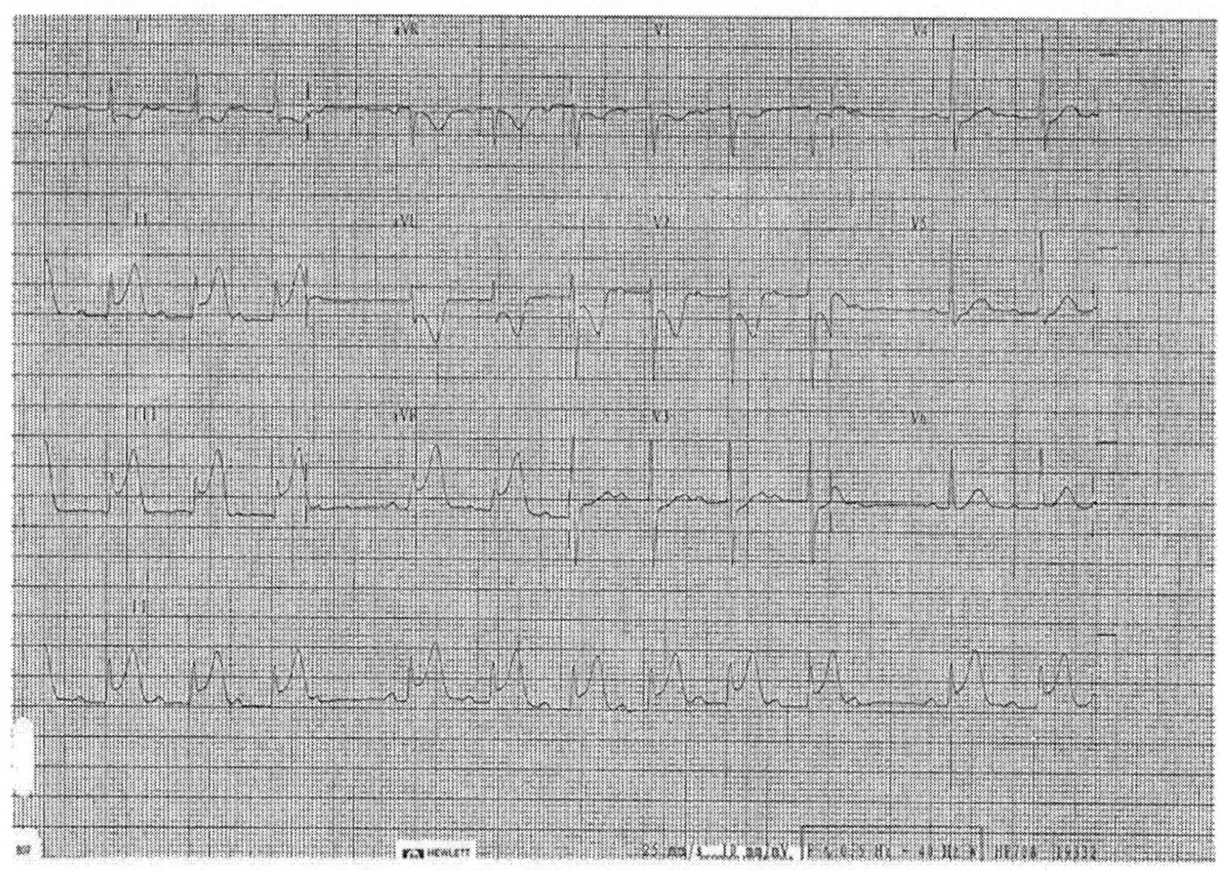

Figure 1.7: Mobitz type 1 in a patient with inferior STEMI. (Reproduced with permission from SW Deanery.)

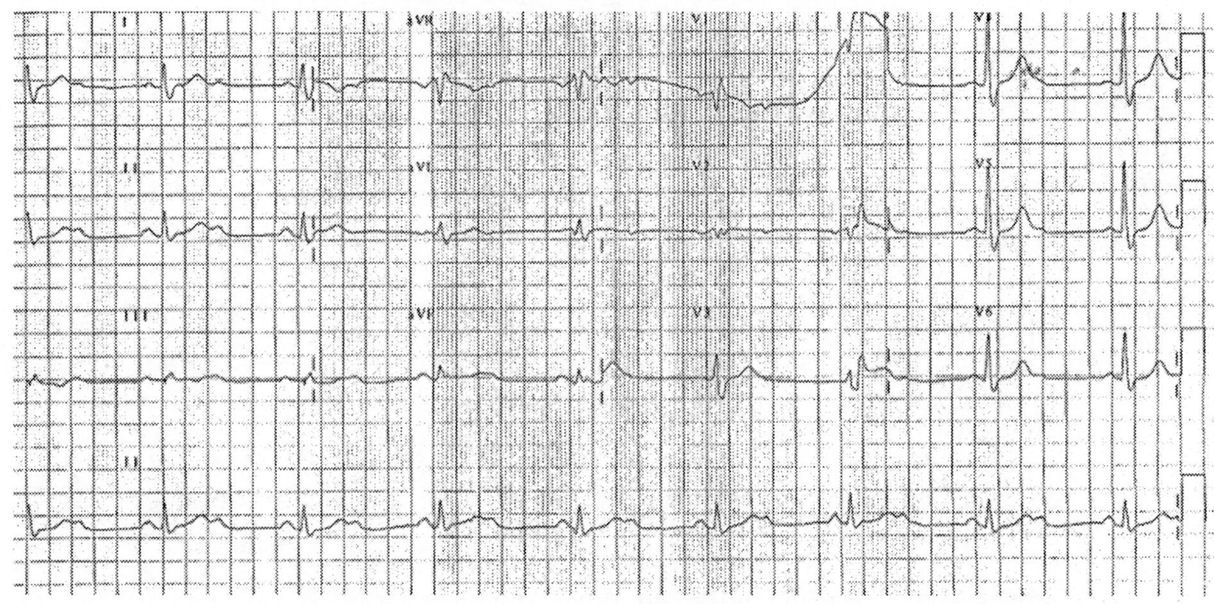

Figure 1.8: Mobitz type 2 AV block. Note P wave at end of T wave and regular PR interval prior to QRS complex. (Reproduced with permission from SW Deanery.)

3rd degree / Complete heart block

- **P** Complete AV dissociation, impulses from atria cannot be conducted to ventricles.
- **A** See 1st degree AV block, can be congenital.
- **S** Bradycardia, hypotension.
- **Sx** Can be asymptomatic SOB, chest pain, pre-syncope/syncope.
- **I** ECG: no association between P waves and ventricular conduction, ECHO.
- **T** Stop offending drugs, TPW, long-term PPM.
- **C** Death, injuries from syncope.
- **Pr** Untreated at high risk of sudden cardiac death, once treated prognosis is good.

ECG abnormalities

Hyperkalaemia

- **P** Raised blood potassium concentration >5.5mmol/L.
- **A** Causes are numerous and are due to increased production (rhabdomyolysis, haemolysis, blood transfusions) and decreased excretion (renal failure, drugs eg ACE inhibitors and aldosterone antagonists, Addison's disease, mineralocorticoid insufficiency).
- **S** Cardiac arrhythmias.
- **Sx** Non-specific eg nausea, malaise, muscle weakness.
- **I** FBC, U&Es, ECG.

  ECG: decreased P wave amplitude, tall tented T waves, widening of QRS complex, sinusoidal waveform, VF and asystole.
- **T** Treat underlying cause.

  K^+ of >6.5 and any degree of hyperkalaemia with ECG change requires urgent treatment.

  Give 10ml 10% IV calcium gluconate which stabilises the myocardium but does not affect potassium level.

  To lower K+ give 15–20U of Insulin in 50mls 50% Dextrose.

  Salbutamol nebs can also lower serum K+.

  Haemodialysis in severe cases.

  In mild cases without ECG changes or chronic cases then calcium resonium can be given.

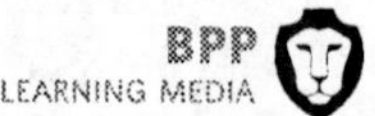

C Sudden death.

Pr Depends on aetiology.

Digoxin toxicity

P Digoxin is widely prescribed however toxicity is rare in comparison, the main route of elimination is via the kidneys.

A Occurs in overdose of digoxin but more commonly occurs in elderly patients with deteriorating renal function.

S Depends on comorbidities.

Bradycardia. Hypotension, cardiogenic shock.

Sx Non-specific: lethargy, xanthopsia (yellow vision), nausea, vomiting and dizziness.

I Digoxin level, magnesium, U&Es especially potassium.

ECG: 'reverse tick' sign, can show bradycardia, AV block, AF, paroxysmal atrial tachycardia, VT, VF.

T Stop digoxin, cardiac monitoring, digibind or digoxin immune fab, TPW.

C Bradycardias, AV block, atrial tachycardia with 2:1 block. VT and in particular 'bidirectional' VT. Digoxin can also initiate AF in patients in SR.

Pr Depends on comorbidities and age.

Hypertension and heart failure

Hypertension

P Elevated systemic arterial blood pressure that confers cardiovascular risk. BP ≥140/90 mmHg and subsequent ambulatory blood pressure daytime average is ≥135/85 mmHg.

A >95% have essential (primary) hypertension, see Table 1.2.

Renal	Endocrine	Other
• Diabetic nephropathy • Renovascular disease • Glomerulonephritis • Vasculitides • Chronic pyelonephritis • Polycystic kidneys	• Conn's syndrome • Cushing's syndrome • Glucocorticoid remediable hypertension • Phaeochromocytoma • Acromegaly • Hyperparathyroidism	• Aortic coarctation • Pregnancy-induced hypertension • Pre-eclampsia • Obesity • Excessive dietary salt or liquorice intake • Drugs (NSAIDs, sympathomimetics, illicit stimulants eg amphetamine, MDMA, and cocaine)

Table 1.2: Secondary causes of hypertension

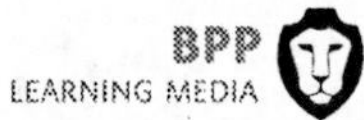

S Signs of underlying cause and evidence of end-organ damage, LVH, heart failure, aortic aneurysm, peripheral vascular disease, and cerebrovascular disease, retinopathy.

Sx Usually asymptomatic, severe hypertension may be associated with headache, drowsiness, confusion, visual symptoms, nausea and vomiting (hypertensive encephalopathy).

I NICE recommends the use of ambulatory (ABPM) and home (HBPM) blood pressure monitoring for diagnosis, and defines stages of hypertension (see Box 1.6).

ECG, full lipid profile, fasting glucose, U&E, urinalysis for blood and protein, and investigations for underlying cause as indicated (which include, but are not limited to, urinary cortisol, plasma renin-aldosterone, renal artery MRA, MAG-3 renogram, 24-hour urinary catecholamines, IGF1, ECHO, CT aortogram).

Stage 1 hypertension: Clinic BP ≥140/90 mmHg and ABPM/HBPM daytime average ≥135/85 mmHg
Stage 2 hypertension: Clinic BP ≥160/100 mmHg and ABPM/HBPM daytime average ≥150/95 mmHg
Severe hypertension: Clinic SBP ≥180 mmHg or clinic DBP ≥110 mmHg

Box 1.6: NICE definitions of hypertension

T Treatment should be offered to everyone with stage 2 hypertension and anyone <80 with stage 1 hypertension and either target organ damage, established CVS disease, renal disease, diabetes or a ten-year CVS risk ≥20% (NICE).

Lifestyle changes: stop smoking, reduce salt, exercise, weight loss.

>55 yrs: Ca^{2+} channel blocker or thiazide 1st line

<55 yrs: ACE-inhibitors 1st line

C Arteriopathy, including ischaemic heart disease, cerebrovascular disease and peripheral vascular disease, LVH and heart failure, retinopathy, nephropathy, encephalopathy.

Pr Large studies have shown that reduction in SBP of 20 mmHg or DBP of 10 mmHg is associated with approximately 50% reduction in risk of death from stroke or ischaemic heart disease.

Heart failure

P A disorder of heart structure or function that impairs its ability to fill and pump blood at a rate proportionate to the body's requirements, resulting in pulmonary or peripheral oedema, graded using the NYHA system (see Box 1.7).

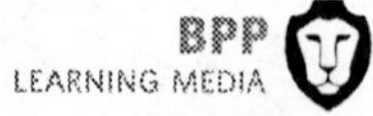

- **NYHA I:** no limitation of physical activity
- **NYHA II:** slight limitation of physical activity. Symptoms with ordinary levels of exertion, such as walking up stairs
- **NYHA III:** marked limitation of physical activity. Symptoms with minimal level of exertion, such as dressing
- **NYHA IV:** symptoms at rest

Box 1.7: NYHA classification of heart failure

A See Box 1.8.

- Ischaemic heart disease
- Dilated cardiomyopathy
- Hypertension
- Valvular heart disease
- Drugs / toxins (especially chemotherapy)
- Radiotherapy
- Pregnancy-related
- Infiltration (amyloid / sarcoid)
- Stress cardiomyopathy
- Post viral
- Alcohol
- Hypothytoidism
- Haemochromatosis
- Familial
- Infections (Chagas disease)
- Nutritional (Beriberi)

Box 1.8: Causes of heart failure

S Dyspnoea, elevated JVP, distended neck veins, pleural effusions, crepitations, hepatomegaly, peripheral oedema, ascites, tachycardia, 3rd heart sound (gallop rhythm), gout, cachexia, low-volume pulse and poor peripheral perfusion, hypotension, displaced apex, RV heave, murmurs.

Sx **LVF**: dyspnoea, reduced exercise tolerance, fatigue, pain, syncope, nocturnal cough.

RVF: weight gain, peripheral oedema, nausea and anorexia, facial engorgement.

Failure of either ventricle can have psychological sequelae, including depression and impotence.

I ECG: arrhythmia, LVH, prolonged QRS, evidence of old infarct.

CXR: cardiomegaly, pleural effusions, upper lobe diversion, alveolar oedema, septal (Kerley B lines) (see Figure 1.9).

ECHO, serum nt-proBNP, FBC, U&E, LFTs, TFTs, uric acid, Troponin.

T *Acute heart failure*: bed rest, fluid and salt restriction, daily weights, IP/OP chart with urinary catheter if needed. Vasodilators and diuretics (a typical combination would be furosemide and isosorbide dinitrate), IV Dopamine or dobutamine in hypotensive patients through a central line.

Chronic heart failure: moderated cardiovascular exercise, low-salt diet, fluid restriction, pneumovax and influenza vaccinations, diuretics, beta blockade and ACE inhibition.

Device therapy: implantable cardiac defibrillators (ICDs) reduce mortality when implanted in patients with LVEF <35%.

Surgical options: bypass grafting, mitral valve repair/replacement, LV reduction surgery, LVADs and transplantation.

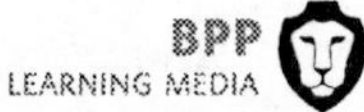

C Treatment can cause numerous side-effects, including nausea, anorexia, gout, impotence, diabetes, weakness, postural hypotension, abnormal taste, and headaches, worsening heart failure, arrhythmias, and death.

Pr Poor, the Framingham study found five-year mortality in men and women to be 62% and 42% respectively.

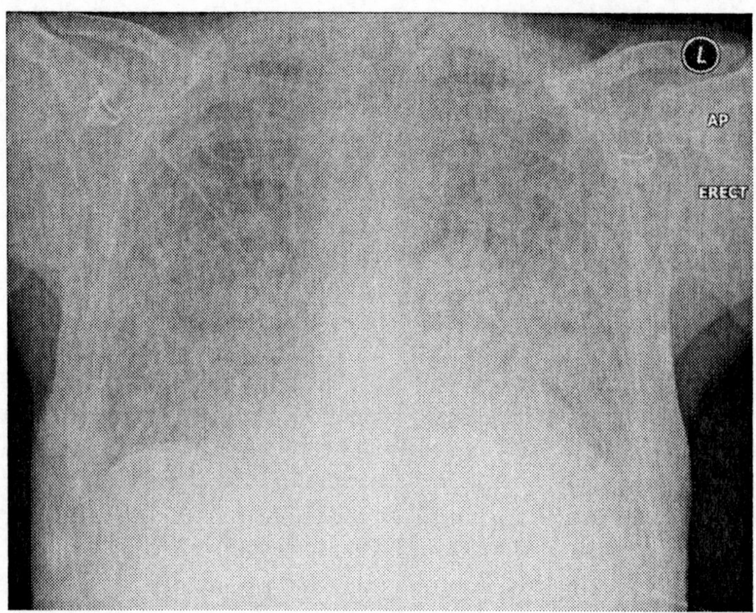

Figure 1.9: Acute pulmonary oedema. (Reproduced with permission from SW Deanery.)

Valve disease

Mitral stenosis (MS)

P MV area < 2 cm^2. LA pressure increases to move blood into LV. High LA pressure causes pulmonary hypertension and symptoms of right-sided heart failure.

A F>M, congenital (rare) or acquired: rheumatic heart disease (most common), endocarditis, SLE.

S Loud S1, low-pitched rumbling mid-diastolic murmur loudest at apex in left lateral position and post exercise, malar flush, AF, pulmonary oedema, raised JVP, may develop pulmonary regurge due to pulmonary HTN leading to early-diastolic Graham-Steell murmur.

Sx Dyspnoea, fatigue, orthopnoea, paroxysmal nocturnal dyspnoea, palpitations.

I ECG: sinus rhythm/AF, LAE (P mitrale), RVH (RAD).

CXR: LAE, pulmonary congestion, pulmonary hemosiderosis, MV calcification.

ECHO (TTE): gold standard, valvular and leaflet anomalies.

Coronary angiography: concurrent CAD in patients if age > 45.

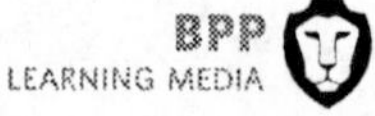

T *Medical*: treat AF (anticoagulation, rate control, cardioversion). Treat right heart failure (diuretics), chronotorops (betablockers) to increase filling time.

Surgical: mitral valve replacement or balloon valvotomy.

C Right-sided heart failure, AF.

Mitral regurgitation (MR)

P Damage to valve at various points leading to regurgitant flow into LA and increased LA & LV pressure.

A See Box 1.9.

- *Annulus:* LV dilatation (CHF, DCM, myocarditis), mitral annular calcification, endocarditis
- *Leaflets:* congenital (eg clefts), myxomatous degeneration (Marfan's), endocarditis, rheumatic heart disease, collagen vascular disease
- *Chordae tendonae:* trauma / tear, myxomatous degeneration, endocarditis, acute MI
- *Papillary muscles & LV*: ischemia / infarction, rupture, aneurysm, HOCM

Box 1.9: Causes of mitral regurgitation

S Hyperdynamic, displaced apex beat (due to LVH), soft S1, panstystolic murmur (radiates to axilla), 3rd heart sound, pulmonary oedema.

Sx Dyspnoea, fatigue, orthopnoea, paroxysmal nocturnal dyspnoea.

I ECG: LAE, left atrial delay (bifid P waves), possible LVH

CXR: LVH, LAE, pulmonary venous HTN.

ECHO: leaflet abnormalties, severity of regurgitation, LV function.

Cardiac catheterisation.

T *Medical*: asymptomatic – serial ECHOs to monitor progress, symptomatic – reduce preload (diuretics) and reduce afterload (ACEI).

Surgery: mitral valve replacement.

C Ventricular ectopics.

Aortic stenosis (AS)

P Narrowed aortic valve orifice leading to LV pressure overload and causing LVH → LVF → pulmonary oedema → CHF.

Normal valve area = 3–4cm^2; severe AS = <1cm^2.

A **Congenital**: bicuspid valve causing calcified degeneration or congenital AS.

Acquired: degenerative calcified AS (most common), 'wear and tear', rheumatic heart disease.

S *Pulse*: narrow pulse pressure, brachial radial delay, slow rising pulse.

Chest: heaving, displaced apex beat (LVH), ejection systolic murmur radiating to carotids and heard loudest over aortic valve area. Soft S2 with splitting of S2 in severe AS, 4th heart sound.

Sx Exertional angina, dyspnoea, syncope, signs and symptoms of CHF if severe (pulmonary oedema, congestive hepatomegaly).

I ECG: LVH and strain +/– LBBB, LAE, AF.

CXR: post-stenotic aortic root dilatation, calcified valve, LVH + LAE, CHF (develops later).

ECHO: valvular area and pressure gradient (assess severity of AS), LVH and LV function.

Cardiac catheterisation: exclude CAD or inconclusive ECHO.

T *Medical*: symptom control – diuretics, beta blocker.

Surgery: aortic valve replacement.

C Ventricular dysrhythmias, sudden death, heart block.

Pr Untreated, symptomatic patients have high mortality rate.

Aortic regurgitation (AR)

P Blood flows back into LV from aorta leading to high pressure in LV, LV dilatation and increased myocardial oxygen demand.

A See Box 1.10.

- Aortic root (with dilatation of ascending aorta): Marfan's syndrome, dissecting aortic aneurysm, systemic HTN, aortic root dilatation, syphilis, connective tissue diseases (both seronegative and rheumatoid arthritis)
- Valve: congenital abnormalities (bicuspid AV, large VSD), connective tissue diseases (SLE, rheumatoid arthritis, etc), rheumatic fever (+/– associated AS), endocarditis, myxomatous degeneration
- Acute AR: infective endocarditis, aortic dissection, acute rheumatic fever, failure of prosthetic valve

Box 1.10: Causes of AR

S See Box 1.11

Chest: heaving, displaced apex beat, high-pitched early diastolic crescendo murmur heard best with patient sitting and leaning forward at lower left sternal border.

Austin-Flint murmur: mid-diastolic rumbling murmur at apex due to fluttering of mitral valve leaflets with regurgitant flow.

Sx Dyspnoea, fatigue, orthopnoea, PND, palpitations.

- Large volume, 'waterhammer' pulse (bounding and rapidly collapsing)
- Wide pulse pressure (due to high systolic and low diastolic BP)
- Bisferiens pulse: twice beating in systole; occurs in presence of combined AS/AR
- de Musset's sign: head bobbing due to increased pulse pressure
- Corrigan's sign: visible carotid pulsations
- Quincke's sign: visible pulsation of nail beds
- Traube's sign: 'pistol shot' diastolic and systolic sounds heard with the stethoscope lightly applied over the femoral arteries
- Duroziez's sign: light proximal compression of femoral artery produces systolic diastolic murmur over femoral artery

Box 1.11 Haemodynamic signs of AR

I ECG: LVH, LAE.

CXR: LV enlargement, LAE, aortic root dilatation.

ECHO (TTE): gold standard, flow and leaflet anomalies.

Radionucleotide imaging: failure to increase EF with exercise suggests decreased LV function.

Cardiac catheterisation.

Coronary angiography indicated if age > 40.

T *Medical*: treat CHF (diuretics), acute AR may require stabilisation with vasodilators.

Surgery: aortic valve replacement.

C Arrhythmias, CHF.

Pr Once symptomatic poor prognosis.

Tricuspid valve disease

P A Tricuspid stenosis (TS): rheumatic, congenital, carcinoid syndrome.

Tricuspid regurgitation (TR): tricuspid annular dilatation (commonest cause due to pulmonary hypertension and RV overload), IE (IV drug users), rheumatic, Ebstein anomaly, AV cushion defects, carcinoid, tricuspid prolapse, trauma.

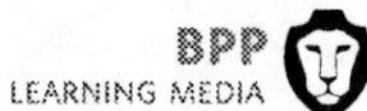

S Sx Raised JVP: prominent 'a' waves in TS and 'cv' waves in TR.

Right-sided heart failure.

I ECG: TS: RAE. TR: RAE, RVH, AF.

CXR: TS: dilatation of RA without pulmonary artery enlargement. TR: RA and RV enlargement.

ECHO.

T Diuretics or valve replacement.

Pulmonary valve disease

P A Pulmonary stenosis (PS): congenital (commonest), rheumatic, carcinoid.

Pulmonary regurgitation (PR): pulmonary HTN, rheumatic, endocarditis.

S Sx Chest pain, syncope, dyspnoea, oedema.

PS: systolic murmur, S4.

PR: early diastolic murmur.

I ECG: RVH.

CXR: prominent pulmonary arteries if pulmonary HTN, enlarged RV.

ECHO: diagnostic – RVH, RV dilatation.

T Treat symptoms or valve surgery.

Infective endocarditis (IE)

P Infection of the endocardium usually lining the heart valves.

Fever and new murmur = endocarditis until proven otherwise.

A Normal heart valves (50%): due to staph aureus from skin.

Risk factors: diabetes, renal failure, immunosuppression.

Abnormal valves: due to strep viridans (35–50%).

Risk factors: aortic/mitral valve disease, IVDU, prosthetic valves.

S See Box 1.12.

Sx Normal valves: acute endocarditis (rapidly progressive).

Abnormal valves: subacute endocarditis (slowly progressive).

Fever, rigors, night sweats, fatigue, anorexia, septic emboli.

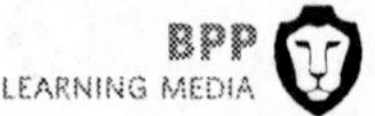

Diagnosed by **2 major** OR **1 major and 3 minor** OR **all 5 minor criteria**

Major criteria
- Blood culture positive for typical organism in two cultures from separate sites or persistently positive cultures >12 hours apart
- Endocardium involvement on ECHO

Minor criteria
- Fever >38
- Predisposition (IVDU or existing cardiac lesion)
- Vascular / immunological phenomena (clubbing, splinter haemorrhages, Osler's nodes, Roth spots)
- Positive blood culture with atypical organism
- Positive ECHO not involving endocardium

Box 1.12: Duke's classification of endocarditis

I Bloods: WCC, CRP, ESR, cultures (three sets at different times from different sites).

Urine: microscopic haematuria.

ECG: long PR.

ECHO (TTE/TOE): vegetations, abscess.

T Early IV broad-spectrum Abx while awaiting cultures.

C Septic emboli.

P 30% mortality with staph.

Rheumatic fever

P Systemic inflammatory disease occurring two to four weeks after pharyngeal infection with beta haemolytic strep, antibody-antigen complex affects heart, joints, skin and brain.

A Peak age 5–15 years.

S Sx See Box 1.13.

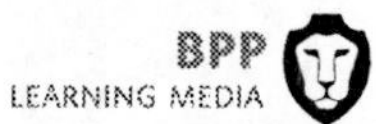

Evidence of **recent strep infection** *plus* **2 major criteria** OR **1 major and 2 minor**

Major criteria (STREP)
Sydenham's chorea
Transient polyarthritis
Rheumatic subcutaneous nodules
Erythema marginatum
Pancarditis

Minor criteria (FRAPP)
Fever
Raised ESR/CRP
Arthralgia
Prolongation of PR interval
Previous rheumatic fever

Box 1.13: Jones criteria for rheumatic fever

I Bloods: raised ESR and CRP.

ECG: long PR.

T Bed rest, analgesia IV Abx haloperidol/benzodiazepine for chorea.

C Valve disease.

Pr 60% with carditis develop chronic rheumatic disease.

Disease of heart muscle

Dilated cardiomyopathy

P Dilated and weakened heart muscle.

A Cause unknown, associated with: alcohol, HTN, viral infection, autoimmune disease.

S Tachycardia, raised JVP, low BP, S3 gallop, pleural effusion.

Sx Dyspnoea, fatigue, AF, VT, RVF.

I CXR: cardiomegaly, pulmonary oedema.

ECG: tachycardia.

ECHO: global dilatation with hypokinesis.

T Bed rest, diuretics, pacing, transplantation.

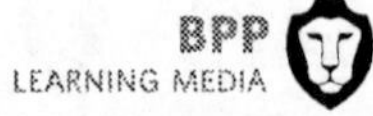

Hypertrophic cardiomyopathy

P Left ventricular outflow tract obstruction due to asymmetrical hypertrophy of the ventricular septum.

A Leading cause of cardiac death in young, autosomal dominant with positive family history but 50% are sporadic.

S 'a' wave in JVP, double apex beat, harsh ejection systolic murmur, jerky pulse.

Sx Cardiac death may be first symptom, syncope, dyspnoea, angina, palpitations.

I ECG: LVH, Q waves, AF, ventricular ectopics.

ECHO: asymmetrical septal hypertrophy.

T *Medical*: beta blockers or verapamil for symptom control.

Surgical: septal myomectomy, implantable defibrillator.

C Sudden death.

Pr 6% mortality/year in those <14 years.

Restrictive cardiomyopathy

P Heart muscle is rigid and is restricted from stretching and filling properly.

A Primary: idiopathic, fibroelastosis.

Secondary: amyloidosis, haemochromatosis, sarcoidosis.

S Sx Features of RVF.

I Cardiac catheterisation.

T Treat underlying cause.

Treat symptoms.

Transplant.

Cardiac myxoma

P Rare, benign cardiac polypoid tumour usually occurs in left atrium adjacent to atrial septum (75%).

A F>M, familial or sporadic.

S 'Tumour plop' 3rd heart sound, clubbing.

Sx May mimic endocarditis or mitral stenosis.

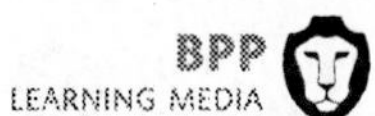

I Bloods: anaemia, raised ESR.

ECHO: visualises tumour.

T Surgical excision.

C Emboli.

Pericardial disease

Acute pericarditis

P Inflammation of the pericardium, usually lasting less than six weeks' duration, it is the commonest pathology of the pericardium.

A See Table 1.3.

Idiopathic	
Infection	Viral (Coxsakievirus), bacteria (Stapyhlococcus or Streptococcus), mycoplasma, fungal, parasitic, infective endocarditis
Radiation	
Neoplasm	Primary (rhabdomyosarcoma), metastatic (lung or breast cancer)
Cardiac	Myocarditis, dissecting aortic aneurysm, Dressler's syndrome (ie post myocardial infarction)
Trauma	Blunt, penetrating, iatrogenic
Autoimmune	Lupus, rheumatoid arthritis, scleroderma, vasculitis
Drugs	Procainamide, isoniazid, Hydralazine
Metabolic	Hypothyroidism, uraemia, ovarian hyperstimulation syndrome

Table 1.3: Causes of acute pericarditis

S Pericardial rub (scratching sound best heard over the left sternal edge), signs of cardiac tamponade.

Sx Chest pain (pleuritic and sharp which may improve on leaning forward or sitting up), fever.

I Blood tests: raised WCC, CRP, ESR.

Acute and convalescent viral titres.

ECG: diffuse concave ST elevation with PR depression.

ECHO: particularly looking for a pericardial effusion.

T Non-steroidal anti-inflammatory drugs (NSAIDs) are first line. Corticosteroids can be used if NSAIDs contraindicated. Colchicine is used for refractory cases.

C Cardiac tamponade or constrictive pericarditis may occur in those with malignancy or tuberculosis as the aetiology.

Pr Usually good for viral pericarditis.

Constrictive pericarditis

P Results from thickening and scarring of the pericardial sac, the fibrotic pericardium therefore loses its elasticity and prevents the heart from expanding.

A Idiopathic, viral, post cardiac surgery, post-radiation therapy (ie after breast cancer), connective tissue disorder, post-infectious (tuberculosis or purulent pericarditis), malignancy, trauma, drugs, asbestosis, sarcoidosis, uraemic pericarditis.

S Sx Elevated JVP (x and y troughs are more prominent than a and v peaks with rapid y descent), Kussmaul's sign (raised JVP on inspiration), pericardial knock, pulsus parodoxus (drop in systemic BP >10 mmHg during inspiration), hepatomegaly and other signs of right heart failure.

I CXR: pericardial calcification or pleural effusions.

ECHO: reduced end-diastolic volumes and raised diastolic pressures, pericardial thickening may be seen.

T Definitive treatment is pericardiectomy. This has a high mortality rate.

Pericardial effusion

P Abnormal collection of fluid around the heart (>50 mLs).

A Transudative (congestive cardiac failure, myxoedema, nephrotic syndrome), exudative (tuberculosis, empyema), haemorrhagic (trauma, aneurysmal rupture), malignant (fluid from metastasis), drugs.

S Sx Chest pain and pressure symptoms, often asymptomatic unless it causes tamponade.

I ECG: low QRS voltage, electrical alternans (beat-to-beat shift in QRS/P waves).

CXR: enlarged cardiac silhouette.

ECHO: specific and sensitive method of detecting a pericardial effusion.

T Monitor, pericardiocentesis.

C Pericardial effusions may progress to cardiac tamponade.

Cardiac tamponade

P Occurs when the pericardial space fills up with fluid faster than it can stretch, resulting in increased pressure within the pericardial sac.

As fluid accumulates less blood enters the ventricles during diastole as the increasing pressure presses on the heart and forces the septum to bend into the left ventricle, this leads to decreased stroke volume and eventually cardiac arrest if left untreated.

A Causes are similar to that of pericardial effusion.

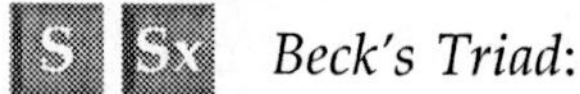

Beck's Triad:

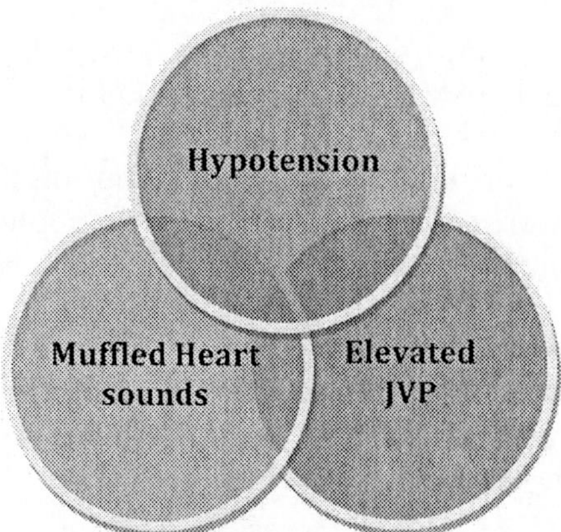

Figure: 1.10: Beck's Triad

Other signs include sinus tachycardia, Kussmaul's sign (raised JVP on inspiration), pericardial rub, and pulsus parodoxus (drop in systemic BP >10 mmHg during inspiration).

I ECG: low QRS voltage, electrical alternans (beat-to-beat shift in QRS/P waves).

CXR: enlarged cardiac silhouette, cardiomegaly only seen with >200 ml of blood.

ECHO: systolic collapse of RA followed by diastolic collapse of RV.

T Removal of pericardial fluid via pericardiocentesis or open surgical drainage with pericardiectomy (pericardial window).

Congenital heart disease

Non-cyanotic congenital heart disease

Atrial septal defect (ASD)

P There are two main types of ASD:

- *Ostium secundum (80%):* defect in centre of atrial septum (foramen ovale)
- *Ostium primum (10%):* defect in lower atrial septum (involving AV valve)

S Soft systolic murmur, upper left sternal edge, fixed splitting of second heart sound.

Sx Commonly asymptomatic, may present with heart failure (poor feeding, failure to thrive, tachypnoea, sweating, vomiting) or recurrent chest infections.

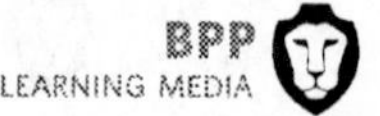

I ECG: sinus rhythm with right axis deviation (due to right ventricular hypertrophy). Partial right bundle branch block.

CXR: cardiomegaly and increased pulmonary vasculature.

ECHO will be required to confirm the defect.

T Surgical closure aged 4–5 years. 90% achieved by insertion of an occlusion device in the catheter laboratory.

C If surgical correction is not undertaken, heart failure may occur.

Ventricular septal defect (VSD)

P A defect in the ventricular septum. Small defects are smaller than the aortic valve and large defects larger than the aortic valve.

S A thrill may be felt at the left lower sternal edge, pansystolic murmur at lower left sternal edge (loud in small defects, quiet or absent in large defects), S2 is quiet/normal in small defects and loud in large defects.

Sx May be asymptomatic if small. Larger defects present early after 1 week of age with symptoms of heart failure or recurrent chest infections.

I ECG: varies from normal to the presence of right ventricular hypertrophy.

CXR: cardiomegaly and increased pulmonary vasculature.

ECHO will be required to confirm the defect.

T Most asymptomatic small VSDs will close spontaneously. Treatment is required for symptoms of heart failure (diuretics +/- ACE inhibitor).

Surgical correction is required by 3–5 months of age for large defects.

C If surgical correction is not performed, heart failure and pulmonary hypertension occur in large defects. Eisenmenger's syndrome may occur secondary to prolonged pulmonary hypertension, producing a right to left shunt with cyanosis.

Patent ductus arteriosus

P The ductus arteriosus connects the pulmonary artery and the descending aorta. It is described to be persistent if it remains open one month after the estimated delivery date. If it remains patent blood flows from the aorta to the pulmonary artery (left to right shunt).

A Common in preterm neonates, due to a defect in the constriction of the duct following birth.

S Continuous murmur beneath the left clavicle, the murmur continues into diastole as the pressure in the pulmonary artery remains lower than that in the aorta throughout the cardiac cycle.

Sx Usually asymptomatic, in large ducts there may be symptoms of heart failure and pulmonary hypertension.

I ECG: usually normal.

CXR: usually normal but in large ducts may have increased pulmonary vasculature.

ECHO will be required to confirm the defect with Doppler ultrasound.

T May close spontaneously.

If symptomatic, treatment for heart failure required (fluid restriction, diuretics or indomethacin – a prostaglandin inhibitor to assist in closure).

Surgical ligation may be required if medical management fails.

C Heart failure, pulmonary hypertension, bacterial endocarditis.

Pr Good prognosis once the PDA has closed.

Coarctation of the aorta

P When the duct closes after birth, the ductal tissue surrounds the aorta and causes narrowing/obstruction of the aorta.

A Commoner in girls (2:1) and associated with Turner syndrome (along with bicuspid aortic valve).

S Sx Severe cases present in the neonate: circulatory collapse, absent femoral pulses, signs of heart failure.

Less severe cases present with signs of heart failure and a murmur radiating to between the shoulder blades. Femoral pulses may be weak.

I Antenatal ultrasound: diagnosis may be made antenatally.

Blood pressure: elevated in blood vessels proximal to coarctation.

ECG: right ventricular hypertrophy.

CXR: may be normal or signs of heart failure and cardiomegaly.

T Resuscitation and prostaglandins to keep the duct patent.

Surgery will be required in cases presenting later in life.

C Premature coronary artery disease, congestive cardiac failure, hypertensive encephalopathy.

Pr Mortality from untreated hypertension is high.

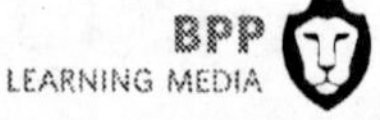

Cyanotic congenital heart disease

Tetralogy of Fallot

P The most common cyanotic congenital heart disease, consisting of:

- Ventricular septal defect
- Pulmonary stenosis
- Overriding aorta
- Right ventricular hypertrophy

S Cyanosis in the first few days of life with a duct-dependant circulation (as the duct closes), others present within the first few months through detection of a murmur.

Harsh murmur heard at the upper sternal edge (due to right ventricular outflow obstruction). Classical description of paroxysmal hypercyanotic spells in late infancy usually associated with excessive crying or irritability and dyspnoea.

Sx Do not usually develop heart failure, although this may be a late feature.

I ECG: normal at birth, later develop right axis deviation and right ventricular hypertrophy.

CXR: boot-shaped heart and decreased pulmonary vasculature (secondary to pulmonary outflow obstruction).

ECHO: required to confirm diagnosis.

T *Hypercyanotic spells*: place in knee-chest position, administer oxygen, morphine and propanolol.

Surgical correction: 10% require a Blalock-Taussig shunt to increased pulmonary blood flow, when infants are symptomatic with cyanosis. Stable patients require corrective surgery at 6–9 months of age, with correction of the VSD and relieving the right outflow obstruction.

C Untreated Tetralogy of Fallot predisposes to cerebral ischaemia, congestive cardiac failure and myocardial ischaemia.

Pr Patients generally remain asymptomatic post surgical correction and have a normal life expectancy.

Transposition of the great arteries

P There are two separate circulations:

- The aorta is connected to right ventricle receiving deoxygenated blood
- The pulmonary artery is connected to the left ventricle receiving oxygenated blood from the lungs

These children are therefore cyanosed and this defect is incompatible with life unless there are separate defects to allow mixing of the blood (ASD, VSD or PDA).

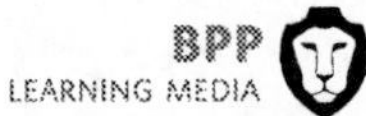

S Cyanosis is the predominant feature with hypoxia. Typical presentation is day 1–2 of life, following spontaneous closure of the ductus arteriosus. Presentation will be delayed if there are other associated defects allowing mixing of the blood.

I Usually diagnosed antenatally via foetal ultrasound.

ECG: often normal.

CXR: classical 'egg on its side' appearance of the heart shadow.

ECHO: required to confirm diagnosis.

T In a sick neonate presenting in the first few days of life, resuscitation may be required alongside prostaglandins in attempt to keep the ductus arteriosus patent.

Balloon atrial septostomy is required to allow mixing of the blood. Ultimately all will require an arterial switch operation, which is carried out in the first two weeks of life.

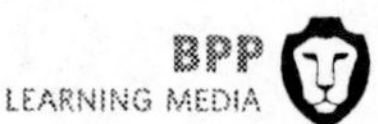

Practice Questions

Single Best Answers

1. Which of the following statements is true regarding bradycardia?

   A It typically accompanies hyperthyroidism
   B It may be a feature of atrial fibrillation
   C If less than 50bpm, it should be treated to prevent renal impairment
   D It is classically associated with multiple small pulmonary emboli

2. Which of the following statements is true regarding hyperkalaemia?

   A It is typically associated with chronic rather than acute renal failure
   B It may be exacerbated by treatment with salbutamol
   C Emergency treatments include pamidronate infusion
   D The T wave amplitude on the ECG tends to increase

3. Which of the following statements is false regarding atrial fibrillation?

   A It is a complication of atrial myxoma
   B It is a typical complication of hypothyroidism
   C It may be caused by alcohol
   D It is associated with fatigue

4. Which of the following statements is false regarding aortic stenosis?

   A Can cause sudden death
   B Is a cause of syncope
   C Needs prophylactic antibiotics in surgery
   D Causes right ventricular hypertrophy

5. Regarding myocardial infarctions which of the following is true:

   A There is ST depression on ECG
   B Pre-existing angina may decrease after the MI
   C Diamorphine is limited by hypotension
   D R waves are pathological

6. Which of the following is a cyanotic congenital heart condition?

   A Tetralogy of Fallot
   B Patent ductus arteriosus
   C Ventricular septal defect
   D Atrial septal defect

7. A waterhammer pulse is palpated in which condition?

   A Aortic stenosis
   B Tricuspid regurgitation
   C Aortic regurgitation
   D Mitral regurgitation

8. In the JVP waveform cannon 'a' waves are observed in

   A Aortic stenosis
   B Complete heart block
   C Tricuspid regurge
   D SVC 1st degree heart block

9. Kussmaul's sign, a paradoxical rise in JVP on inspiration, is seen in

   A Dilated cardiomyopathy
   B Atrial myxoma
   C Constrictive pericarditis
   D Transposition of the great arteries

10. The following causes a 'reverse tick' ST appearance on ECG

   A Hypokalaemia
   B Hyperkalaemia
   C Digoxin
   D Hypothermia

Extended Matching Questions

Chest pain

A Angina
B MI
C Acute aortic dissection
D Pericarditis
E Reflux oesophagitis
F Peptic ulcer disease
G Pneumonia
H Pulmonary embolism
I Pneumothorax
J Rib fracture
K Costochondritis

Match the patient description with one of the above diagnoses.

1. A 55-year-old obese female complains of an occasional burning pain behind the sternum. The pain is worse after large meals and when drinking hot liquids.

2. A 50-year-old female presents with a sharp chest pain which is worse on inspiration. Her temperature is 380°C and she has a history of a recent viral infection. Her pulse is much weaker on inspiration and the JVP is found to be raised.

3. A 26-year-old racing driver is brought to A&E following an RTA. He is dyspnoeic, has a BP of 105/60 and pulse 95. On examination the trachea is deviated to the left and there is decreased expansion of the left side relative to the right.

4. A 70-year-old man with history of hypertension presents with sudden tearing chest pain radiating to the back. The peripheral pulses are absent and there is a widened mediastinum on CXR.

5. A 65-year-old male complains of a severe crushing pain in his chest. He is sweating, short of breath, says he feels sick and appears very drowsy. The pain is not relieved by the GTN spray he was given by his GP.

Dyspnoea

A Alcohol heart muscle disease
B Aortic valve disease
C Atrial septal defect
D Cardiac arrhythmia
E Dilated cardiomyopathy
F Hypertension
G Infective endocarditis
H Mitral regurgitation
I Pericardial effusion
J Pulmonary fibrosis
K Tuberculosis
L Viral myopericarditis

Which diagnosis do you think is the cause of the breathlessness in each patient?

6. An 18-year-old girl has felt unwell for about three weeks, complaining of chest pains, which are worse when she lies flat. She has now become short of breath. She is admitted to hospital where she is found to be in acute pulmonary oedema.

7. During the month following his acute inferior myocardial infarction, a 56-year-old man has become progressively more breathless. On examination he has a loud pan-systolic murmur.

8. A 24-year-old Asian man who has come to work as a chef in an Indian restaurant has a two-month history of cough, fever, night sweats and weight loss. He has been treated with a number of antibiotics by the GP but remains unwell. He is admitted with shortness of breath and haemoptysis. On chest X-ray his heart size is normal.

9. A 42-year-old man is admitted with peripheral oedema and breathlessness. A routine medical examination six months before, was normal. He has no murmurs, but his heart is enlarged both on clinical examination and chest X-ray. Investigations include normal liver function tests and normal C-reactive protein.

10. A 55-year-old man with known carcinoma of the lungs develops shortness of breath over a few days. He has a large cardiac silhouette on his CXR but no pulmonary oedema.

Chest pain

A Angina
B Pericarditis
C Myocardial infarction
D Pulmonary embolism
E Oesophageal spasm
F Dissecting aortic aneurysm
G Anxiety
H Coronary artery disease
I Tietze's syndrome
J Hiatus hernia

Match the patient description with one of the above diagnoses.

11. A 49-year-old man with recent history of long-haul travel presents with shortness of breath and haemoptysis. He also complains of chest pain and ECG shows sinus tachycardia.

12. A 53-year-old lady complains of central 'crushing' chest pain, sudden onset and spontaneous remission, with no attributable cause. She has no history of hypertension, current BP is 116/76.

13. A 73-year-old gentleman presents to A&E with sudden 'tearing' chest pain, radiating to the back. The house officer on duty notices unequal arm pulses and BP.

14. A 63-year-old gentleman develops acute central chest pain, radiating down the left arm. He appears very pale and sweaty, and has a strong family history of ishaemic heart disease.

15. A 67-year-old man recovering from an inferior MI complains of sharp retrosternal chest pain. He comments that leaning forward provides relief of the pain. The attending medical student claims to have heard a 'rub' on auscultation.

Diagnosis of valvular heart disease and murmurs

A Aortic stenosis
B Aortic regurgitation
C Mitral stenosis – rheumatic
D Mitral regurgitation – rheumatic
E Mitral regurgitation – non-rheumatic
F Infective endocarditis
G Innocent murmur
H Mixed aortic valve disease
I Mixed mitral valve disease
J Mixed mitral and aortic valve disease
K Prolapsing mitral valve
L Congenital aortic stenosis
M Hypertrophic obstructive cardiomyopathy

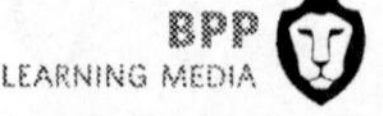

For each situation below, choose the **single** most likely diagnosis from the above list of options.

16. A 30-year-old man attends for a routine pre-employment medical. On examination of the cardiovascular system, the doctor finds a soft (grade 2/6) ejection systolic murmur at the apex. He has no previous cardiac or respiratory problems, and has normal pulse and BP.

17. A 60-year-old Irish woman comes to see you with a progressive one-year history of shortness of breath and recent onset of paroxysmal nocturnal dyspnoea. She has been previously well apart from Sydenham's chorea as a child. She had six normal pregnancies. On examination she has plethoric cheeks, the pulse is rapid (110/min), irregular and small volume. BP 128/80 JVP normal. The apex is in the 5th mid clavicular line and tapping in nature. The 1st heart sound is loud and P2 accentuated. A low pitched mid-diastolic murmur 2/4 is heard in the apex.

18. A 50-year-old man attends A&E with shortness of breath, fever and hyperdynamic regular pulse of 100 beats per minute. BP 160/60. He has an early diastolic murmur at the left sternal edge. On further enquiry it is found that he attended for a routine dental procedure two months ago.

19. An 80-year-old woman presents with recent onset of effort-related chest pain. On examination of the cardiovascular system she is found to have a loud ejection systolic murmur and a low pulse pressure with slow rising pulse.

20. A 65-year-old man had an inferior MI 10 days ago. His initial course was uncomplicated. He suddenly deteriorates with acute left ventricular failure. On examination the pulse is regular 100/min and normal volume and character. BP 110/60. The apex beat is dynamic. There is a loud grade 6/6, apical pansystolic murmur which radiates to the axilla.

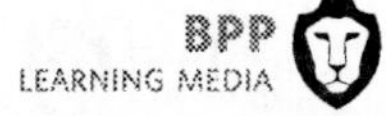

Answers

SBAs		EMQs	
1	B	1	E
2	D	2	D
3	B	3	I
4	D	4	C
5	B	5	B
6	A	6	L
7	C	7	H
8	B	8	K
9	C	9	E
10	C	10	I
		11	D
		12	G
		13	F
		14	C
		15	B
		16	G
		17	C
		18	F
		19	A
		20	E

Chapter 2

Respiratory

Dr Philip Mitchelmore and
Dr Rahul Shrimanker

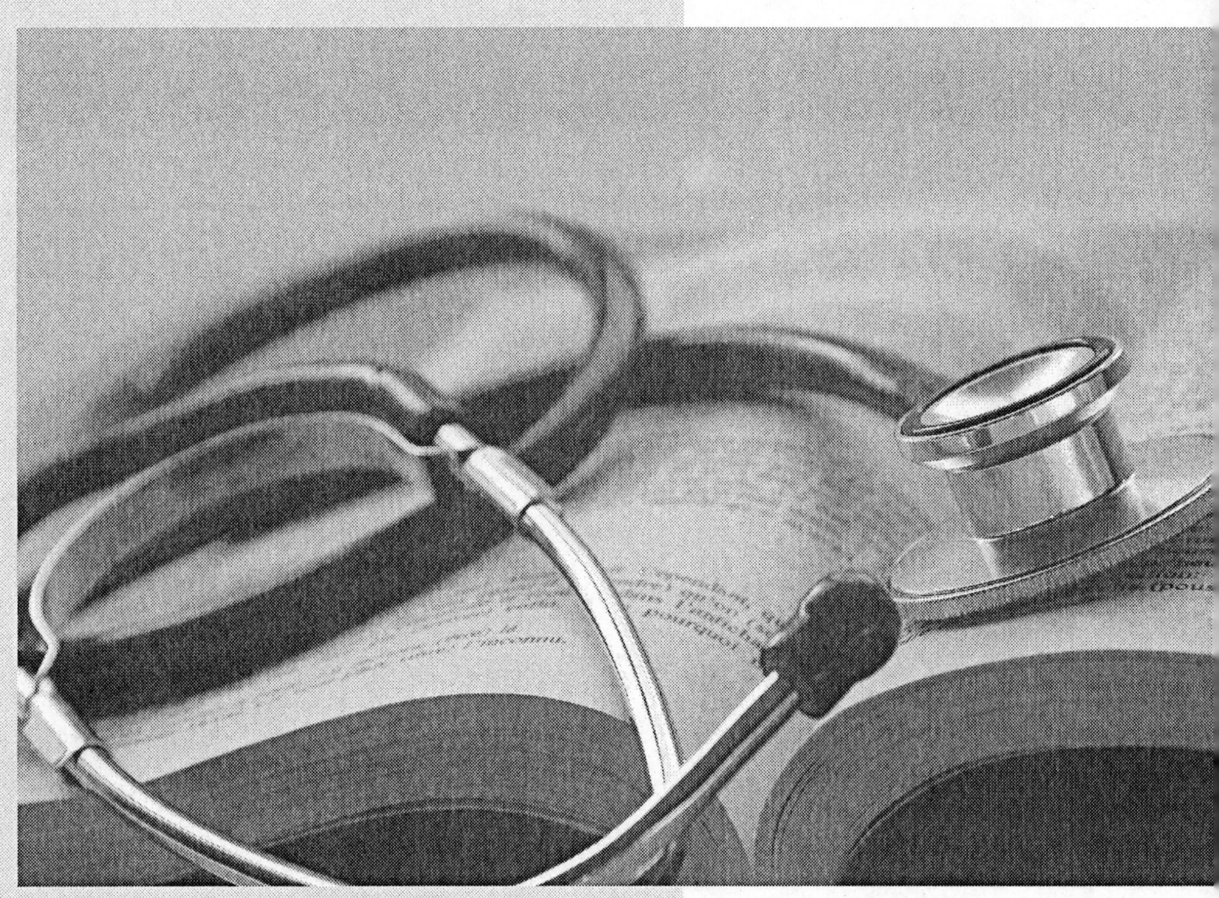

Respiratory failure

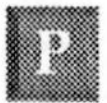

Term used to describe failure to maintain oxygenation (usually a PaO_2 of 8.0kPa is the cut-off).

Type 1: hypoxia (PaO_2 <8.0kPa) normal CO_2. This a due to a ventilation/perfusion (V/Q) mismatch (eg pulmonary embolus, pneumonia, fibrosis).

Type 2: hypoxia (PaO_2 <8.0kPa) plus hypercapnia ($PaCO_2$ >6.0kPa). Due to alveolar hypoventilation (eg COPD, neuromuscular disease, sedation).

- *Pulmonary disease:* asthma, COPD, pneumonia, pulmonary fibrosis, obstructive sleep apnoea, tumour, ARDS
- *Thoracic wall:* flail chest, kyphoscoliosis
- *Reduced respiratory drive:* sedatives, CNS disorder, brainstem stroke
- *Neuromuscular:* cervical cord lesions, diaphragm paralysis, poliomyelitis, Guillain-Barré, myasthenia gravis

Box 2.1: Causes of respiratory failure

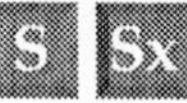

Type 1 (hypoxia): agitation, dyspnoea, tachycardia and confusion.

Type 2 (hypoxia plus hypercapnia): sleepy/confused, metabolic flap, bounding pulse, vasodilated.

ABG: hypoxia, +/- hypercapnia, respiratory acidosis.

ABC with appropriate oxygen delivery (beware hypoxic drive in type 2 respiratory failure – aim for sats of 88–90%).

Treat underlying cause.

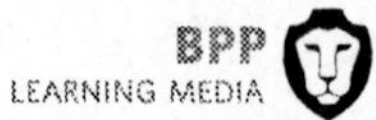

Infection

Pneumonia

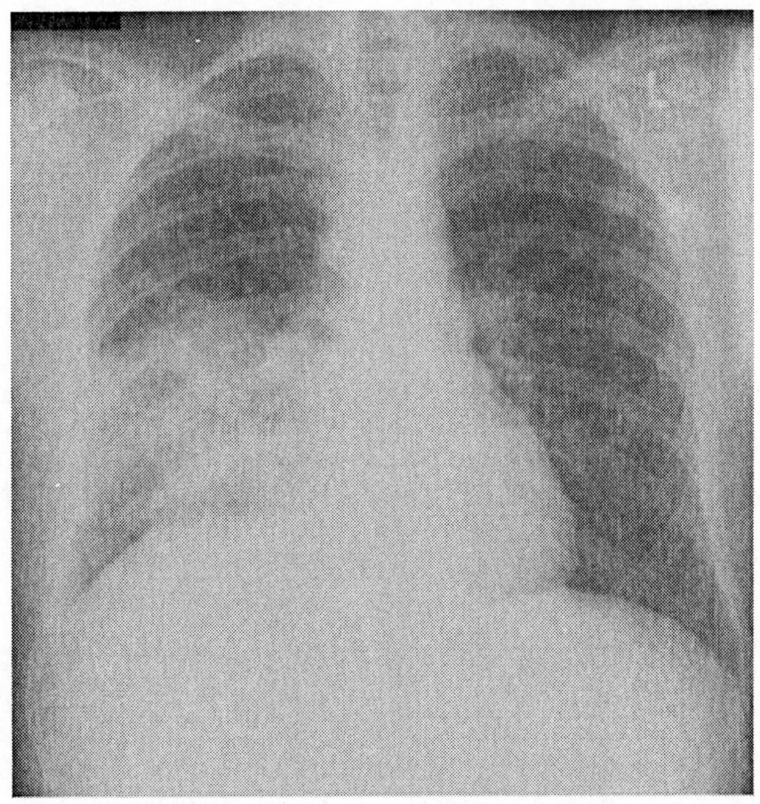

Figure 2.1: Right lower lobe pneumonia. (Reproduced with permission from SW Deanery.)

P Inflammation of the lung parenchyma as a result of an infection. Community acquired (CAP) or hospital acquired (HAP) developing 48 hours after admission.

A See Box 2.2. Certain groups are at increased risk of pneumonia: diabetics, COPD, previous splenectomy, underlying cardiorespiratory disease, the elderly and HIV infected patients.

CAP organisms	HAP organisms
• Streptococcus pneumonia (65%) • H. Influenza, • Mycoplasma pneumonia • Chlamydophilia pneumonia	• Gram – ve bacteria • Staphylococcus aureus • Streptococcus pneumonia

Box 2.2: Common causative organisms in pneumonia

S Pyrexia, dyspnea, tachypnoea, confusion, cough with purulent sputum. Auscultation may reveal crackles and bronchial breathing. A dull percussion note may be present.

Sx Pleuritic pain, cough (productive), rigors and shortness of breath. Atypical pneumonias see Box 2.3.

- *Mycoplasma pneumonia:* epidemics every four years in UK. Associated with erythema multiforme ('target lesions'), erythema nodosum and DIC
- *Klebsiella:* affects homeless and carers. CXR: bulging of horizontal fissure
- *Legionella:* flu-like symptoms. Urine tested for antigen. Tx clarithromycin and rifampicin

Box 2.3: Atypical organisms (produce atypical symptoms)

I Chest X-ray: reveals areas of consolidation and potentially pleural effusions.

Bloods: FBC, U&E, CRP and liver function tests, ABG, blood cultures.

Sputum culture and gram stain: in suspected cases of TB, samples can be sent for acid fast bacilli.

Urine antigen: for pneumococcal (in moderate to high severity), legionella (high severity or suspected).

Bronchoscopy: in persistent cases post course of antibiotics.

1 point for each of the following '**CURB-65**'	Prognosis – based on CURB-65 score
Confusion, **U**rea >7.1mmol/L **R**espiratory Rate >30/min **B**lood Pressure <90 systolic or <60 diastolic Over **65**	0–1 = Mortality <3% admission unnecessary 2 = Mortality 9% should be admitted 3–5 = Mortality 15–40% urgent admission

Box 2.4: CURB-65 score for community acquired pneumonia

T *Oxygen:* aim for oxygen saturations of 94–98%.

Intravenous Fluids: patient's fluid balance should be assessed and supplemented appropriately.

IV/PO antibiotics: follow local policy. Eg amoxicillin for non-severe, Tazocin for severe.

Nutrition and chest physio: this is very important in prolonged illness.

C Septicaemia, para-pneumonic effusions, empyema and cavity formation.

Pr See Box 2.4.

Post discharge, patients should have a follow up CXR at six weeks.

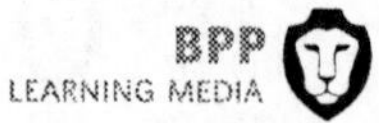

Pulmonary tuberculosis

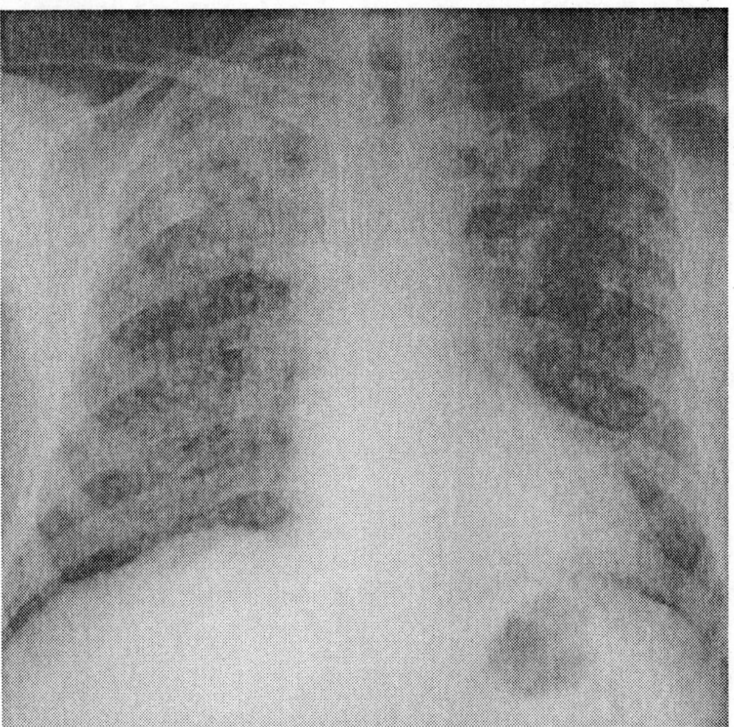

Figure 2.2: Left upper lob cavitating consolidation on miliary TB background. (Reproduced with permission from SW Deanery.)

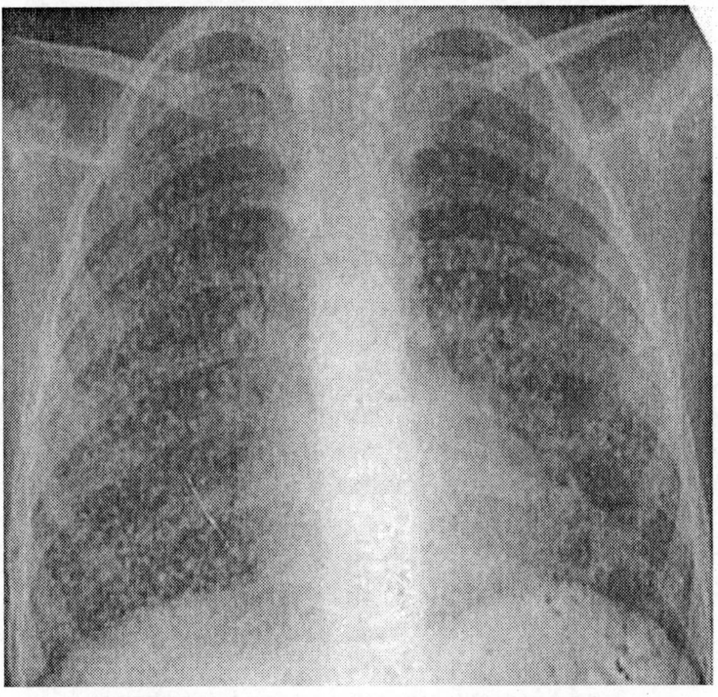

Figure 2.3: Miliary TB (like millet seeds). (Reproduced with permission from SW Deanery.)

P Caseating granulomatous disease.

Inhalation of infection through aerosol → alveoar macrophage engulfs bacterium, → local replication, → granuloma formation and enlargement of draining lymph nodes (the Ghon complex).

Miliary TB is due to haematogenous spread.

A Due to *mycobacterium tuberculosis,* increasing incidence in UK.

S May have relatively few signs.

Severe disease: marked wasting and weight loss, may have lymphadenopathy, splenomegaly, erythema nodosum.

Chest: dull upper zones with crackles.

Sx Cough lasting > 3 weeks unresponsive to antibiotics, creamy white sputum, haemoptysis, upper lobe cavitation/patchy consolidation and fibrosis, fever, night sweats, weight loss.

I CXR: miliary shadowing, hilar lymphadenopathy, pleural effusion, cavitating patchy consolidation in upper lobes, Ghon complex, signs of old healed TB.

Mantoux (tuberculin skin test): becomes positive after four to eight weeks on development of cell mediated immune response.

Sputum culture: AFB (acid fast bacilli) on ZN staining.

Tissue for histology: caseating granulomas with or without AFB on staining.

T See Box 2.5 and contact tracing.

Six months' anti-tuberculous chemotherapy in fully sensitive uncomplicated TB.

Induction phase **two months' RIPE**

- Rifampicin: hepatitis, orange urine, flu-like symptoms, inactivates OCP
- Isoniazid: hepatitis, neuropathy, agranulocytosis (daily pyridoxine protects)
- Pyrazinamide: hepatitis, arthralgia
- Ethambutol: optic neuritis (ishihara test)

Continuation phase **four months**

- Rifampicin
- Isoniazid

Box 2.5: Anti-tuberculous drugs and side effects

C Cavitation in lungs leading to massive haemotysis: Razmussen's aneurysm (where bronchial artery runs close to cavity and is eroded), drug side effects.

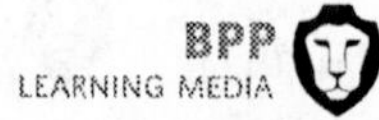

Pleural disease

Pleural effusion

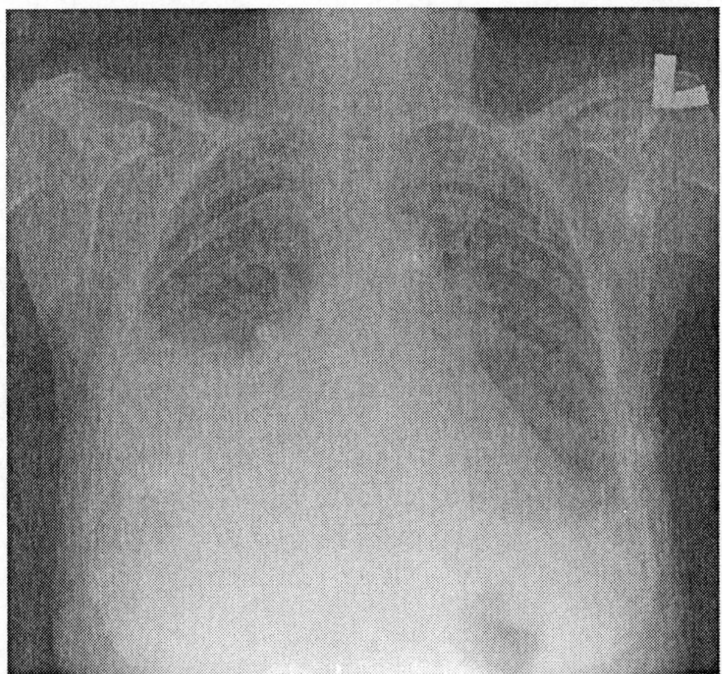

Figure 2.4: Large right and small left pleural effusions. (Reproduced with permission from SW Deanery.)

P Increase in fluid formation and/or absorption in the pleural space. The pathology is dependent on aetiology and divided into transudates and exudates.

A *Exudate* (protein >35g/L) due to ↑ microvascular permeability following disease or injury:

- Malignancy eg metastatic carcinoma, mesothelioma
- Infection eg TB, parapneumonic, empyema
- Inflammation eg SLE, rheumatoid arthritis, post-CABG, benign asbestos effusion and drugs

Transudate (protein <35g/L) due to ↑ hydrostatic pressure or ↓ osmotic pressure:

- Cardiac eg LVF, mitral stenosis, constrictive pericarditis
- Renal eg peritoneal dialysis, nephrotic syndrome
- Liver eg cirrhosis, ascites, hypoalbuminaemia

Light's criteria for protein 25-35g/L. See Box 2.6.

For pleural protein 25–35g/L sample is an *exudate* if at least one of the following is met:

- Sample protein divided by serum protein is >0.5
- Sample LDH divided by serum LDH is >0.6
- Sample LDH >2/3 upper limit of normal for serum LDH

Box 2.6: Light's criteria for pleural effusions

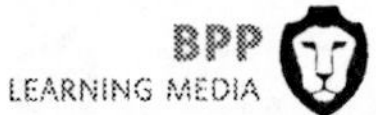

S Trachea displaced away from effusion, reduced chest movement on affected side, stony dull percussion note, reduced vocal fremitus and resonance, pleural friction rub, reduced breath sounds.

Sx Shortness of breath, occasional pleuritic pain.

I *Imaging:* CXR (see Figure 2.4), ultrasound, CT chest.

Pleural fluid: via diagnostic aspiration.

Pleural biopsy: eg Abram's needle, radiologically guided, video-assisted thoracoscopy.

Samples for: LDH and protein, M,C&S, AFB and TB culture if TB suspected.

T Treat underlying cause.

Therapeutic aspiration of 1–1.5L can be performed for symptomatic effusions.

C Breathlessness, empyema.

Pr Dependant of cause.

Pneumothorax

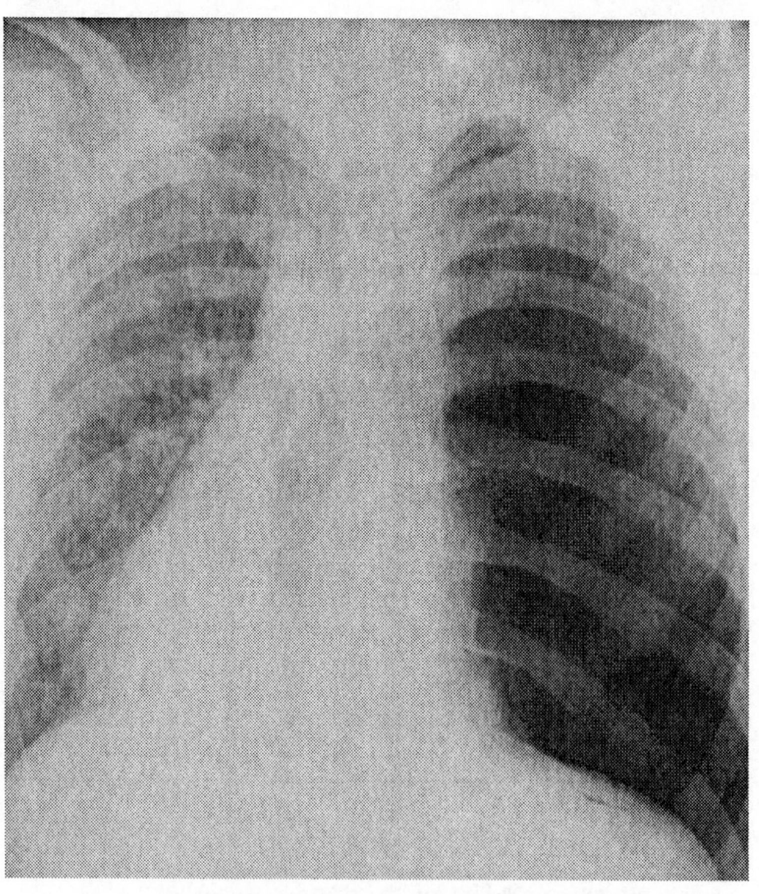

Figure 2.5: Left tension pneumothorax.
(Reproduced with permission from SW Deanery.)

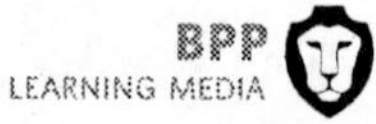

P The presence of air in the pleural cavity.

Spontaneous pneumothorax: primary (occurring in otherwise healthy patients) or secondary (associated with underlying lung disease, eg ruptured subpleural bleb or bullae in COPD).

Open pneumothorax: a 'sucking chest wound' – an open wound in the chest draws air in leading to tension pneumothorax.

Tension pneumothorax: a one-way valve develops allowing air into the pleural cavity but not to leave it. Intrapleural pressure rises, venous return and cardiac output become impaired and hypoxaemia and haemodynamic instability develops.

A *Primary spontaneous:* smoking, taller patients.

Secondary spontaneous: COPD, asthma, pulmonary fibrosis.

Trauma: blunt and penetrating chest trauma.

Iatrogenic: invasive ventilation, post-CPR, post-chest drain, post-central line insertion.

S Reduced chest expansion, reduced breath sounds, hyper-resonant percussion note.

Tension pneumothorax: cyanosis, severe tachypnoea, tachycardia and hypotension, mediastinal shift away from affected side.

Sx Chest pain, dyspnoea.

I CXR: aids diagnosis and sizing of pneumothorax.

CT: useful for uncertainty or complex cases.

T *Spontaneous pneumothorax:* see Box 2.7.

Tension pneumothorax: 100% oxygen and immediate needle decompression with needle/venflon into 2nd intercostal space in the mid-clavicular line (converting to simple pneumothorax) then proceed to chest drain insertion.

Open pneumothorax: an occlusive dressing is applied to the open wound and taped down on three sides allowing air to escape but not enter preventing progression to tension pneumothorax then chest drain insertion.

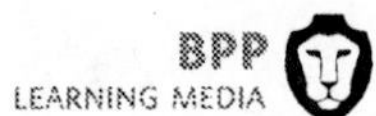

Primary

- Patient breathless or pneumothorax >2cm: aspirate up to 2.5L
  - If reduced to <2cm and breathing improved: consider discharge with out-patient review
  - If no improvement repeat aspiration or consider chest drain insertion
- Patient is not breathless or pneumothorax <2cm: consider discharge with out-patient review

Secondary

- Patient breathless or pneumothorax >2cm: chest drain insertion
- Patient not breathless and pneumothorax <1cm: observe for 24 hours with high flow oxygen
- Patient not breathless and pneumothorax 1–2cm: aspirate up to 2.5L
  - If reduced to <1cm: observe for 24 hours
  - If not reduced proceed to chest drain insertion

Box 2.7: Treatment of spontaneous pneumothorax

Chemical pleurodesis: not as effective as surgical options. Can be considered for recurrent pneumothoraces in patients who cannot tolerate surgery.

Surgical input: considered in patients with persistent air-leak. Options include open thoracotomy and pleurectomy.

C Reoccurrence, persistent air leak, re-expansion pulmonary oedema.

Pr Reoccurrence rates in primary spontaneous (five years): 28–32%.

Secondary spontaneous (five years): 43%.

Mortality rates variable, based on environment, treatment and pathology.

Pulmonary embolus

P Embolus in the pulmonary vasculature that has classically travelled from a deep vein of the leg (DVT) via the right heart.

A From a DVT or from right atrial thrombus in AF.

Virchow's Triad:

- *Venous stasis* eg immobility, congestive cardiac failure, dehydration and venous obstruction
- *Damage to a vein* eg trauma, inflammation and previous thrombosis
- *Hypercoaguable state* eg malignancy, oestrogen therapy, surgery and abnormalities of the clotting cascade

S *Acute minor:* hyperventilation, haemoptysis, hypoxia, fever, effusion.

Acute major: as above + hypotension, cyanosis, engorged neck veins and sudden collapse.

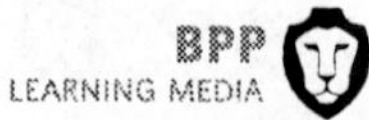

Sub-acute/chronic: hyperventilation, raised JVP.

Sx *Acute minor:* pleuritic pain, dyspnoea.

Acute major: central chest pain, dyspnoea.

Sub-acute/chronic: progressive dyspnoea.

I CXR: often normal. Elevation of a hemi-diaphram and linear atelectasis may be suggestive. Small effusions or wedged shaped infarcts may be present.

ECG: may just show sinus tachycardia, right heart strain may be present with S1Q3T3.

ABG: low PaO_2 and $PaCO_2$.

D-dimer blood test: if clinical probability is high then the test should not be performed. If the probability is intermediate or low then a negative d-dimer is a reliable rule-out of thromboembolic disease.

Pulmonary angiography: definitive test but invasive and rarely performed.

CTPA: non-invasive imaging modality, accepted as the recommended initial investigation for non-massive PEs.

V/Q scan: rarely performed.

T Thrombolysis: reserved for those with clinically massive PE and marked haemodynamic compromise.

Anticoagulation: low molecular weight heparin acutely then Warfarin with a target INR of 2.0–3.0.

IVC filter: aims to prevent further clot from DVT reaching the pulmonary vasculature. May be of use when anti-coagulation is contraindicated.

C Pulmonary haemorrhage, pulmonary hypertension, congestive cardiac failure, recurrent episodes.

Pr Massive PE 30–60% mortality. Most occur in the first one to two hours of care.

Airway disease

Asthma

P Chronic, reversible inflammation of the airways, which causes obstruction to airflow due to increased sensitivity to a variety of stimuli.

Two phases:

- Early reaction (minutes): bronchospasm
- Late reaction (three to five hours): oedema and mucus

A Genetic: probable polygenic inheritance, atopy.

Environmental: house dust mites, pet-derived allergens, smoke, pollen and work place agents, NSAIDs, beta-blockers, cold.

S Polyphonic wheeze on auscultation, tachypnoea, diurnal variation.

Sx Wheeze, shortness of breath, cough, chest tightness.

I Spirometry: >15% improvement after B_2 agonist/steroid trial.

Peak Expiratory Flow (PEF): >20% diurnal variation for >3 days.

Airway responsiveness testing: eg exercise testing, methacoline provocation test.

Hypersensitivity testing: eg skin prick tests, RAST, total IgE level.

CXR: exclusion of other diagnoses, pneumothorax, infection.

- Moderate:
  - PEF 50–75% of best / predicted
  - Increasing symptoms
- Acute severe:
  - PEF 33–50% of best / predicted
  - Tachypnoea (resp rate >25)
  - Tachycardia (pulse rate >110)
  - Inability to complete a sentence in one breath
- Life-threatening: **33-92-CHEST**
  - PEF **<33%** best or predicted
  - Sats **<92%**
  - **C**yanosis
  - **H**ypotension
  - **E**xhaustion / confusion
  - **S**ilent chest
  - **T**achy / bradycardia

Box 2.8: Assessment of acute asthma severity

T *Acute:* assessment of severity, including peak flow.

Supplementary oxygen to keep sats 94–98%.

B_2 agonist bronchodilators: inhaled or nebulised. (IV delivery if inhalation not achievable).

Ipratropium bromide: add in nebulised form if acute severe, life-threatening or poor response to B_2 agonist.

Steroids: give in all cases of acute asthma.

Magnesium sulphate: consider a single dose in near fatal or life-threatening asthma.

ITU: to be reviewed for intensive care if has life-threatening or near-fatal asthma which is failing to respond to initial therapy.

Chronic: see Box 2.9.

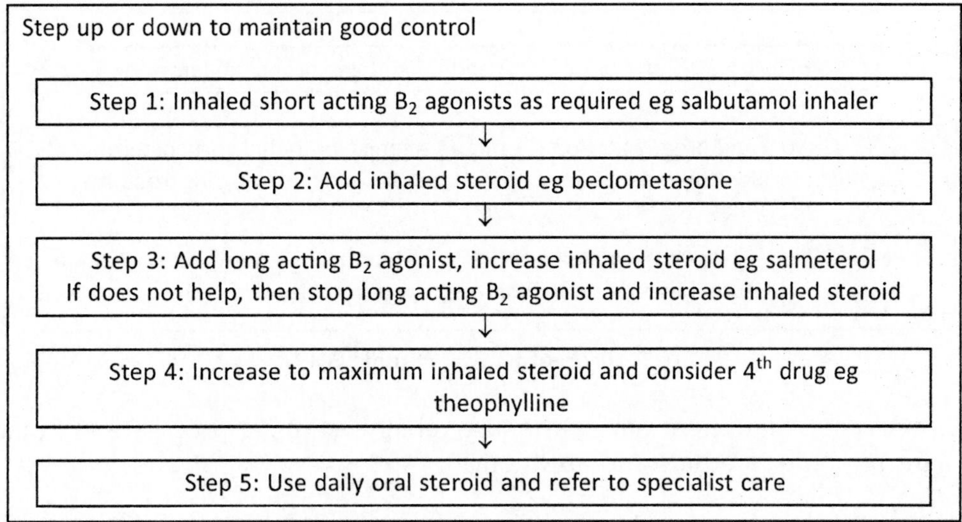

Box 2.9: Treatment of chronic asthma

C Persistent symptoms, cough, decreased activity, infections, pneumothorax, fixed airway disease, long-term steroid therapy, bronchietasis.

Pr Generally very good.

Chronic obstructive pulmonary disease (COPD)

P Progressive airway obstruction with little to no reversibility. Due to chronic bronchitis and emphysema.

Emphysema: dilatation and destruction of terminal air spaces. *Chronic bronchitis:* productive cough on most days for at least three months of two successive years. It is a hypersecretory disorder.

A Tobacco smoking, occupational environments, alpha-1 anti-trypsin deficiency.

S Tachypneoa, hyperinflated thorax, lip pursing, plethoric, cyanosis, use of accessory muscles, quiet breath sounds.

Sx Cough, sputum production, breathlessness and wheeze.

I Spirometry: airflow obstruction on post-bronchodilator therapy.

Transfer factor: reduced in emphysema.

CXR: hyperinflation, bullae.

HRCT: gives an indication of the extent of emphysema.

T *Acute:* oxygen, oral steroids, antibiotics, nebulisers if required, BIPAP for uncompensated respiratory acidosis not responding to treatment.

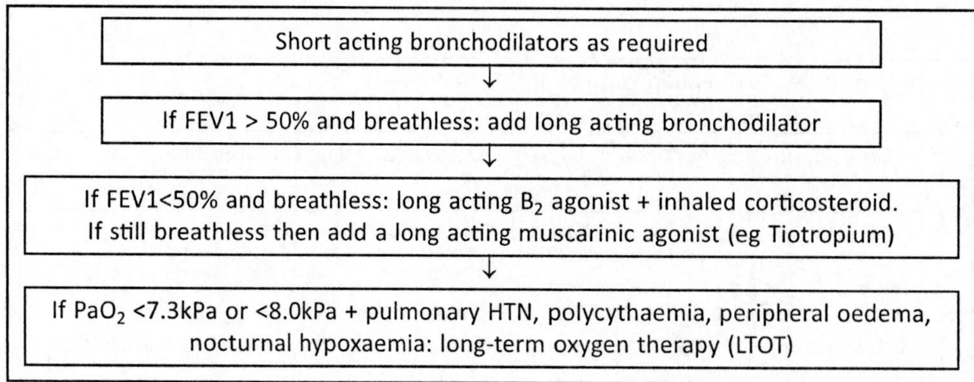

Box 2.10: Treatment of chronic COPD

Chronic: smoking cessation, pulmonary rehabilitation, appropriate self management plans (eg home steroids and antibiotics).

Appropropriate oxygen therapy if needed.

C Infective exacerbations, pneumothorax, cor pulmonale, pulmonary hypertension, immobility, weight loss, ventilator failure.

Pr Only stopping smoking and long-term oxygen therapy (LTOT) improve prognosis.

Adult respiratory distress syndrome (ARDS)

P Acute respiratory failure with oedematous lung field resulting from inflammatory events without a raised left atrial pressure.

The oedema arises due to increased alveolar permeability.

A See Box 2.11.

ARDS is often a complication of another insult

- Pulmonary insult
  - Pneumonia
  - Aspiration
  - Inhalation injury (eg smoke)
  - Lung contusion
- Non-pulmonary insult
  - Sepsis
  - Trauma
  - Burns
  - Pancreatitis
  - Blood transfusion

Box 2.11: Causes of ARDS

S Tachypnoea, confusion secondary to hypoxia.

Sx Shortness of breath, agitation.

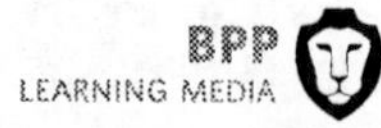

I CXR: bilateral infiltrates.

ABG: PaO_2/FiO_2 <26.7kPa (<200mmHg).

Pulmonary artery wedge pressure: <18mmHg.

T The underlying cause must be treated if possible. Good supportive care is key.

C The complications are based on the effects of a severe illness and potentially a prolonged period of mechanical ventilation.

Pr Mortality rate 50–60%.

Interstitial lung disease

Pulmonary fibrosis

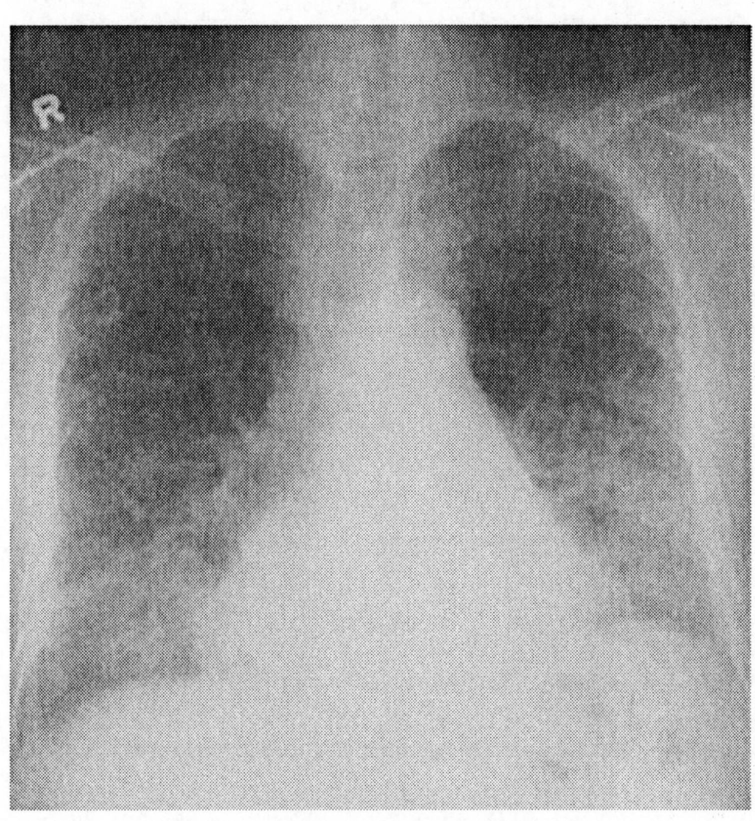

Figure 2.6: Bilateral lower zone fibrosis. (Reproduced with permission from SW Deanery.)

P Fibrosis and remodeling of the interstitium following chronic inflammation.

A See Box 2.12.

Upper zone fibrosis	Lower zone fibrosis
BREAST **B**erylliosis **R**adiation **E**xtrinsic allergic alveolitis **A**nkylosing spondylitis **S**arcoidosis **T**uberculosis	Connective tissue disorders: • SLE • RA • Scleroderma Drugs: • Amiodarone • Nitrofurantoin • Methotrexate • Bleomycin • Cyclophosphamide Occupational lung disease: • Asbestosis • Silicosis

Box 2.12: Causes of pulmonary fibrosis

S Dyspnoea, hypoxia, clubbing, late inspiratory crackles on auscultation, raised JVP and peripheral oedema.

Sx Shortness of breath on exertion, dry cough.

I CT: reticulation and honeycombing suggest fibrosis while ground glass suggests inflammation.

Spirometry, lung volumes and gas transfer: classically a restrictive pattern.

Lung biopsy: can be via bronchoscope or surgical biopsy.

T Avoidance of aetiology.

Steroids: more likely to help if there is more inflammation and less fibrosis.

Immunosuppressants: eg azathioprine.

Lung transplantation: should be considered in the young with advanced unresponsive disease.

Palliation: important in end-stage disease.

C End-stage fibrosis.

Pr Variable, depending on the conditions. Overall five-year survival rate is around 50%.

Idiopathic pulmonary fibrosis

P Inflammatory infiltrate and fibrosis of unknown cause.

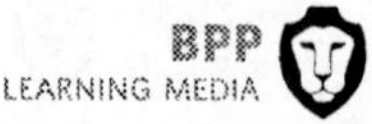

A Commonest cause of interstitial lung disease (ILD).

Also known as cryptogenic fibrosing alveolitis (CFA).

S **Sx** Bilateral fine end-inspiratory crackles ('velcro-like') in 90%, clubbing (60%), dry cough, exertional dyspnea.

I Clinical, exclude other diagnoses.

T Steroids, azathioprine, cyclophosphamide, transplant.

C 10% develop lung tumour.

Pr 50% at five years.

Extrinsic allergic alveolitis

P Hypersensitivity reaction to inhaled allergens.

Acute phase: inflammation.

Chronic exposure: granuloma formation, bronchiolitis obliterans.

A Multiple allergens: bird fancier's lung, pigeon fancier's lung, farmer's lung (micropolyspora faeni), malt worker's lung (aspergillus clavatus) amongst others.

S Crackles, fever, weight loss if chronic process.

Sx *Acute (four to six hours post-exposure):* dry cough, dyspnoea, fever, rigors, myalgia.

Chronic: progressive dyspnoea, weight loss, cor pulmonale.

I FBC: ↑ WCC (neutrophils), ↑ CRP/ESR.

CXR: bilateral mid-zone shadowing.

Spirometry: restrictive defect, allergen testing.

T Remove offending allergen, in the acute phase give oxygen if hypoxic and steroids.

C May progress to permanent lung damage if chronic exposure, type 1 respiratory failure, cor-pulmonale.

Pr Resolves if allergen removed +/- steroids in the acute period.

Sarcoidosis

P Inflammatory disorder with accumulation of T-cells and granulomas that can affect many systems, most commonly the pulmonary system.

A Cause is unknown. Most commonly affects younger adults (30–40 years), female > male.

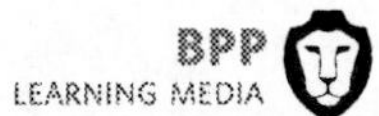

S Erythema nodosum and bilateral hilar lymphadenopathy is pathognomic, fine crackles on inspiration, uveitis, hypercalcaemia, polyarthralgia.

Sx Up to 40% may be asymptomatic, dry cough, increasing dyspnoea, rash, ocular symptoms, neuropathy.

I CXR: bilateral hilar lymphadenopathy (90%), infiltrates.

Bloods: ↑ serum ACE, ↑ ESR, ↑ Ca^{2+}

Spirometry: reduced lung volumes and/or a restrictive defect. Tissue sample from affected organ eg transbronchial lung biopsy: histology shows non-caseating granulomata.

T May resolve spontaneously.

If symptoms persist then treatment with 6–12 months of oral steroids (prednisolone).

C Can progress to lung fibrosis, respiratory failure, cor-pulmonale.

Pr 60% recover in <2 years. Monitor with CXR, lung function and clinical review.

Industrial lung disease

P Lung fibrosis secondary to inflammation caused by inhaled particles.

A Coal workers pneumoconiosis: coal dust particles.

Silicosis: silica particles, found in many industries including metal mining, quarrying and ceramics manufacturing.

Asbestosis: asbestosis fibres, previously used as a common material for fireproofing and insulation.

S Finger clubbing, end inspiratory crackles.

Sx May be asymptomatic, progressive dyspnoea.

I Spirometry: restrictive defect.

CXR: interstitial changes, pleural plaques with asbestos exposure.

T Avoid causative particles, otherwise supportive treatment.

C Patients exposed to asbestos are at a much greater risk of developing bronchial carcinoma and malignant mesothelioma. Patients with silicosis are at increased risk of developing tuberculosis.

Pr Depends on degree of fibrosis.

Patients with industrial lung disease are often eligible to claim compensation through the Industrial Injuries Act.

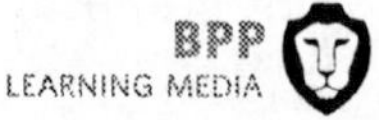

Suppurative lung disease

Bronchiectasis

P Abnormal and permanently dilated airways with increased mucus production, decreased mucus clearance and recurrent infections.

A Post infection, immune overactivity (ABPA) and underactivity (hypogammaglobulinaemia), cystic fibrosis, Kartagener's Syndrome (situs inversus and ciliary dysfunction), bronchial obstruction, rheumatoid arthritis, idopathic.

S Finger clubbing, coarse inspiratory crackles over the affected area, halitosis, wheeze.

Sx Persistent, productive cough with large volumes of purulent sputum, haemoptysis, dyspnoea, recurrent infections, weight loss.

I CXR: may be normal.

HRCT: bronchial damage.

Lung function tests, sputum cultures, test for cystic fibrosis if <40 years/suspicion of CF.

T Physiotherapy for sputum clearance.

Antibiotics to treat infections.

Treat co-existing lung disease.

C Recurrent infections causing progressive lung damage and respiratory failure.

Pr Generally deteriorate over time/with exacerbations. Rate of decline linked to organisms in sputum.

Cystic fibrosis

P Abnormal viscosity of mucus produced at the epithelial surfaces causing recurrent infections and bronchiectasis in lungs.

Patients also have pancreatic insufficiency amongst other secretory problems.

A Autosomal recessive defect in the cystic fibrosis transmembrane conductance regulator (CFTR) gene located on the long arm of chromosome 7. CFTR controls chloride channel behaviour causing defective chloride secretion and increased sodium absorption altering the composition of mucus secretions.

S As those with bronchiectasis, usually presenting in the first years of life, malnourishment. Males are infertile due to the absence of the vas deferens.

Sx As those of bronchiectasis, failure to thrive and steatorrhoea secondary to pancreatic insufficiency.

I Sweat test to look for excess sweat sodium (Cl^-/Na^+ channel reversed in skin epithelium), DNA analysis, CXR, HRCT, pulmonary function tests.

T Physiotherapy for sputum clearance, good nutrition and supplemental vitamins and pancreatic enzymes.

Antibiotics for chest infections, mucolytics, nebulised antibiotics, lung/heart-lung transplant.

C Recurrent infections, respiratory failure.

Pr Had improved greatly over the last few decades, most children survive to their teens. Median survival is around 40 years.

Lung tumours

P Neoplastic growth in the respiratory tract.

Bronchial carcinoma accounts for 95% of all primary cancers of the lung, with alveolar cell carcinoma accounting for 2% and other tumours accounting for 3%.

Histology can be split into non-small cell and small cell. See Box 2.13.

A Smoking (including passive smoking) is the largest causative factor. Other factors include occupational exposures to substances such as asbestos.

Small cell (30%):	Non-small cell:
• ADH secreted produces dilutional hyponatraemia • ACTH-like peptide produces Cushing's symptoms (pigmentation, proximal myopathy)	• Squamous cell (40%) – PTH-like peptide produces hypercalcaemia • Adenocarcinoma (10%)
70% metastasize	40% metastasize

Box 2.13: Types of bronchial carcinoma and endocrine secretions

S May have no signs. Supraclavicular lymphadenopathy, signs of pleural effusion (unilateral).

Sx Cough, haemoptysis, chest pain, lethargy, weight loss, dyspnoea, hoarse voice (due to involvement of the recurrent laryngeal nerve eg Pancoast's tumour which can also cause Horner's syndrome).

I CXR: lesion/mass, pleural effusion and/or signs of lobar collapse.

CT chest: stage the disease (tumour, node, metastasis (TNM) staging system).

Bronchoscopy +/- biopsy if endobronchial lesion, CT guided biopsy to obtain tissue to histology.

T Limited, curable disease: surgical resection, radical radiotherapy or combination treatment.

Non-curable disease (most common): systemic treatment with chemotherapy, localised treatment with radiotherapy for local disease control/symptomatic relief, palliative care input for symptom control and support.

C Invasion of local structures: eg nerves, bones, muscles, blood vessels, occlusion of bronchus.

Metastatic spread: can metastasise to any site, commonly '**Brain BALL**': **brain**, **b**one, **a**drenal, **l**iver, **l**ymph nodes.

Pr Dependent of type and stage of lung cancer but overall prognosis is poor.

Overall five-year survival is less than 10% as most cancers are inoperable by time of presentation/diagnosis.

Other lung conditions

Obstructive sleep apnoea (OSA)

P Episodes of apnoea during sleep caused by collapse/obstruction of the pharyngeal airways. Terminated by partial waking resulting in fragmented sleep.

A Most commonly seen in overweight, middle-aged men and is made worse by alcohol. Upper airways abnormalities eg large tonsils, can sometimes be the cause.

S Overweight.

Sx Daytime sleepiness, morning headaches, disturbed sleep, decreased libido, partners will report snoring and apnoeas.

I Overnight pulse oximetry will show frequent desaturations which quickly resolve when partially wakens. Full sleep studies (polysomnography) may be needed if overnight oximetry is not diagnostic.

T Reduce weight and avoid alcohol. Continuous positive airways pressure (CPAP) overnight is an effective treatment.

Surgery is sometimes used to correct upper airways abnormalities.

C Pulmonary hypertension leading to cor pulmonale, hypertension, type 2 respiratory failure.

Pr Dependant on the development of vascular complications. Can resolve if sufficient weight loss.

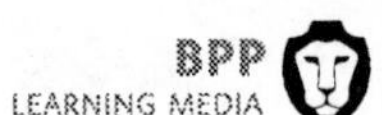

Cor pulmonale

P Right heart failure due to chronic pulmonary hypertension.

A Any cause of pulmonary hypertension.

Pulmonary vascular disease: acute pulmonary embolism, primary pulmonary hypertension, chronic pulmonary embolism, parasitic infection.

Lung disease: COPD, asthma, pulmonary fibrosis, bronchiectasis.

Chronic hypoventilation: motor neurone disease, myasthenia gravis, kyphosis, scoliosis, OSA.

S Peripheral oedema, raised JVP, right ventricular heave, cyanosis, tricuspid regurgitation, hepatomegaly, cyanosis.

Sx Dyspnoea, fatigue, anorexia, weight loss.

I ECG: right ventricular hypertrophy and right axis deviation, P pulmonale.

CXR: right atrial enlargement, cardiomegaly.

FBC: polycythaemia.

ECHO: right ventricular dysfunction, tricuspid regurgitation and estimation of right sided pressures.

T Treat the underlying cause. Oxygen if hypoxic. Diuretics for oedema. Younger patients (<55 years old) can be considered for heart-lung transplantation.

C Arrhythmia, liver failure.

Pr Poor, 50% five-year mortality.

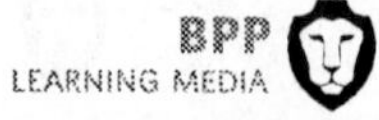

Practice Questions

Single Best Answers

1. Which of these are most commonly associated with sarcoidosis?

   A Erythema nodosum
   B Erythema multi form
   C Gout
   D Pyoderma gangrinosa

2. Which of these is not a cause of bronchiectasis?

   A Cystic fibrosis
   B Bronchial obstruction
   C Immunodefiency
   D Ramipril

3. Which of the following does not have a routine role in the management of CF?

   A Dietary advice
   B Supplemental pancreatic enzymes
   C Steroids
   D Antibiotics

4. Which of the following is associated with the greatest risk of lung cancer?

   A Asbestos
   B Sillica particles
   C Coal dust particles
   D Aspergillus clavatus

5. Which of the following is not associated with obstructive sleep apnoea?

   A Morning headaches
   B Daytime sleepiness
   C Obstructive defect on spirometry
   D Decreased libido

6. Which of the following is not a cause of pulmonary hypertension?

   A COPD
   B PE
   C Myocardial infarction
   D Motor neuron disease

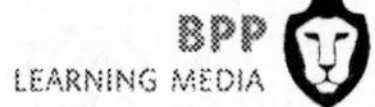

7. Which of the following is the most common type of lung cancer?

   A Squamous cell carcinoma
   B Adenocarcinoma
   C Small cell lung cancer
   D Alveolar cell carcinoma

8. Which of the following is needed to make a diagnosis of COPD?

   A CXR
   B High resolution CT scan
   C Spirometry
   D Peak flow

9. A 67-year-old man is diagnosed with pneumonia. He has a respiratory rate of 28 breaths per minute, a blood pressure of 91/58 mmHg, he is not confused, has a urea of 7.9 mmol/L and a C-reactive protein of 258. His CURB-65 score is:

   A 0
   B 1
   C 2
   D 3

10. Which of the following pleural fluid analysis is suggestive of an exudate?

    A Sample protein 30g/L with a serum protein 62g/L
    B Sample protein 29g/L with a serum protein 57g/L
    C Sample LDH half the upper limit of normal for serum LDH
    D Sample pH 7.4

11. Which of the following arterial blood gases is most compatible with acute pulmonary embolism?

    A PaO_2 11 kPa, PCO_2 5.9 kPa – on 24% oxygen
    B PaO_2 7.1 kPa, PCO_2 8.3 kPa – FiO_2 0.4
    C PaO_2 8.1 kPa, PCO_2 3.7 kPa – on room air
    D PaO_2 14.1, PCO_2 5.0 – on 24% oxygen

12. Features of a pneumothorax include:

    A A dull percussion note
    B Pleural rub
    C Decreased breath sounds on auscultation
    D Increased vocal fremitus

13. Patient presents with a peak expiratory flow rate which is 40% of their predicted value, a respiratory rate of 24 breaths per minute, pulse of 108 beats per minute and oxygen saturations of 93% on air. How would you class the severity of this exacerbation of their asthma?

    A Moderate
    B Acute severe
    C Life threatening
    D Near fatal

14. Which of the following spirometry results demonstrates airflow obstruction?

    A FEV1 1.5 L, FVC 2.0 L
    B FEV1 2.5 L, FVC 3.0 L
    C FEV1 0.7, FVC 1.8 L
    D FEV1 0.8, FVC 1.1 L

15. Which of the following has shown benefit in the management of ARDS?

    A Ventilation at 6mls/kg
    B Ventilation at 12mls/kg
    C Antibiotics
    D ACE inhibitors

Extended Matching Questions

Breathlessness on exertion

A Bronchopneumonia
B IDA
C Congestive cardiac failure
D Pulmonary tuberculosis
E Sarcoidosis
F Pulmonary embolus
G AML
H COPD
I Pulmonary fibrosis
J CLL

Match the description of the patient with the most likely diagnosis.

1. A 70-year-old retired boilermaker gives a five-year history of exertional dyspnoea, and a dry cough. The patient is a non-smoker. On examination, fine crackles are heard at the base of both lung fields.

2. A 25-year-old HIV positive man who has had a productive cough for the last three months with haemoptysis and night sweats. Chest X-ray shows hilar lymphadenopathy.

3. A 76-year-old lady seven days post-total hip replacement suddenly drops her sats to 80%. The nurses note that her right leg had looked red and swollen.

4. A 60-year-old publican who smokes 20 cigarettes a day has a ten-year history of having a 'smoker's morning cough' when he expectorates clear sputum. This is worse in the winter when it sometimes turns green and he has to go to his general practitioner for antibiotics. On examination, he has poor air entry over both lung fields and his Peak Expiratory Flow Rate is 210l/min (reduced by 80%).

5. A 35-year-old lady with shortness of breath and tiredness over six weeks. She had decided to consult her doctor when multiple mauve lesions 1–3cm in diameter appeared over both shins. Chest X-ray shows hilar lymphadenopathy.

Causes of cough

A Bronchiectasis
B Postnasal drip
C Asthma
D Carcinoma of the bronchus
E Oesophageal reflux
F Foreign body
G COPD
H Drug adverse effect
I Sarcoidosis

For each patient below, choose the **single** most likely diagnosis from the above list of options.

6. A 58-year-old man, who smoked 30 cigarettes a day, presents with a six-week history of cough, malaise, anorexia and weight loss.

7. A 45-year-old woman with essential hypertension is prescribed lisinopril. Two weeks later she complains of a constant dry cough which keeps her awake. There are no systemic symptoms.

8. A 40-year-old Afro-Caribbean woman presents with bilateral parotid swelling, and painful nodules on the front of her shins. She has a dry cough and slight shortness of breath on exertion.

9. An 18-year-old man presents with a night-time cough and shortness of breath while playing football. This has got progressively worse over the previous two months.

10. A 30-year-old man, lifelong non-smoker, presents with a history of at least six months of purulent sputum. He has had an infection since an attack of measles at the age of 14.

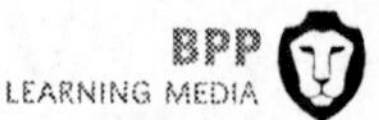

Causes of cough

A Tuberculosis
B Bronchial carcinoma
C Asthma
D Pneumonia
E Extrinsic allergic alveolitis
F Influenza
G Chronic bronchitis
H ACE inhibitor therapy
I Fibrosing alveolitis
J Left ventricular failure

For each of the following patients choose the **single** most likely diagnosis from the above list of options.

11. A 50-year-old male smoker presents with a three-month history of cough, haemoptysis and weight loss. Chest examination is unremarkable.

12. A five-year-old child coughs most nights. He has frequent courses of antibiotics for a 'bad chest' especially in the winter. He also has eczema.

13. A 50-year-old male smoker has a cough productive of clear sputum most days especially in the winter. He has not lost weight. On examination, he has a hyper-expanded chest and a few scattered wheezes and crackles.

14. A 40-year-old Asian man has a two-month history of cough, haemoptysis, weight loss and night sweats. He has swollen cervical lymph nodes and his trachea is deviated to the left.

15. A 40-year-old man has a history of hypertension. His anti-hypertensive medication was recently changed due to ankle swelling. He has now developed a dry cough.

Causes of dyspnoea

A Anaemia
B Valvular disease
C Bronchial asthma
D Atelectasis
E Atypical pneumonia
F Bronchial carcinoma
G Acute pulmonary oedema
H Pulmonary embolus
I Exacerbation of chronic bronchitis
J Metastatic carcinoma

From each patient below, choose the **single** most likely diagnosis from the above list of options.

16. An obese 33-year-old man, one day post open cholecystectomy becomes acutely short of breath.

17. A 65-year-old man with a history of chronic productive cough now presents to A&E short of breath and drowsy.

18. A 60-year-old woman presents with dyspnoea. On examination, she has a firm mass in the left breast and decreased breath sounds in the right lower lung fields. Chest X-ray reveals a pleural effusion.

19. A 50-year-old male patient on the ward awakes with dyspnoea and frothy sputum. He had suffered an MI a week earlier. On examination, he is cyanosed and tachypnoeic. Auscultation of the lung reveals creps.

20. A 40-year-old man presents with cough and breathlessness. Chest X-ray demonstrates diffuse consolidation of the right lower lobe. Despite treatment with IV augmentin, the fever persists. Chest X-ray shows expansion.

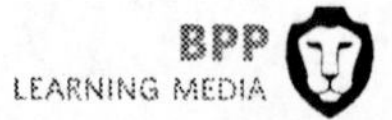

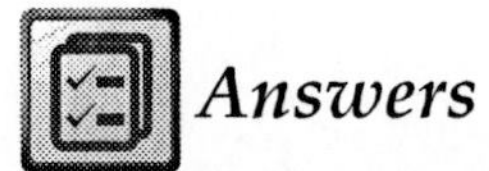

Answers

SBAs		EMQs	
1	A	1	I
2	D	2	D
3	C	3	F
4	A	4	H
5	C	5	E
6	C	6	D
7	A	7	H
8	C	8	I
9	D	9	C
10	B	10	A
11	C	11	B
12	C	12	C
13	B	13	G
14	C	14	A
15	A	15	H
		16	D
		17	I
		18	J
		19	G
		20	E

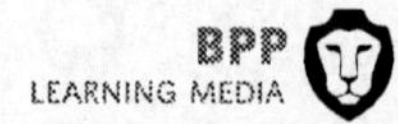

Chapter 3

Gastroenterology

Dr Utti Chelvaratnam and
Dr Barnaby Hole

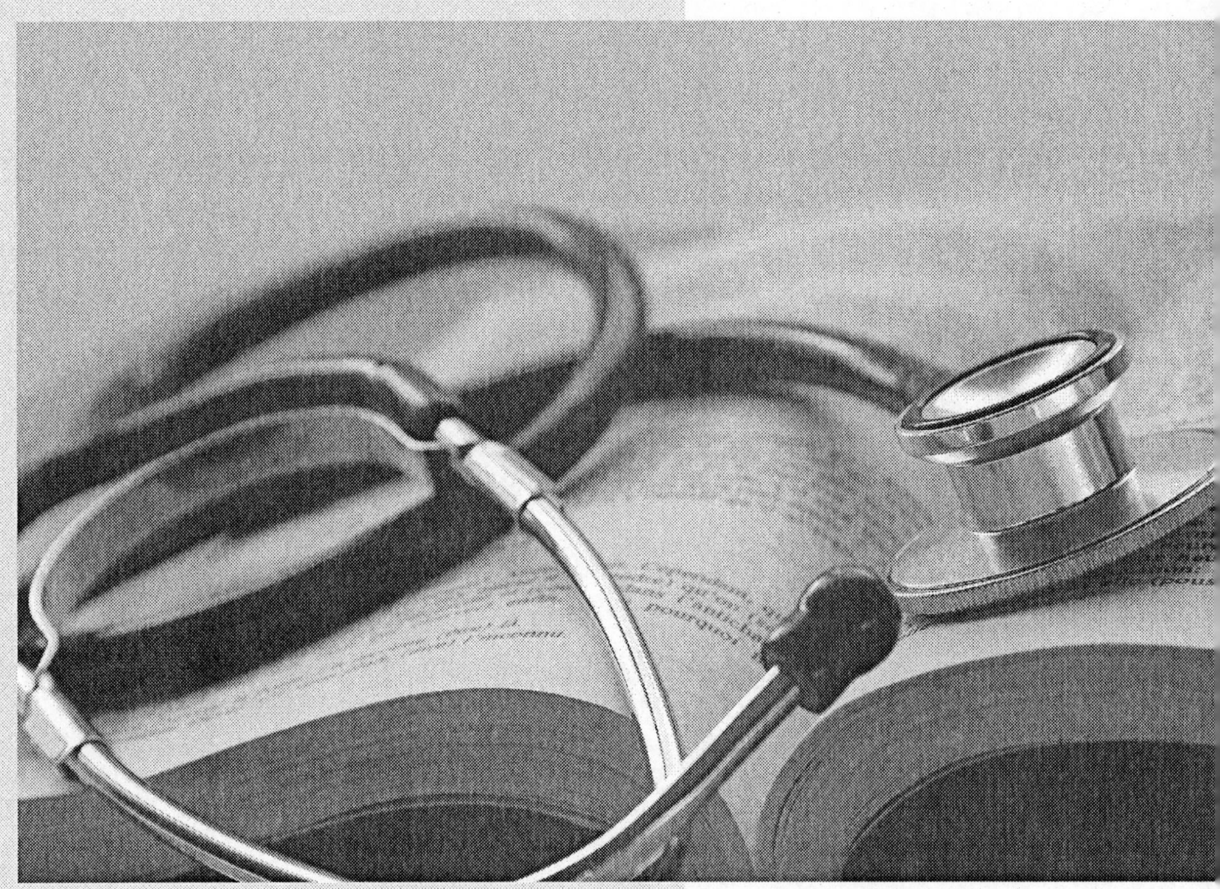

Key investigations

- **Barium swallow**: patient swallows contrast and flouroscopy images are taken at a rate of two to three frames per second to highlight any oeosphageal abnormality
- **Barium follow through**: as above however further image capture allows imaging of small bowel
- **Barium enema**: application of contrast by rectal enema and X-rays images of the colon performed
- **Video fluoroscopy**: real-time image capture allows functional as well as anatomical assessment to be made
- **CT colonography**: computerised tomography imaging of large bowel with contrast and air insufflation; think 3D barium enema
- **USS abdomen**: low cost and risk assessment useful for assessing for cirrhosis and biliary tree obstruction
- **Oesophageal gastroduodenoscopy (OGD)**: endoscopic examination of the upper GI tract
- **Endoscopic retrograde cholangiopancreatography (ERCP)**: endoscopic examination of the stomach and duodenum and injection of contrast into the biliary tree. This allows extraction of gallstones and placement of stents
- **Colonoscopy**: endoscopic examination of the whole of the large bowel
- **Flexible sigmoidoscopy**: endoscopic examination of the left side of the colon
- **Alpha-fetoprotein**: tumour marker associated with hepatocellular carcinoma
- **CA 19-9**: tumour marker associated with pancreatic cancer

Oesophagus and stomach

Dysphagia

P Symptom of difficulty in swallowing.

A *Neurological:* stroke, Parkinson's disease, MND, MS, myasthenia gravis, muscular dystrophy, thyroxicosis, steroid myopathy.

Structural: malignancy, benign oesophageal stricture, oesophageal web, oesophageal dysmotility eg achalasia, scleroderma, extrinsic compression (eg lung malignancy).

S Odynophagia, regurgitation, retrosternal chest pain.

I OGD: malignancy, web.

Barium swallow: malignancy, dysmotility.

CT head: neurological causes.

Video fluoroscopy: oropharyngeal dysphagia, swallow safety.

T *Structural:* if malignancy – may be resectable. Other options are OGD and dilatation / stenting.

Neurological: treatment of underlying condition (ie pyridostigmine in myasthenia gravis). If dysphagia results in unsafe swallowing and risk of aspiration, PEG may be inserted for nutrition.

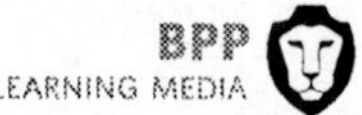

Dyspepsia

P Defined as epigastric burning or pain.

A Gastro-oesophageal reflux disease, gastric ulcer (10% associated with H. pylori infection), duodenal ulcer (90 % associated with H. pylori infection).

S Epigastric tenderness.

Sx If any red flags patient **must** to be investigated further.

- Dysphagia
- Weight loss
- Vomiting
- Epigastric mass
- Iron deficient anaemia

Box 3.1: Dyspepsia red flags

I Helicobacter pylori serology, OGD: gastritis, oesophagitis, malignancy.

T *Lifestyle advice:* sleeping propped up with more pillows at night time, reducing caffeine intake, reduce late night alcohol and caffeine, losing weight.

Medical: antacid (eg calcium carbonate and alginates), proton pump inhibitors or H2 receptor antagonists, if H. pylori +ve then eradication therapy with PPI and antibiotics.

Gastro oesophageal reflux disease (GORD)

P Oesophagitis, gastritis or duodenitis due to reflux.

A Lax lower oesophageal sphincter tone H. pylori infection.

Sx Dyspepsia, acid brash, odynophagia, dysphagia.

I OGD: gastritis, oesophagitis, malignancy.

Barium swallow: irregularity of oesophageal mucosa reflux of barium.

T *Medical*: lifestyle advice, antacids, PPI, H_2 receptor antagonist, pro-kinetic medications.

Surgical: if refractory to medications and patient's premorbid state allows, then surgical treatment may be an option.

C Due to recurrent insults to the GI mucosa: ulceration, benign stricture, barrett's oesophagus (low risk 1% per year of progressing to malignancy).

Nausea and vomiting

A Drugs: antibiotics, chemotherapy and digoxin.

Infections: viral gastroenteritis, labyrinthitis, food poisoning.

Mechanical: pyloric stenosis, gastric outlet obstruction, oesophageal malignancy, alcoholism.

Metabolic: Addison's disease, diabetes, hypercalcaemia, hyperthyroidism.

Cranial: brain tumour, encephalitis, meningitis, stroke, migraine, functional vomiting.

Pregnancy (including hyperemesis gravidum).

I U&Es: ↓ K ↓ Ur ↑ Creat ↑ Bicarbonate.

OGD: pyloric stenosis, gastric outlet obstruction.

Cortisol/Short Synacthen test: Addison's disease.

CT head: space occupying lesion.

T Treatment of underlying condition. Antiemetics and prokinetics may help if no pathology found.

Upper GI bleeding

P Bleeding originating **proximal** to the ligament of Treitz (suspensory muscle of duodenum, inserts into distal duodenum) in the GI tract.

A *Oesophagus:* oesophageal ulcer (aspirin, NSAIDs), oesophageal varices (secondary to portal hypertension), malignancy, Mallory-Weiss tear.

Gastric: gastric ulcer (H. pylori / aspirin / NSAIDs / malignancy), gastric adenocarcinoma, gastric varices (secondary to portal hypertension), angiodysplasia.

Duodenum: duodenal ulcer (H. pylori /aspirin / NSAIDs / malignancy), duodenal varices (secondary to portal hypertension), malignancy, angiodysplasia.

S Haematemesis, melaena, shock.

Stigmata of liver disease (suggestive of variceal bleeding): jaundice, ascites, spider naevi, caput medusae, splenomegaly if portal hypertension.

Sx If oesophageal aetiology: dysphagia, odynophagia, dyspepsia. Mallory-Weiss tear: recurrent vomiting with normal vomitus followed by vomiting blood.

Gastric ulcer: abdominal pain, worsens on eating.

Duodenal ulcer: abdominal pain, improves on eating.

I FBC: ↓ Hb ↓ Hct ↓ MCV (chronic blood loss); U&Es: ↓ Ur (protein meal from blood) ↓ Creat (shock); clotting.

OGD: ulcers, bleeding tumours, varices, can apply therapy to ulcers and varices to stop bleeding.

CT angiography: show bleeding vessel and embolise it to stop bleeding.

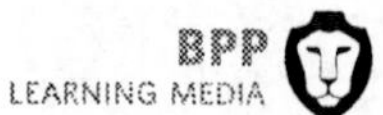

T Medical: PPI, correct coagulopathy, transfuse with blood.

OGD: treat ulcers to stop bleeding. CT angiography: embolisation of bleeding vessel. Surgery: if bleeding refractory to above.

Radiotherapy: if secondary to ooze from malignant mucosa.

C Hypovolaemic shock, renal failure, death.

Pr The Rockall score is used to risk stratify mortality and rebleeding risk of UGI bleeds. It incorporates endoscopic findings for the full score but pre-endoscopy score is often used to calculate risks. Score > 3 is high risk UGI bleeding

	Score 0	Score 1	Score 2	Score 3
Age	< 60	60–79	> 80	
Shock	No shock	HR > 100 SBP > 100	SBP < 100	
Co-morbidity	Nil major		CCF, IHD, major morbidity	Renal failure, liver failure, metastic cancer
Diagnosis	Mallory-Weiss			
Evidence of bleeding	None		Blood, adherent clot, spurting vessel	

Table 3.1: Rockall score

Liver and bile ducts

Liver disease

Jaundice

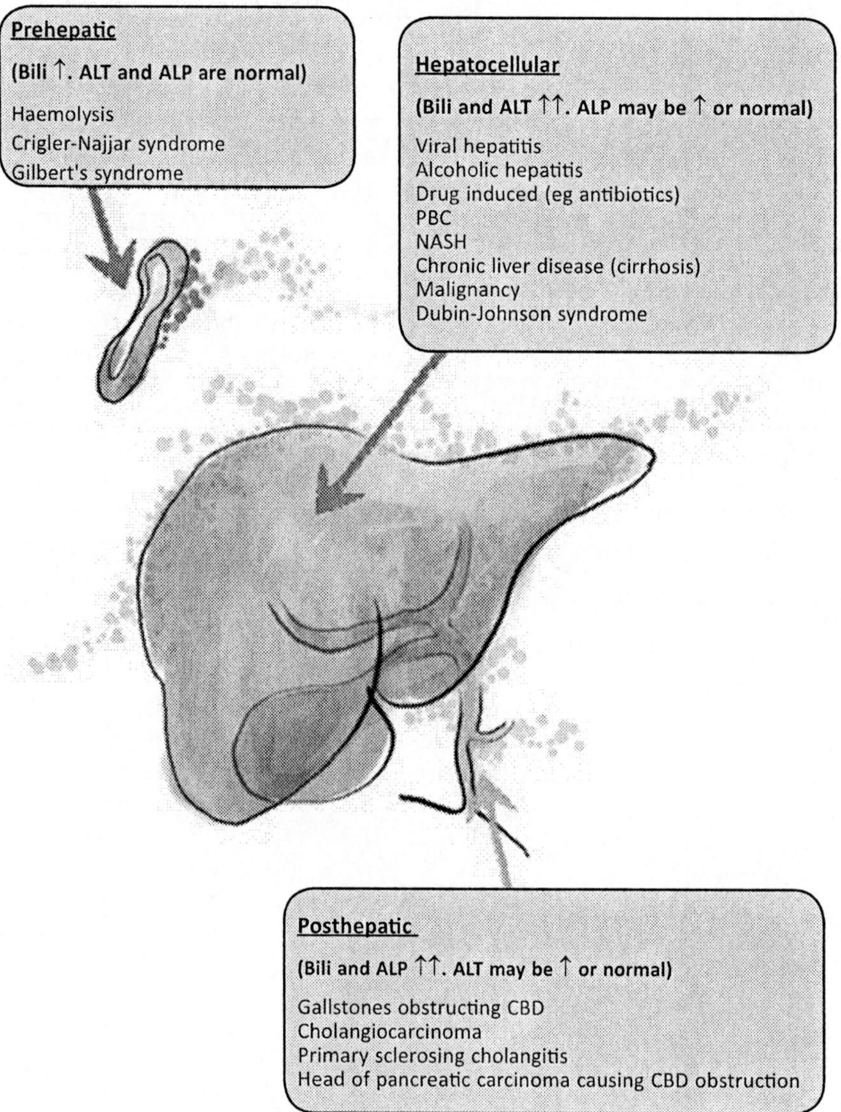

Figure 3.1: Causes of jaundice

Haemolysis: Hb may be ↓, unconjugated bilirubin > conjugated.

Gilbert's syndrome: benign condition, impaired uptake of unconjugated bilirubin by hepatocytes, unconjugated bilirubin > conjugated.

Crigler-Najjar syndrome: very rare. Type I do not survive into infancy without liver transplantation. Type II normal life expectancy, unconjugated > conjugated.

Dubin-Johnson syndrome: impaired excretion of conjugated bilirubin from liver, benign condition.

Gallstones: USS abdomen shows dilated common bile duct, treated with ERCP to remove stones.

Liver failure

P Abnormal liver function associated with coagulopathy **and** hepatic encephalopathy in a previously normal liver with onset within a six-month period.

A Drugs: paracetamol overdose (commonest in UK), antibiotics (augmentin, rifampicin), mushroom ingestion (amanita phalloides), acute Wilson's disease (rare), autoimmune hepatitis, thrombosis of hepatic vein (Budd-Chiari), Hepatitis B (rare), idiopathic, malignancy (infiltrative eg lymphoma, metastatic malignancy).

S Jaundice, ascites, bruising, asterixis (liver flap).

Sx Drowsiness, confusion (hepatic encephalopathy), abdominal pain, abdominal distension (ascites) vomiting, easy bruising (coagulopathy).

I LFTs: ↑ bilirubin, ↑ ALP, ↑ ALT, ↓ albumin; clotting, paracetmol level, hepatitis viral serology, autoimmune profile.

USS abdo: normal, no blood flow in hepatic vein in Budd-Chiari.

T Paracetamol: N-acetylcysteine (Parvolex®).

Drugs: supportive, stop causative agent.

Mushroom ingestion, Wilson's disease and Budd Chiari: supportive, may require liver transplant.

Autoimmune: high dose steroids.

Hepatitis B: supportive treatment.

C GI bleeding, sepsis.

Pr Usually poor without liver transplantation. Paracetamol, autoimmune hepatitis, antibiotic related most likely to improve without transplant.

Liver cirrhosis

P Irreversible liver fibrosis with liver architecture disrupted by regenerative nodules, caused by persistent insults to the liver from a number of causes.

A Alcohol (commonest in UK), non-alcoholic steatohepatitis, haemochromatosis, Wilson's disease, alpha-1 antitrypsin deficiency, autoimmune hepatitis, PBC, PSC, Hepatitis C, idiopathic.

S Spider naevi (central arteriole with vessels branching from it, blanch), ascites, peripheral oedema, jaundice, asterixis, caput medusae, splenomegaly.

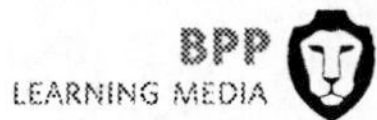

Sx Abdominal swelling (ascites).

I FBC: ↑ MCV suggests alcohol, ↓ PLTs due to splenomegaly and sequestration of platelets in spleen, LFTs: ↑ bilirubin, ALP may be ↑, ↓ albumin, U&Es: ↓ Na ↓ Urea ↓ Creat, clotting.

USS abdo: irregular small liver (can be large in early cirrhosis), splenomegaly, OGD: varicies.

T Ascites: diuretics (frusemide and spironolactone).

Hepatic encephalopathy: lactulose.

C See below.

Pr Child-Pugh classification assesses severity of liver disease by taking into account ascites, extent of jaundice, albumin, INR and presence of encephalopathy to produce a score.

	Score 1	Score 2	Score 3
Bilirubin (umol/L)	<34	34–50	>50
Albumin g/L	>35	28–35	<28
INR	<1.7	1.71–2.2	>2.2
Ascites	None	Controlled with diuretics	Refractory to diuretics
Hepatic encephalopathy	Grade 1	Grade 2	Grade 3–4
	Child Pugh A 5–6 points	**Child Pugh B** 7–9 points	**Child Pugh C** 10–15 points
One-year survival	100%	81%	45%
Two-year survival	85%	57%	35%

Table 3.2: Child-Pugh score

C The three cardinal signs of decompensated cirrhotic lever disease are encephalopathy, fluid retention (ascites/oedema) and jaundice.

Complications of liver failure

Hepatic encephalopathy

P High ammonia levels results in confusion, drowsiness, asterixis (liver flap).

A Can be caused by infection, drugs, alcoholic binge, variceal bleeding and constipation in cirrhotic patients.

T Lactulose is given to ensure bowels opening daily.

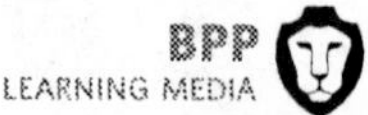

Ascites / Oedema

P Due to inability to excrete sodium resulting in water retention.

A Ascites is commonest complication in cirrhosis.

T Diuretics (spironolactone and frusemide), dietary sodium restriction, daily weights.

Patients who still accumulate ascites despite medical therapy may also require regular ascitic drainage.

Varices

P Increased portal venous pressure leads to collateral vessel formation in oesophagus, stomach, duodenum and rectum.

T Beta blockers or variceal banding if bleeding. All cirrhotic patients should have an OGD to look for varices.

Hepatorenal syndrome

P Renal impairment secondary to severe or advanced hepatic dysfunction.

Pathophysiology unclear but likely due to renal vasoconstriction and hypoperfusion.

HRS is a diagnosis of exclusion and when established there is a high mortality.

T Terlipressin (a vasopressin analogue) and daily human albumin solution intravenously.

Hepatocellular carcinoma

P Primary liver tumour which usually occurs in the context of chronic liver disease (ie cirrhosis).

T Patients with cirrhosis are screened yearly with abdominal USS and serum alpha-fetoprotein.

Metabolic liver disease

Alcoholic liver disease

P Alcohol excess can cause inflammation resulting in fat being deposited in the liver.

Steatosis, steatohepatitis, fibrosis, cirrhosis.

S Of chronic liver disease, Dupytren's contracture.

Sx Of chronic liver disease.

I FBC: ↑ MCV; LFTs: ↑ ALT; USS abdo: fatty liver, hepatomegaly.

T Cessation of alcohol.

C Can progress to cirrhosis if drinking continues.

Non-alcoholic fatty liver disease

P Similar pathologically to alcoholic liver disease.

A Associated with diabetes, obesity, metabolic syndrome.

S Asymptomatic.

Sx Asymptomatic.

I LFT: ↑ ALT; USS abdo: fatty liver, can have hepatomegaly.

T Weight loss, control hypertension, improve diabetic control.

C Can progress to fibrosis then cirrhosis.

Alpha-1 antitrypsin deficiency

P Liver disease due to the accumulation of mutant alpha-1 antitrypsin molecules in hepatocytes.

A Increased risk of cirrhosis in patients with alpha-1 antitrypsin deficiency in alleles Z and M (Pi*ZZ or Pi*MM).

S Can be asymptomatic or have hepatomegaly or signs of cirrhosis. Respiratory signs.

I Alpha-1 antitrypsin genotyping.

T Supportive, in patients with established cirrhosis, treatment is as per cirrhosis.

C Cirrhosis, hepatocellular carcinoma.

Hereditary haemochromatosis

P Iron is deposited in liver, myocardium, pituitary and pancreas resulting in abnormal liver function tests, heart failure, pituitary failure and diabetes mellitus.

A Autosomal recessive genetic condition where mutations in the HFE gene causes excess iron absorption resulting in iron overload.

S Signs of chronic liver disease, signs of congestive cardiac failure, signs of hypogonadism, 'bronze' diabetes (skin pigmentation from iron deposition and increased melanin).

Sx Liver: symptoms of cirrhosis; CCF: shortness of breath, peripheral oedema; diabetes: polydipsia, polyuria; arthopathy.

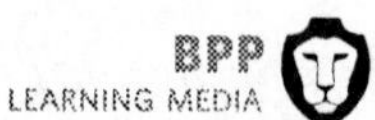

I ↑↑ ferritin: (can be over 1,000); ↑ transferrin saturation; liver biopsy: iron overload.

HFE gene analysis: C282Y (most symptomatic), H63D.

T Regular venesection (preferred) or iron chelation with medications.

C Hepatocellular carcinoma, cardiovascular risks from heart failure and diabetes.

Wilson's disease

P Copper accumulation in liver and brain.

A Autosomal recessive condition, which causes impaired cellular copper transportation, usually young (usually around 16 years old).

S Jaundice, Kayser-Fleischer rings, tremor, parkinsonism, cerebellar and pyramidal signs.

Sx Depression, tremor, jaundice if cirrhotic.

I ↓ Serum caeruloplasmin, ↑ 24-hour urinary copper collection; liver biopsy: ↑ hepatic copper concentration.

T Copper chelators (penicillamine and trientine) lifelong.

C Cirrhosis, psychiatric illness, liver failure.

Autoimmune liver disease

Autoimmune hepatitis

P Chronic hepatitis of autoimmune origin.

A Unknown, association with other autoimmune diseases.

S Asymptomatic, jaundice.

Sx Lethargy, pruritus.

I LFT: ↑ bilirubin ↑ ALT, anti-smooth muscle antibody +ve, anti nuclear antibody +ve.

USS abdo: normal, cirrhosis if advanced.

T Steroids (prednisolone) and immunosuppression with azathioprine.

C Cirrhosis, liver failure.

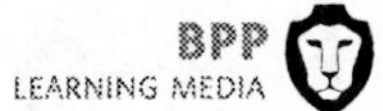

Primary bilary cirrhosis

P Destruction of intralobular bile ducts of the liver. This causes cholestasis resulting eventually in cirrhosis.

A Autoimmune condition, commonest in women aged 30 to 65.

Associated with other autoimmune conditions.

S Scratch marks due to pruritus, jaundice, xanthoma due to hyperlipidaemia, if progresses to cirrhosis patients may have signs of chronic liver disease.

Sx Often diagnosed when patient is asymptomatic with abnormal LFTs. Other symptoms include lethargy, pruritus (often early symptom).

I LFT: ↑ bilirubin, ↑ ALP.

Autoimmune: antimitochondrial antibody (AMA) +ve.

Lipids: ↑ cholesterol (usually HDL ↑ and LDL ↓ so no increased risk of atherolosclerosis).

USS abdo: normal, cirrhosis if advanced.

T Ursodeoxycholic acid, steroids if UCDA not working, liver transplantation if cirrhotic.

Pr If respond to UCDA have normal life expectancy.

Primary sclerosing cholangitis

P Inflammation and stricturing autoimmune disease of the *intra and extra hepatic* bile ducts.

A Autoimmune, higher incidence in men, associated with IBD (UC > Crohns, but associated with both).

S Excoriations from pruritus, jaundice if late.

Sx Pruritus, lethargy, symptoms of IBD.

I LFT: ↑ bilirubin ↑ ALP.

Autoimmune: ANCA +ve.

USS abdo: usually normal, can show bile duct dilatation.

T ERCP if become jaundiced, liver transplantation.

C Increased risk of cholangiocarcinoma, increased risk of colonic carcinoma if has IBD, cholangitis.

Pr Median survival 12 years from diagnosis.

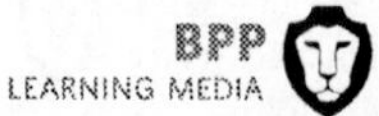

	PSC	PBC
Affects	Men > women	Women > men, 30–65 years
Assoc	IBD	Hypothyroidism
Pathology	Intra /extrahepatic bile ducts	Intralobular bile ducts
Autoimmune	ANCA +ve	AMA +ve

Table 3.3: PBC versus PSC

Liver infections

Liver abscess

P Commonest sites are bowel and biliary (ie cholangitis).

Common bacteria are s. aureus, s. pyogenes, strep milleri (associated with bowel carcinoma), E. coli, amboiesis (if travelled overseas).

A Usually a result of haematological spread of a bacterial infection.

S RUQ tenderness, hepatomegaly, jaundice, fever, signs of sepsis (hypotension, tachycardia).

Sx Fever, RUQ pain, rigors.

I Bloods: ↑ WCC, ↑ CRP. LFT: ↑ ALT, ↑ ALP, bilirubin can be ↑.

Blood cultures, aspiration of abscess.

USS abdo: liver lesion; CT abdo: liver lesion.

T Antibiotics, drainage of abscess.

Hydatid disease

P Cysts due to echinococcus granulosa.

A Consider in UK farmers, endemic in the Mediterranean, Australia, New Zealand, the Middle East, South America, Iceland and part of Africa.

S Hepatomegaly.

Sx Can be asymptomatic, RUQ pain.

I USS abdo: hepatic cysts, hydatid serology +ve.

T Nil if asymptomatic, albenazole (anthelmintic), surgery or aspiration if symptomatic.

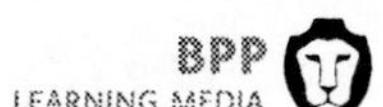

Viral hepatitis

Hepatitis A

P RNA virus.

A Faeco-orally (contaminated food, water).

S Sx Incubation time two to four weeks.

Malaise, jaundice, diarrhoeal illness and fever.

I HAV IgM +ve.

T Usually self-limiting.

Hepatitis B

P DNA virus, endemic in Asia, China and South America.

A Exchange of body fluids: sexual intercourse, vertical transmission from mother to baby, needle sharing.

S Sx Incubation two to six months, can be asymptomatic.

I Hep B serology (see Table 3.4).

	Acute infection	Carrier	Past infection	Vaccinated
HBsAg	**+ve**	**+ve**	-ve	-ve
HBeAg	**+ve**	+/-	-ve	-ve
Anti-HBs	-ve	-ve	**+ve**	**+ve**
Anti-HBe	-ve	+/-	+/-	-ve
Anti-HBc IgM	**+ve**	**+ve**	**+ve**	-ve

Table 3.4: Hepatitis B serology

T Interferon-alpha and lamuvidine.

Vaccination of those at risk of exposure.

C Hepatocellular carcinoma.

Pr 1% develop acute liver failure.

90–95 % clear spontaneously.

5–10 % become carriers.

Hepatitis C

P RNA virus.

A Exchange of body fluids: needle sharing, less commonly vertical transmission (mother to baby) and sexual intercourse.

S Sx Incubation six to eight weeks. Usually asymptomatic.

I Hepatitis C PCR, viral load and genotyping.

T Interferon-alpha and ribavirin.

C Risk of hepatocellular carcinoma and cirrhosis.

Pr 60–90 % become carriers.

Hepatitis D

P RNA virus.

Incubation 6–20 weeks.

Can only affect carriers of Hepatitis B as virus is dysfunctional as a lone pathogen.

Mainly associated with high risk activities such as drug abuse.

Hepatitis E

P RNA virus, endemic in Asia, Africa and Middle East.

A Faeco-orally.

S Sx Incubation of six weeks, jaundice.

Pr Can cause significant mortality in pregnant women (20%).

Liver tumours

Hepatic adenoma

P Benign liver lesion, which has some malignant potential.

A Associations include the oral contraceptive pill.

T Surgical resection if this is possible.

Hepatocellular carcinoma

P Primary liver tumour which usually occurs in the presence of cirrhosis.

A Cirrhosis (secondary to any cause), hepatitis B.

I ↑ alpha-fetoprotein; USS abdo: liver lesion.

T Liver resection if possible or liver transplantation are curative Radiofrequency ablation (insertion of a probe percutaneously into the tumour and application of heat directly) or transarterial chemoembolisation (injection of chemotherapy into hepatic artery to directly reach tumour) are palliative procedures.

Pr Median survival is 6 to 20 months.

Cholangiocarcinoma

P Cancer that arises from epithelial cells of the bile ducts.

A Increased incidence in patients with PSC.

Usually patients are asymptomatic until they become jaundiced due to obstruction.

S Jaundice when malignancy results in bile duct obstruction.

Sx Bile duct obstruction results in pruritis, steatorrhoea.

I LFT: ↑ bilirubin ↑ ALP.

USS abdo: dilated bile ducts; MRCP: dilated bile ducts; ERCP: tissue biopsy.

T ERCP to insert stent in bile duct and relieve obstruction. Surgery if possible.

Pr Poor, frequently due to late presentation, the malignancy may have already metastasised to lymph nodes or liver.

The pancreas

Pancreatic carcinoma

P Can be an exocrine tumour (adenocarcinoma) or endocrine (eg insulinoma, VIPoma, gastrinoma).

This section concerns only exocrine tumours which are more common.

A Exocrine tumours more common in patients with chronic pancreatitis and smokers.

S Jaundice, steatorrhoea, sometimes epigastric mass.

Sx Classically painless jaundice and steatorrhoea, can however present with epigastric pain, usually symptoms with head of pancreas tumours.

I LFT: ↑ Bilirubin, ↑ ALP, ↑ CA 19-9.

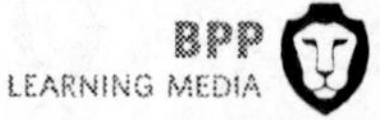

USS abdo: dilated biliary tree, pancreatic mass; CT abdo: pancreatic mass; CT or OGD guided biopsy.

T If resectable, usually treated with Whipple's pancreatoduodenectomy.

If unresectable, treatment is chemotherapy.

Pr Often diagnosed late so prognosis is poor.

Survival post Whipple's procedure (*curative* intent) averages 24 months.

Median survival with advanced disease is 8 to 12 months and metastatic disease is 3 to 6 months.

Chronic pancreatitis

P Chronic inflammation of the pancreas resulting in disruption of pancreatic architecture. This causes impaired endocrine and exocrine function.

A Alcohol excess is commonest, other causes are genetic, SLE, autoimmune and idiopathic.

Sx Epigastric pain, radiating to the back, chronic pain, exocrine dysfunction results in steatorrhoea, fat malabsorption and diarrhoea. Endocrine dysfunction results in diabetes.

I AXR: calcification of the pancreas; CT abdo: calcification of the pancreas, may have pseudocysts.

↓ Faecal elastase.

T Analgesia for chronic pain, pancreatic enzyme supplements with meals for exocrine function and insulin if patient has diabetes.

C Pancreatic carcinoma, fat soluble vitamin deficiency.

The bowel

Malabsorption

Acute diarrhoea

P Defined as loose, watery stools of less than 14 days, can be bloody or non-bloody.

A Usually infective. Infective causes of bloody diarrhoea are E. coli, shigella, campylobacter, yersinia, amoebic dysentry, salmonella.

Causes of non-bloody acute diarrhoea are viral (Norovirus) or bacterial clostridium difficile, giardia, strongyloides, E. coli, cholera or malaria.

S **Sx** Fever, systemically unwell, abdominal pain.

I Bloods: ↑ WCC, ↑ CRP; stool cultures; AXR.

T Rehydration, antibiotics for infection: erythromycin, ciprofloxacin or metronidazole.

C If lasts longer than four to six weeks **or** patient is systemically unwell then should be considered for flexible sigmoidoscopy.

Chronic diarrhoea

P Watery stools lasting longer than two weeks.

A See Box 3.2.

- Colon: IBD, malignancy, IBS
- Small bowel: coeliac disease, Crohn's disease, Whipple's disease, giardiasis, tropical sprue, bacterial overgrowth
- Pancreas insufficiency
- Other: medications (eg metformin, omeprazole), laxative abuse, alcohol, thyrotoxicosis, carcinoid syndrome

Box 3.2: Causes of chronic diarrhoea

I See Table 3.5.

Investigations	Looking for
FBC	Hb ↓ in IBD / malignancy / coeliac MCV ↓ malignancy MCV ↑ coeliac / alcohol / terminal ileal Crohn's disease Plts ↑ in IBD (inflammatory reaction)
U&Es	↓ K+ in chronic diarrhoea
LFTs	↓ albumin in IBD / malignancy
CRP	↓ in IBD / malignancy
Ferritin	↓ in coeliac / malignancy
tTG[1] / anti-endomysial antibodies	+ve in coeliac disease
Stool cultures	Giardiasis
Stool faecal elastase[2]	↓ in pancreatic insufficiency
OGD and duodenal biopsies	Coeliac disease, Whipple's disease, tropical sprue
Colonoscopy / flexible sigmoidoscopy	Malignancy / IBD / normal in IBS
CT abdomen	Colonic malignancy, chronic pancreatitis

[1] tissue transglutaminase antibodies

[2] measure of pancreatic elastase in stool. Correlates to exocrine pancreatic function.

Table 3.5: Investigations for chronic diarrhoea

Coeliac disease

P Immune-mediated destruction of villi in the proximal small bowel due to exposure to gluten, usually diagnosed in childhood, can present in adulthood with anaemia or new onset diarrhoea in adulthood.

A Commonest in white Europeans.

S Pallor due to anaemia, dermatitis herpetiformis (itchy rash on extensor surfaces).

- Rice
- Meat
- Cheese
- Vegetables
- Potato
- Fish
- Milk
- Pulses (peas, beans and lentils)
- Corn
- Eggs
- Fruit

Box 3.3: Gluten-free foods

Sx Lethargy due to anaemia, steatorrhoea, diarrhoea, weight loss, vitamin deficiency, iron deficiency, oesteoporosis.

I ↓ Hb, ↓/↑ MCV, ↓ K, Autoantibodies: tTG +ve , anti-endomyseal antibodies.

OGD: duodenal biopsies show villous atrophy.

T Gluten-free diet (avoidance of bread and cereals).

C If poor compliance with gluten-free diet osteoporosis, small bowel lymphoma.

Pr Normal if gluten-free. Small proportion do not respond to gluten-free diet and require steroids.

Irritable bowel syndrome

P Chronic relapsing functional bowel disorder. Constipation predominant, diarrhoea predominant or alternate between the two. One must exclude organic pathology in patients over the age of 50.

A Unknown, IBS is common, highest prevalence in young women. Altered motility and visceral hypersensitivity are implicated in causing the symptoms of IBS.

S See Box 3.4.

Diagnostic criteria are recent abdominal pain or discomfort at least three days per month in the last three months associated with two or more of:

- Improvement of pain on defecation
- Onset associated with change in frequency of stool
- Onset associated with change in appearance of stool

Box 3.4: ROME III criteria for IBS

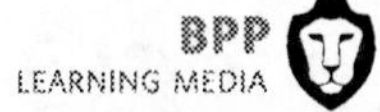

Sx Diarrhoea, constipation, abdominal pain, bloating, relieved by defecation, passing mucous, increased flatulence.

I Performed to rule out organic pathology, all patients should have coeliac disease ruled out with tTG testing.

T Antispasmodics for pain, antidiarrhoeal agents for diarrhoea or laxatives for constipation.

In more difficult to treat patients, tricyclic antidepressants, biofeedback, hypnotherapy and cognitive behavioural therapy all have a role to play in pain control. Probiotics may help with bloating.

Constipation

P Defined as hard stools with straining on defecation, sensation of incomplete evacuation and fewer than three defecations per week.

T *Lifestyle:* smoking cessation. (Stopping smoking is as effective as medications in reducing rate of relapse). Elemental diet can induce remission in small bowel Crohn's disease but is poorly tolerated in adults.

Medical: steroids to induce remission, maintenance is 5-aminosalicylates (eg mesalazine, sulphasalazine), azathiaprine or 6-mercaptopurine. Biologic agents such as infliximab and adalimumab are second line.

Surgery: for strictures resulting in bowel obstruction, laying open of fistulas, resection of diseased bowel.

C Abscesses, fistula formation (colo-vesicular, colo-vaginal), small bowel obstruction, toxic megacolon (transverse colon >5.5cm or caecum >9cm), short bowel syndrome (in patients who have had recurrent small bowel resections), malignancy, primary sclerosing cholangitis (in those with pan-colitis).

Pr 80% of patients will have surgery at some stage. Overall mortality is slightly higher than normal population.

HR ↑, Temp ↑, Hb ↓, stool frequency ↑

- Requires inpatient treatment

Treatment:

- IV hydrocortisone
- Metronidazole / ciprofloxacin
- IV fluids and electrolyte replacement
- Converted to oral steroids when improving
- Infliximab if not improving

Box 3.5: Severe Crohn's disease

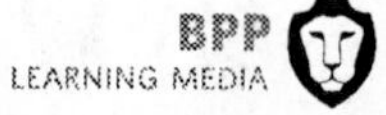

Inflammatory bowel disease

Ulcerative colitis

P *Macroscopic:* continuous from rectum and extending proximally, shallow ulceration.

Microscopic: crypt abscesses, goblet cell depletion.

A Unknown, increased incidence in those with relatives with IBD, decreased incidence in smokers.

S Abdominal tenderness.

Sx Bloody diarrhoea, malaise, urgency.

I ↓ Hb, ↑ CRP and ESR, ↓ albumin, stool cultures.

AXR: toxic dilatation.

Colonoscopy: continuous erythematous mucosa, shallow ulcers.

T *Medical:* steroids to induce remission, 5-aminosalicylates (mesazaline) orally or topically as enemas and suppositories, azathioprine is used as a steroid sparing agent.

Surgery: colectomy in resistant disease and toxic dilatation.

C Toxic dilatation (transverse colon > 5.5cm), perforation, malignancy, primary sclerosing cholangitis.

Pr 20–30% with pancolitis have a colectomy.

Severe disease:

- Defined as HR >90, Temp >37.8, Hb 10.5 g/dl
- Stool frequency >6/day, ESR >30
- (Truelove and Witts criteria)
- Requires inpatient treatment

Treatment:

- IV hydrocortisone
- IV fluids and electrolyte replacement
- Converted to oral steroids when improving
- Ciclosporin or colectomy if not improving

Box 3.6: Severity of ulcerative colitis

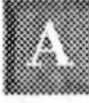

- Common: increased age, inadequate fibre, drugs (opiates, anticholinergics, iron)
- Motility: slow transit constipation, spinal cord lesions, Hirschsprung's disease, Chagas disease, autonomic neuropathy
- Endocrine: hypothyroidism, hypercalcaemia, hypopituitarism, Addison's disease

Box 3.7: Causes of constipation

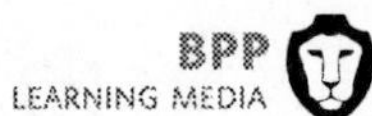

Sx Straining, sensation of incomplete evacuation, requiring manoeuvres to open bowels, manual evacuation.

I To rule out organic cause, colonic transit studies show slow movement of radiologically opaque markers through the colon on X-ray in slow transit constipation.

T Laxatives, increased dietary fibre.

Crohn's disease

P *Macroscopic:* usually rectal-sparing, transmural, deep ulceration, fissures, strictures, fistulating, apthous ulceration, skip lesions.

Microscopic: non-caseating granulomas.

A Unknown aetiology but increased incidence in those with relatives with IBD and increased incidence in smokers.

S Abdominal tenderness (RIF if terminal ileum affected), perianal fistulas, anal skin tags, extra-intestinal manifestations such as pyoderma gangrenosum, clubbing, apthous ulcers, iritis and erythema nodosum.

Sx Abdominal pain, fever, malaise, diarrhoea, weight loss, joint pain, back pain (due to sacroilitis).

I ↓ Hb, ↓ MCV, ↓ Ferritin, ↑ CRP / ESR, ↓ albumin, stool cultures.

AXR: colonic dilatation in acute flares.

Colonoscopy: for large bowel and terminal ileal disease

Barium follow-through: small bowel strictures.

MRI small bowel: thickening, stricturing for small bowel disease.

MRI pelvis: in perianal disease, looking for abcesses or fistulas.

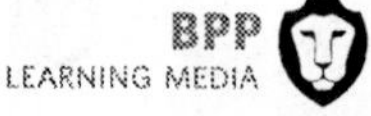

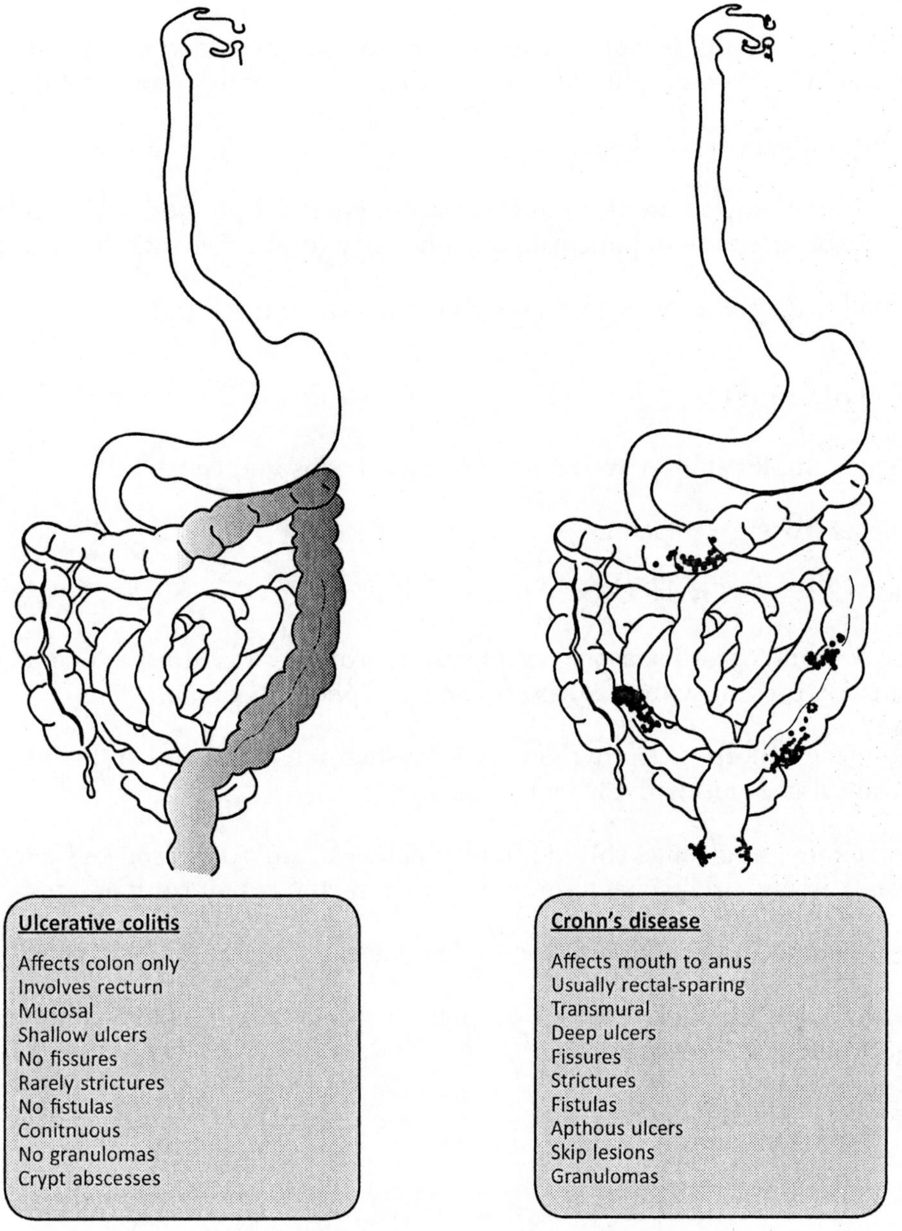

Figure 3.2: Crohn's disease versus ulcerative colitis

Nutritional disorders

Vitamin A (Retinol)

P Fat soluble vitamin, found in liver, kidney, eggs and green vegetables. Role in corneal and conjunctival development.

A Rare in the industrialised world but more common in developing countries.

Can occur in diseases causing malabsorption including chronic pancreatitis, coeliac disease, Crohn's disease (if small bowel is affected) and cystic fibrosis due to fat malabsorption.

S Sx Deficiency results in xeropthalmia (due to impaired lacrimal gland function and results in dry eyes, night blindness and can even result in total blindness).

I Clinical diagnosis.

T Vitamin A supplements, pancreatic enzyme supplements if secondary to fat malabsorption due to pancreatic insufficiency (cystic fibrosis, chronic pancreatitis).

Pr Usually reversible, advanced xeropthalmia can be irreversible.

Vitamin B1 (Thiamine)

P Water soluble vitamin, found in pork, rice, beans and cereals.

Role as enzyme co-factor.

A Alcohol excess (in the UK).

S Sx Beriberi: motor and sensory peripheral neuropathy resulting in pain and weakness. Can also present with CCF, ascites and peripheral oedema.

Wernicke's encephalopathy: confusion, nystagmus, ataxia and opthalmoplegia, almost always associated with alcohol excess.

Korsakoff's syndrome: chronic state which is a result of Wernicke's encephalopathy, results in impaired short term memory characterised by confabulation.

T IV thiamine and oral thiamine supplements.

Pr Beriberi and Wernicke's encephalopathy reverse with supplementation. Korsakoff's syndrome is irreversible.

Vitamin B3 (Nicotinic acid)

P Water soluble, found in yeast, meat, beans, role as an enzyme cofactor.

A Alcohol excess, anorexia nervosa, malabsorption.

S Sx Pellagra: symmetrical photosensitive hyperpigmented rash, red tongue.

T Supplements.

Pr Reversible.

Vitamin C (Ascorbic acid)

P Water soluble vitamin, found in citrus fruits, tomatoes, cabbage and spinach. Roles include co-factor and antioxidant.

A Dietary: seen in malnourished individuals.

S Sx Scurvy: bleeding gums, poor wound healing, weakness, malaise, oedema, neuropathy and depression.

T Vitamin C supplementation.

Pr Reversible.

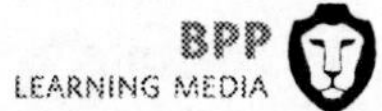

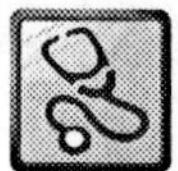

Practice Questions

Single Best Answers

1. A 63-year-old female is admitted on the medical take with six weeks of bloody diarrhoea and abdominal pain. She has a CRP of 100 (<5). Which test is most likely to confirm diagnosis?

   A Abdominal ultrasound
   B Abdominal X-ray
   C CT abdomen
   D Flexible sigmoidoscopy and biopsies

2. A 46-year-old man is admitted with four days of melaena and coffee ground vomiting. He is found to have a haemoglobin of 10g/dL (normal = 13g/dL). He recently injured his knee playing football. Which of the following is the most likely cause of his GI bleeding?

   A Angiodysplasia
   B Gastritis
   C Gastric ulcer
   D Mallory-Weiss tear

3. A 70-year-old man presents with three weeks of dyspepsia, weight loss and odynophagia. The next best investigation is:

   A Abdominal X-ray
   B Barium swallow
   C CT abdomen
   D Oesophogastroduodenoscopy

4. A 19-year-old male attends ED having noticed his skin has gained a yellowish tinge following a cold. He is concerned as his uncle died from cirrhosis. His liver function tests are Bili 62 ALP 85 ALT 32 Alb 39. The most likely diagnosis is:

   A Crigler-Najjer type 1
   B Gilbert's syndrome
   C Haemachromatosis
   D Hepatitis C

5. A 56-year-old lady visits her GP due to pruritus and jaundice. Liver function tests reveal a high alkaline phosphatase. You suspect primary biliary cirrhosis. Which of the following is pathognomonic?

   A Anti-mitochondrial antibody
   B Anti-nuclear antibody
   C Anti-smooth muscle antibody
   D pANCA

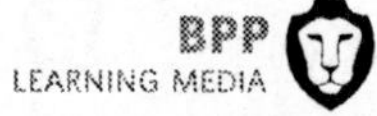

6. You are asked to see an 18-year-old girl in ED who was referred by her GP after becoming jaundiced. She is confused and drowsy on arrival. Blood tests show abnormal liver function tests with a elevated prothrombin time. Which is the most common cause of her current condition?

   A Autoimmune hepatitis
   B Hepatitis B
   C Mushroom poisoning
   D Paracetamol overdose

7. A 62-year-old man with known bowel cancer is admitted into hospital with a liver abscess. The most likely organism to be grown on blood cultures is:

   A Clostridium difficile
   B Entamoeba histolytica
   C Escherichia coli
   D Streptoccus milleri

8. A 22-year-old male has a colonoscopy and biopsies for suspected Crohn's disease. What would you expect to see on histology to confirm the diagnosis?

   A Crypt abscesses
   B Goblet cell depletion
   C Non-caseating granulomas
   D Inclusion bodies

9. A 42-year-old male with a history of alcohol excess is admitted with confusion. On examination he is found to be ataxic with nystagmus and opthalmoplegia. Which of the following would be the next most appropriate treatment option?

   A Intravenous antibiotics
   B Intravenous N-acetylcysteine
   C Intravenous thiamine
   D Chlordiazepoxide

10. A 26-year-old female with ulcerative colitis attends ED with acute onset of bloody diarrhoea. She is opening her bowels 14 times daily. Her observations show she is tachycardic at 100 bpm. Relevant blood tests include Hb 10.4 (12g/dL) and ESR 45. Which is the next most appropriate treatment?

   A Intravenous antibiotics
   B Intravenous hydrocortisone
   C Oral 5-aminosalicylates
   D Prednisolone

11. You are the on call house officer and are bleeped to the gastroenterology ward as a patient has had an episode of large volume haematemesis. On arrival the patient appears clammy and pale. His pulse is thready. He appears jaundiced and has a slightly distended abdomen. Which is the most likely source of bleeding in this gentleman?

    A Duodenal ulcer
    B Gastric ulcer
    C Mallory-Weiss tear
    D Oesophageal varices

12. A barium follow through shows stricturing disease of the terminal ileum. This is most consistent with a diagnosis of

    A Coeliac disease
    B Crohn's disease
    C Ulcerative colitis with reflux ileitis
    D Small bowel bacterial overgrowth

13. A 62-year-old male is referred to ED with jaundice. He denies any pain but states he has noticed that his stools have become pale and his urine dark. He feels itchy all the time. Which of the following would you expect to be elevated?

    A AFP
    B CA 125
    C CA 19-9
    D CEA

14. A 26-year-old male has been low in mood and withdrawn for six months. On examination he has a tremor of the upper limbs and has a shuffling gait. You note a yellow-brown ring around the iris. Which of the following would be the diagnostic?

    A Alpha-1 antitrypsin
    B Caeruloplasmin and urinary copper
    C Ferritin and transferrin saturations
    D Haemoglobin electrophoresis

15. A 21-year-old female is admitted to ED hypoglycaemic, hypotensive and hypothermic. On further history taking, she reports nausea and vomiting for three months. The likely diagnosis is:

    A Addison's disease
    B Alcohol excess
    C Hyperemesis gravidum
    D Hypothyroidism

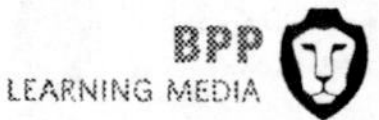

Extended Matching Questions

Upper gastrointestinal tract

A Oesophagitis
B Oesophageal carcinoma
C Duodenal ulcer disease
D Mallory-Weiss tear
E Variceal bleeding
F Barrett's oesophagus
G Gastric ulcer disease

Match the following descriptions with the most likely answer.

1. Erosion of the mucosa which is associated with Helicobacter pylori infection in 90% of cases.

2. Mucosal inflammation, which can be secondary to acid reflux, lax sphincter tone or H. pylori infection.

3. Haematemesis due to mucosal tearing from recurrent retching and vomiting.

4. Transformation of stratified columnar epithelium to columnar epithelium.

5. Haematemesis associated with chronic liver disease.

Diarrhoea

A Campylobacter
B Norovirus
C Cholera
D Clostridium difficile
E Coeliac disease
F Laxative abuse

Match the following scenarios with the most likely diagnosis.

6. A 50-year-old female inpatient who develops profuse watery diarrhoea after four days of treatment for community acquired pneumonia.

7. A 17-year-old male presents acutely unwell with profuse watery diarrhoea with mucous flecks appearing like rice water. Mainstay of treatment is oral rehydration therapy and tetracycline antibiotics.

8. A 25-year-old house officer develops myalgia, diarrhoea and vomiting lasting for 48 hours.

9. A 60-year-old male presents with 24 hours of severe cramping abdominal pain with bloody diarrhoea following a meal of sweet and sour chicken at a restaurant. He is treated with erythromicin.

10. A 19-year-old ballet dancer presents with five months of loose pale stools which are difficult to flush and weight loss of one stone.

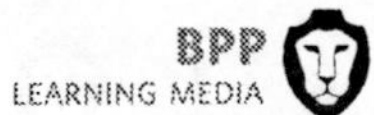

Diarrhoea

A Chronic pancreatitis
B Ulcerative colitis
C Crohn's disease
D Ischaemic colitis
E Irritable bowel syndrome
F Drug induced diarrhoea

Match the following scenarios with the most likely diagnosis.

11. A 27-year-old male presents with six weeks of bloody diarrhoea. Flexible sigmoidoscopy shows erythematous colonic mucosa extending from the rectum with shallow ulceration.

12. A 54-year-old male with a history of alcohol excess presents with abdominal pain and pale hard to flush stools.

13. A 23-year-old female medical student approaching her final examinations presents with a four-month history of loose stools, bloating, abdominal pain and increased flatulence. Blood tests are normal.

14. A 19-year-old female presents with right iliac fossa pain and loose stool. Colonoscopy shows non-confluent erythema with apthous ulceration.

15. A 60-year-old male presents with recent onset of frequent, loose stools. He denies any abdominal discomfort. He was diagnosed with Type 2 diabetes mellitus one month ago.

Liver

A Haemachromatosis
B Wilson's disease
C Alcoholic liver disease
D Non-alcoholic fatty liver disease
E Hepatitis B
F Hepatitis C

Match the following scenarios with the most likely diagnosis.

16. A 62-year-old male with a BMI of 31 and Type 2 diabetes mellitus presents with abnormal liver function tests showing an elevated ALT.

17. A 42-year-old male presents complaining of a loss of libido, polydipsia and polyuria. He appears tanned.

18. A 22-year-old female is admitted to a psychiatric unit with acutepsychosis. Blood tests show an elevated ALT, elevated prothrombintime and lowalbumin.

19. A 56-year-old chief executive presents to ED with acute jaundice and abdominal pain. He has just returned from a business trip to Bangkok.

20. A 49-year-old female presents to ED with jaundice, abdominal distension and palmar erythema. She appears tremulous and agitated.

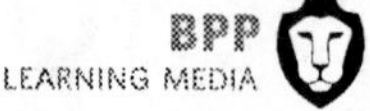

Jaundice

A Pancreatic head carcinoma
B Gilbert's syndrome
C Primary biliary cirrhosis
D Crigler-Najjer syndrome
E Metastatic malignancy
F Primary sclerosing cholangitis

Match the following descriptions with the most likely answer.

21. Benign condition due to impaired uptake of unconjugated bilirubin by hepatocytes.

22. Post hepatic jaundice due to extrinsic compression of the common bile duct.

23. Autoimmune condition most commonly seen in middle aged women with symptoms of pruritis and lethargy.

24. Autoimmune disease resulting in intra and extrahepatic duct inflammation. Associated with ulcerative colitis.

25. Defect of bilirubin conjugation which results in death in infancy in its most severe form.

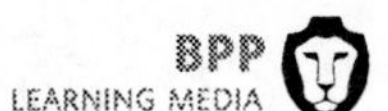

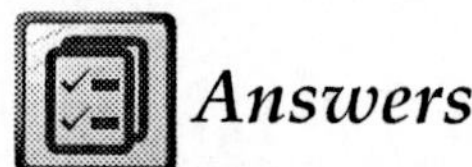

Answers

SBAs		EMQs	
1	D	1	C
2	C	2	A
3	D	3	D
4	B	4	F
5	A	5	E
6	D	6	D
7	D	7	C
8	C	8	B
9	C	9	A
10	B	10	E
11	D	11	B
12	B	12	A
13	C	13	E
14	B	14	C
15	A	15	F
		16	D
		17	A
		18	B
		19	E
		20	C
		21	B
		22	A
		23	C
		24	F
		25	D

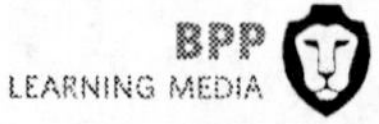

Chapter 4

Renal

Dr Duncan Whitehead

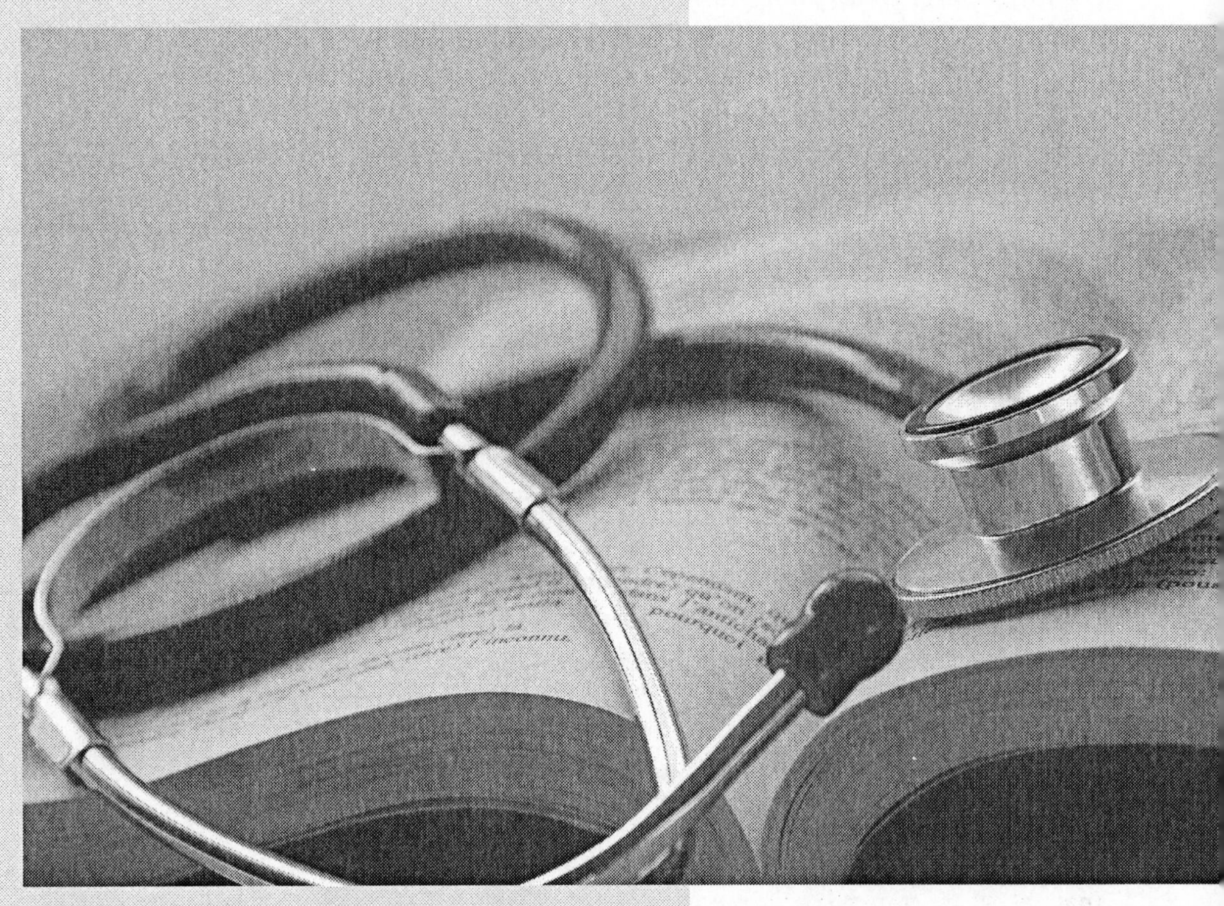

Key investigations

- **Urine dipstick**: gives a rapid indication of blood, protein, leucocytes and nitrites in the urine demonstrating if there is likely urinary tract pathology. It is rare to have active glomerular disease without either blood or protein present in the urine.
- **Urine protein to creatinine ratio**: a spot urine sample, which gives a rapid and good estimation of the 24-hour protein excretion.
- **Serum creatinine**: is a breakdown product from muscle also absorbed in a meat-containing diet from the GI tract. It is filtered by the glomeruli. There is some secretion by the proximal tubule. It is an imperfect marker of renal function especially in the setting of AKI.
- **eGFR**: creatinine is used to generate an estimated glomerular filtration rate (eGFR) most commonly using the Modified Diet in Renal Disease (MDRD) equation. This is reasonable when renal function is stable in individuals of average size and muscle bulk. The Cockcroft-Gault formula includes weight, which is more accurate at the extremes of size.
- **Ultrasound**: the initial imaging of choice for excluding obstructive causes of renal failure. It is also useful to confirm normal renal anatomy and structure.
- **Renal biopsy** is essential to diagnose glomerulonephritides and is normally indicated in the setting of nephrotic syndrome. It is performed with ultrasound guidance using local anaesthetic. The main complication is bleeding

Diuretics

All promote an increase in water losse from the kidneys. The mechanisms to achieve this differ as does the potency and side effect profile.

Osmotic diuretics (eg mannitol)

Action: filtered by the glomerulus but not reabsorbed so they increase the osmolarity of the ultra-filtrate and reduce water reabsorption as it passes through the tubule.

Clinical use: most commonly used for the reduction of cerebral oedema in specific circumstances under the guidance of a specialist.

It should also be noted that glucose and calcium also act as osmotic diuretics and this is the reason why patients with hyperglycaemia and hypercalcaemia are often significantly hypovolaemic at presentation.

Loop diuretics (eg frusemide, bumetanide)

Action: in the thick ascending limb of the loop of Henle on the $Na^+ K^+ 2 Cl^-$ co-transporter.

Clinical uses: they reduce sodium reabsorption from the loop of Henle so can cause a very potent diuresis. They are used to correct states of fluid overload, for example pulmonary oedema from left ventricular failure, maintaining euvolaemia in patients with chronic kidney disease (CKD) and in nephrotic syndrome.

Complications: hypovolaemia. They can also cause hyponatraemia and hypokalaemia.

Thiazide diuretics (eg bendrofluazide)

Action: distal convoluted tubule inhibiting the Na^+/Cl^- symporter, so as to cause a naturesis and associated diuresis, although relatively mild compared to loop diuretics.

Clinical uses: they are one of the most commonly used anti-hypertensives and are favoured in part due to being inexpensive.

Complications: can cause profound hyponatraemia and significant hypokalaemia, gout.

Potassium sparing diuretics (eg amiloride)

Action: collecting ducts on the epithelial sodium channel, as such they reduce potassium loss within the urine but when used in isolation are weak diuretics.

Clinical uses: in combination with loop or thiazide diuretics to maintain normal serum potassium levels. Used in some potassium wasting conditions such as Gitelman syndrome.

Complications: hyperkalaemia especially when used in combination with ACE inhibiters, angiotensin II receptor antagonists or potassium supplements.

Aldosterone antagonists (eg spironolactone)

Action: blocks the mineralocorticoid effects on the collecting ducts and distal convulted tubule.

Clinical uses: cardiac failure, ascites secondary to decompensated liver failure, resistant hypertension. They are also useful in conjunction with loop diuretics in fluid overloaded patients to maintain normal serum potassium and enhanced diuresis.

Complications: hyperkalaemia, gynaecomastia in men.

Renal failure

Acute kidney injury (AKI)

P An all-encompassing term for patients with a rapid deterioration of renal function defined by a creatinine rise ≥26.4μmol/l within a 48-hour period or a urine output <0.5 ml/kg/hour sustained for >6 hours.

A See Box 4.1.

Pre-renal

- Hypovolaemia: CCF, liver cirrhosis, renal artery stenosis, blood loss

Renal

- Acute tubular necrosis: nephrotoxins, rhabdomyolysis, myeloma
- Acute glomerulonephritis
- Interstitial nephritis
- Vasculitis

Post-renal

- Blocked catheter, enlarged prostate, retroperitoneal fibrosis

Box 4.1: Causes of AKI

S Varied depending on cause, can have no signs until severe (see symptoms below). A uraemic frost and pericardial effusion are rare late features of uraemia.

Sx Varied on cause and state of renal function, it is common to have no symptoms of mild or moderate AKI. In severe cases nausea, vomiting, confusion, lethargy, pruritus, uraemic jerks and coma can arise – in this context these symptoms are termed 'features of uraemia' and can be indicates for renal replacement therapy.

I U&Es, FBC, urine dipstick. Then consider: USS renal tract, CRP, ANCA, anti-GBM, ANA, DS DNA, RhF, complement, immunoglobulins, electrophoresis, free light chains, LDH, blood film, cryoglobulins. Renal biopsy is indicated in a few following discussion with nephrologist.

T Fluid resuscitation, stop aggravating medications and dose adjust continuing medications, treat urinary tract obstruction if present. More specific treatments required for some causes.

C Hyperkalaemia, fluid overload, uraemia and a high anion gap metabolic acidosis. Ultimately any one of these may result in the need to commence renal replacement therapy.

Pr 50–60% of patients admitted to ITU have AKI. There is a significant increase in length of hospital stay and increased mortality in patients who develop AKI – this is more profound the worse the renal function becomes. The majority make a good renal recovery; those with CKD prior to the AKI have a worse renal prognosis.

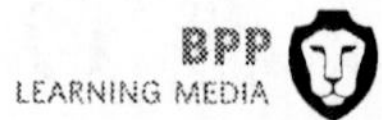

Chronic kidney disease (CKD)

P Progressive, irreversible renal disease with abnormal eGFR for >3 months.

eGFR (ml/min/1.73m^3 surface area)	CKD stage	Comment
>90	1	Only if other evidence of kidney disease
60–90	2	
30–60	3	
15–30	4	
<15	5	End stage renal failure

Table 4.1: eGFR and CKD

A Many different causes. The commonest include ischaemic nephropathy, diabetic nephropathy, autosomal dominant polycystic kidney disease and IgA nephropathy. CKD is not a primary diagnosis (there is always an underlying cause).

S Dependent on underlying diagnosis.

Sx Often none until develop stage 5 CKD. The symptoms that can occur include lethargy, poor concentration, pruritus, fluid retention, reduced appetite, nausea and vomiting, dyspnoea in very advance stages (due to metabolic acidosis, anaemia and fluid overload). Reduced consciousness and uraemic jerks can occur and ultimately death if renal replacement therapy isn't initiated.

I Serial serum creatinines to gauge rate of deterioration, if proteinuria present on dipstick quantification with a protein creatinine ratio. Further investigations depend on the clinical picture but renal tract ultrasound scan, myeloma screem and autoantibodies as for AKI may be appropriate and where the cause is unclear or deterioration rapid a renal biopsy may be indicated.

FBC, phosphate, calcium, potassium, bicarbonate, PTH are appropriate to look for complications of the CKD (see below).

T Divided into four key areas. See Box 4.2.

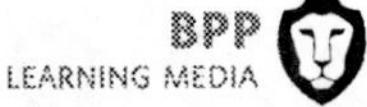

- **Fluid overload and hypertension**: as kidney failure progresses it is not uncommon that the normal fluid homeostasis starts to go awry, as the kidneys fail to control the salt and water balance. This is one of several mechanisms that leads to hypertension developing in CKD. Another prominent mechanism is through the renin-angiotensin system. Fluid control needs to be achieved with fluid restriction or commonly loop diuretics. This will help blood pressure control, but often these patients require multiple agents to achieve target blood pressures <130/80 or <125/75 if proteinuria is present with the CKD

- **Renal anaemia**: generally seen in CKD stages 4 and 5 although can this occur in stage 3 patients. Classically a normocytic anaemia, treatment is with iron supplementation often intravenous and erythropoietin injections may be required

- **Renal bone and mineral disease**: hyperphosphataemia due to reduced renal clearance, reduction of 1 alpha-hydroxylation of vitamin D leads to secondary hyperparathyroidism developing. This progressive disruption of calcium and phosphate homeostasis is implicated as a major contributor towards premature vascular calcification and increased cardiac death rates in CKD patients

  Treatment is with a low phosphate diet, phosphate binders with meals and 1 alphacalcidol supplementation

- **Hyperkalaemia**: dietary restriction of high potassium containing foods, treatment of acidosis, attention to drugs which can raise potassium (eg ACEi)

Box 4.2: Treatment and complications of CKD

Pr CKD is a significant risk factor for cardiovascular disease and most patients with CKD die from a cardiovascular cause before requiring dialysis or transplantation. A major component of managing patients with CKD is targeting modifiable cardiovascular risk factors, eg smoking cessation, hypertension control (slows rate of renal deterioration as well), treating hypercholesterolemia and weight management.

Infection

Urinary tract infection (UTI)

P Bacterial or fungal infection of the urinary tract.

A E. coli, enterocci, pseudomonas and candida are the commonest pathogens.

S Supra-pubic tenderness, fever, confusion and systemic sepsis can occur.

Sx Cystitis, urinary frequency, visible haematuria, odorous and cloudy urine.

I Urine dipstick, mid-stream urine for microscopy, culture and sensitivity, FBC, CRP, U&Es, blood cultures if systemically unwell.

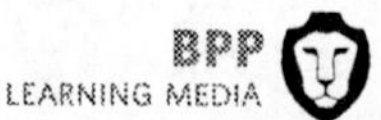

Consider bladder scan or ultrasound scan if looking at urinary retention as a cause or consequence.

T Antibiotics as sensitivities – trimethoprim, amoxicillin and nitrofurantion most commonly used. If systemically unwell consider IV gentamicin, augmentin or ciprofloxacin.

C Systemic sepsis which can cause multi-organ failure.

Pr Normally a full and rapid recovery occurs. However in those who are delirious or develop sepsis as a consequence it can be fatal.

Glomerulonephritis

IgA nephropathy

P IgA nephropathy is a histological diagnosis. IgA can be demonstrated to be deposited within the glomerulus.

A It is currently unclear what causes IgA nephropathy despite it being the commonest primary glomerulonephritis world wide.

S High blood pressure and invisible haematuria +/- proteinuria are the commonest findings.

Sx Frequently none, recurrent visible haematuria within a few days of developing upper airway infections.

Henoch-Schonlein purpura: non-blanching purpuric rash classically over legs and buttocks, abdominal pains can also be present.

I Serial U&Es, urine dipstick and protein: creatinine ratio, serum IgA can be elevated in around 50% of affected individuals, renal biopsy is the definitive investigation.

T Blood pressure control with ACEi is the mainstay of therapy, fish oils may be beneficial and aren't harmful. In the minority with progressive disease and crescentic glomerulonephritis on biopsy immunosuppression may be initiated.

C Hypertension and the cardiovascular consequences, end stage renal failure in the minority of patients.

Pr A gradual deterioration in renal function over many years with about a third developing end stage renal failure.

Anti-glomerular basement membrane disease (Goodpasture's syndrome)

P Anti-glomerular basement membrane (anti-GBM) antibodies can be detected in the serum. Renal biopsy demonstrates a crescentic glomerulonephritis.

A It is unclear what triggers anti-GBM antibody production. They bind to the alpha-3 chain of type IV collagen. This is found in the alveolar basement membrane as well as the glomerular basement membrane. It is a rare but life threatening condition.

S Hypertension, invisible haematuria +/- proteinuria and respiratory findings consistent with alveolar haemorrhage, alongside features of renal failure may all be present at initial presentation.

Sx Haemoptysis, shortness of breath, lethargy, nausea and anuria may be present.

I U&E, FBC, CRP (raised), anti-GBM antibodies, urine dipstick, renal biopsy (ANCA antibodies as this presents similarly).

T Plasma exchange, cyclophosphamide. Prednisolone is the mainstay of treatment. Stop smoking.

C End stage renal failure, pulmonary haemorrhage. Infections secondary to the immunosuppressive treatment can also be life threatening.

Pr Depends on the initial renal function and extent of lung involvement and speed of appropriate treatment so prompt diagnosis is key.

ANCA-associated glomerulonephritis

P Auto-immune condition, immunological testing of blood reveals pANCA or cANCA positive and on ELISA testing MPO or PR3 positivity found. Renal biopsy most commonly shows a crescentic glomerulonephritis. On immunological testing this is pauci-immune (meaning no deposition of IgA, IgG, IgM, C3 or C4 is seen).

A Various theories exist to explain the mechanism for developing an ANCA associated vasculitis None is yet proven beyond doubt.

S Hypertension, invisible haematuria +/- proteinuria, rapidly rising creatinine and may have a reduced urine output. Pulmonary-renal syndrome with aveolar haemorrhage and haemoptysis, vasculitic non-blanching purpuric rash, mononeuritis, CNS involvement, saddle nose, sinus congestion and epistaxsis.

Sx As signs above would suggest, shortness of breath features of AKI can be present. Rarely a diverse range of neurology can be associated with the initial presentation.

T Plasma exchange, cyclophosphamide and steriods are again the mainstay of initial induction treatment. Mycophenolate mofetil and rituximb in some patients, maintenance treatment with steroids and azathioprine.

C End stage renal failure, relapse requiring further significant immunosuppression.

Pr Early diagnosis results in better outcomes. The condition is varied, from a multi-systems disease running a very aggressive course requiring ITU admission for organ support, to renal limited disease with a steadily progressive deterioration in renal function, until diagnosed and treated.

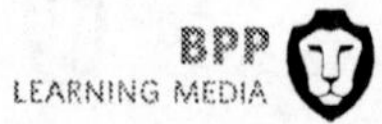

Nephrotic syndrome

P Classic triad of:

- Proteinuria >3g/24 hours,
- Hypoalbuminaemia <30g/l and
- Oedema also an associated hypercholestrolaemia

A Membranous nephropathy is the commonest cause in adults. Other common causes include focal segmental glomerulosclerosis (FSGS), renal amyloid, diabetic nephropathy, and minimal change disease is seen in all age groups, and is the commonest cause in children.

S Marked pitting oedema, ascites and pleural effusions sometimes present.

Sx Swollen legs, weight gain, lethargy, shortness of breath.

I U&Es, FBC, cholesterol, LFTs, glucose, myeloma screen, ANA, urine dipstick and protein: creatinine ratio, renal biopsy.

T ACEi, loop diuretics, statin specific treatments depend on the underlying cause (eg minimal change disease normally responds to steriods).

C A catabolic state can ensue from protein loss so muscle wasting and weakness. A hypercoagulable state may occur increasing risk of thrombotic events, infections are more common.

Pr Varied and dependent on the underlying cause and response to treatments. Persistent heavy proteinuria is associated with progressive renal failure and a worse outcome.

Post streptococcal glomerulonephritis

P Following group A streptococci infection an immune complex is deposited in the glomerulus.

A In children after a streptococcal infection.

S Gross haematuria, oedema, hypertension and fever.

Sx Malaise, anorexia, abdominal pain.

I Urine: proteinuria and RBC casts.

Bloods: increased urea and creatinine, decreased C3.

Serum ASO titre to confirm recent streptococcal infection.

T Sodium restriction, diuretics, antihypertensives, penicillin orally for ten days.

C Encephalopathy.

Pr Haematuria, proteinuria and hypertension can last for weeks. 95% make a full recovery.

Interstitial nephritis

P Inflammatory cells infiltrate the interstitium of the kidney, with sparing of the glomeruli.

A It is most often caused by a drug reaction, most commonly in the UK penicillins and proton pump inhibitors. It can also result secondary to infection.

S Often none present, a minority of patients have a skin rash in association with the drug reaction. May have signs of an infection, viral or otherwise.

Sx Normally vague or none present, loin pains occasionally, lethargy, reduced appetite. If advanced renal failure results the symptoms of end stage renal failure may be present.

I U&Es, FBC: eosinophilia sometimes present.

Urine dipstick: negative or small amounts of blood and protein present.

Renal biopsy.

T Withdraw any possible causative drugs, treat underlying infections, monitor renal function.

If significant AKI or worsening may warrant renal biopsy prior to initiation of steroids, if there isn't excessive scarring and diagnosis confirmed.

C Interstitial nephritis can progress resulting in scarring and ultimately end stage renal failure. Those with AKI may require short-term renal replacement therapy prior to a degree of recovery of renal function.

Pr Most will improve with withdrawal of causative agent, but may be left with a component of CKD. A minority will require steroids, and a few will develop end stage renal failure and require long-term renal replacement therapy.

Renal replacement therapy

Indications for acute dialysis

- Persistent hyperkalaemia (>6.5mmol/l)
- Severe metabolic acidosis (pH <7.2)
- Refractory pulmonary oedema
- Signs of uraemic encephalopathy
- Signs of uraemic pericarditis

Dialysis is also used in patients with chronic renal failure and creatinine clearance of <5ml/min.

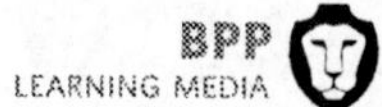

Haemodialysis

Mechanism: Blood interfaces with dialysis fluid across a semi-permeable membrane. Small solutes diffuse easily by diffusion, larger solutes less easily. May be continuous or intermittent.

Complications: Dysequilibrium syndrome (cerebral oedema and headaches due to sudden changes in osmolality), hypotension, immune reactions, hypoxia, line sepsis, fistula thrombosis / stenosis / aneurysm / steal.

Haemofiltration

Mechanism: Blood is filtered continuously across a permeable membrane with waste removed by convection and fluid removed replaced with a buffered physiological solution. Good at removing larger solutes. More costly and takes longer than haemodialysis but also more haemodynamically stable so good for critically ill patients.

Complications: As for haemodialysis but more haemodynamically stable.

Peritoneal dialysis

Mechanism: Dialysis fluid is introduced into the abdominal cavity via a Tenckhoff catheter and filtered across the peritoneal membrane. Allows for continuous ambulatory peritoneal dialysis (CAPD) or automated peritoneal dialysis requiring minimal equipment and is more convenient for patients.

Complications: Peritonitis, catheter-site infection, incisional hernias, catheter blockage, membrane dysfunction.

See Box 4.3.

Haemodialysis	**Peritoneal dialysis**
• Created by anastomosis of artery and vein: commonly radio-cephalic or brachio-cephalic • Complications include: thrombosis, infection, venous stasis and aneurysm formation	• Tenckhoff catheter into abdomen • More convenient • Less expensive • Minimises time off work • Risk of peritonitis

Box 4.3: Renal replacement therapy

Other renal disease

Renal artery stenosis

P Narrowing of the renal artery.

A Atherosclerosis (80%), fibromuscular dysplasia (10%, younger patients), scar formation.

Risk factors: smoking, diabetes, obseity, peripheral vascular disease, coronary artery disease, carotid artery disease.

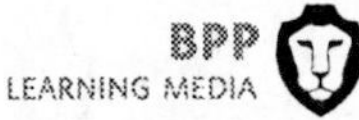

S Hypertension, 'flash' pulmonary oedema (sudden onset without LV impairment), renal artery bruit.

Sx Renal failure.

I Angiogram (gold standard but invasive), MRA, renal USS (affected kidney is smaller).

T Artery stenting, angioplasty, anti-hypertensives.

C CRF, pulmonary oedema, malignant hypertension.

Haemolytic uraemic syndrome

P Endothelial damage triggers deposition of fibrin, which damages passing red blood cells causing:

Triad of: AKI, thrombocytopenia and haemolysis with red cell fragmentation (microangiopathic haemolytic anaemia).

A Post-infections: classically E. coli 0157.

S Sx ARF.

I FBC, U&Es.

T Supportive: IVI fluids, dialysis.

C CCRF, hypertension.

Inherited renal disease

Autosomal dominant polycystic kidney disease (ADPCKD)

P Multiple cysts develop within both kidneys. Normally first seen in 20s, these can become very bulky and uncomfortable leading to progressive CKD in the majority of affected individuals.

A Mutation in PKD-1(chromosome 16) or PKD-2 (chromosome 4) lead to a defect in synthesis of polycystin-1 or polycystin-2.

S ADPCKD may have ballotable large kidneys +/- enlarged cystic liver (more common in women).

Sx Abdominal swelling, early satiety, pain in loins (bleeding into cysts), recurrent infection in cysts in some. Otherwise as in CKD.

I Renal tract ultrasound scanning in early 20s normally confirms the diagnosis, genetic screening can be done but is rarely needed and is expensive.

T Blood pressure control normal using ACE inhibiters, treatment of CKD complications.

C Bleeding into cysts, infected cysts, hypertension, intra cerebral aneurysms leading to subarachnoid haemorrhage and mitral valve prolapse. Aortic regurgitation and diverticular disease are all more common in patients with ADPCKD.

Pr A significant number never need renal replacement therapy – rate of deterioration varies even within a family. Those who do require dialysis generally have a better prognosis than most dialysis patients.

Alport's syndrome

P Genetic disorder characterised by glomerulonephritis, end-stage kidney disease and hearing loss.

A Second commonest inherited renal disease most commonly X-linked, this affects the production of the alpha 3, 4 or 5 chains of type IV collagen. Interestingly it is the same collagen subtype affected by the anti-GBM anti-bodies in anti-GBM disease.

S Sx Persistent haematuria, bilateral sensorineural hearing loss of gradual onset, lenticonus (bulging of lens in eye), symptoms of end-stage renal disease as above.

I USS kidneys, hearing and eye testing, immunohistology of basement membrane.

T Symptomatic treatment with ACE-inhibitors and dialysis as required.

C End-stage renal disease.

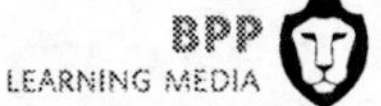

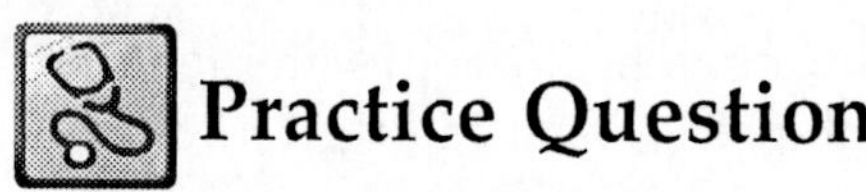

Practice Questions

Single Best Answers

1. Which of these diuretics has a side effect of hyperkalaemia?

   A Mannitol
   B Amiloride
   C Furosemide
   D Bendroflumethiazide

2. Which of these is a cause of AKI?

   A Vasculitis
   B Hypovolaemia
   C Glomerulonephritis
   D All of the above

3. Which of these is not a typical sign / symptom of a UTI?

   A Urinary frequency
   B Suprapubic tenderness
   C Headache
   D Dysuria

4. The following acts on the distal convoluted tubule inhibiting the Na^+/Cl^- symporter.

   A Thiazide diuretcis
   B Loop diuretics
   C Aldosterone antagonists
   D Potassium sparring diuretics

5. Proteinuria, hypoalbuminaemia and oedema are characteristic of

   A IgA nephropathy
   B Goodpasture's syndrome
   C Nephrotic syndrome
   D Interstitial nephritis

6. The triad of AKI, thrombocytopenia and red cell haemolysis is seen in

   A Haemolytic uraemic syndrome
   B Renal artery stenosis
   C Goodpasture's syndrome
   D ANCA associated glomerulonephritis

7. Anti-GBM antibodies are detected in which of the following conditions?

   A ANCA associated glomerulonephritis
   B Goodpasture's syndrome
   C IgA nephropathy
   D Hameolytic uraemic syndrome

8. A Tenckhoff catheter is used in which of the following?

   A Peritoneal dialysis
   B Difficult urinary catheterisation
   C Haemofiltration
   D Renal artery angioplasty

9. Which of the following is not an indication for acute dialysis?

   A Severe metabolic alkalosis (pH >7.5)
   B Refractory pulmonary oedema
   C Persistent hyperkalaemia
   D Uraemic encephalopathy

10. Haemolytic uraemic syndrome classically follows infection with which organism?

    A E. coli
    B Group A strep
    C CMV
    D Listeria

Extended Matching Questions

A UTI
B AKI
C Peritoneal dialysis
D Autosomal dominant polycystic kidney disease
E Goodpasture's syndrome
F Aldosterone antagonist
G Loop diuretic
H Haemodialysis
I ANCA associated glomerulonephritis
J IgA nephropathy
K Renal artery stenosis
L Haemolytic uraemic syndrome
M Thiazide diuretic

Match the following scenarios to the most appropriate answer.

1. Possible complications include exacerbation of gout and insulin resistance.

2. A 30-year-old male who has been complaining of severe bloody diarrhoea. His FBC reveals low platelets.

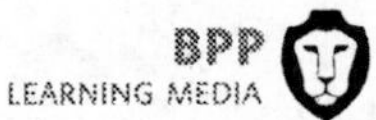

3. A gentleman with a BP 170/110. He also complains of haemoptysis. ANCA –ve. Anti GBM antibodies +ve.

4. An elderly lady is admitted to MAU 'off legs'. On examination she has mild suprapubic tenderness. Urine dip reveals nitrites and leucocytes.

5. Angiogram is the gold standard to diagnose this condition.

6. An elderly lady comes into MAU following three days of diarrhoea and vomiting. On examination she looks dehydrated. Her U&Es reveal urea 12.5 and creatinine 180 (baseline urea 5.0 and creat 90).

7. A 40-year-old man presents to A&E with a sudden collapse and is currently GCS 3. On examination he has bilateral palpable masses in both his loins.

8. A 60-year-old male smoker is admitted with 'flash' pulmonary oedema, an audible renal bruit is heard on auscultation.

9. Spironolactone is in this class of drugs.

10. A 40-year-old woman presents with haemoptysis, epistaxis, a non-blanching purpuric rash and a rapidly rising creatinine. Bloods reveal high ANCA titre and renal biopsy reveals a crescentic glomerulonephritis.

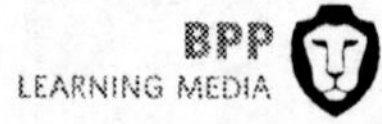

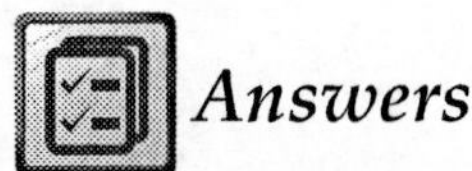

Answers

SBAs		EMQs	
1	B	1	M
2	D	2	L
3	C	3	E
4	A	4	A
5	C	5	K
6	A	6	B
7	B	7	D
8	A	8	K
9	A	9	F
10	A	10	I

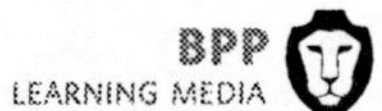

Chapter 5

Endocrinology

Dr Rajeev Raghavan

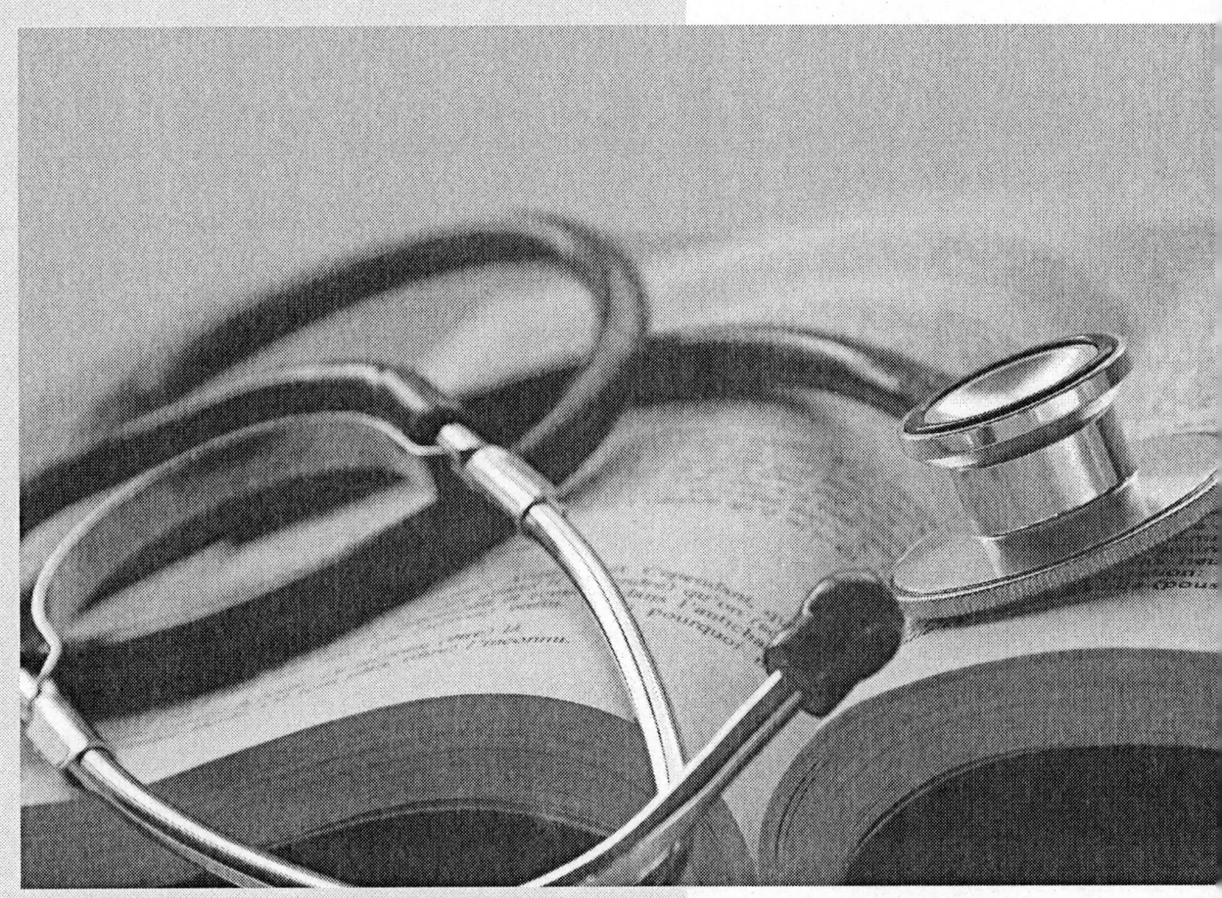

Diabetes mellitus

	Normal	Impaired glucose tolerance	Diabetes
Fasting glucose	<6.0	<7.0	>7.0
Oral glucose tolerance test	<7.8	7.8–11.0	>11.0

Table 5.1: Diabetes and elevation of blood glucose

Type 1 diabetes

P Absolute lack of insulin secretion > impaired glucose metabolism.

Autoimmune destruction of β pancreatic islet cells.

A Primary 90% associated with HLD-DR3/4, peak age of onset <25 years.

Secondary due to destruction of pancreas.

S Acutely: low BMI, dehydration, 'pear drop'/fruity odour on breath.

Chronic: peripheral neuropathy, decreased vision, lack of hypo awareness.

Sx Polyuria, polydipsia, weight loss, lethargy, blurred vision, thrush.

I Plasma glucose, serum ketones, blood gas for PH and bicarbonate, anti-GAD and islet cell antibodies, c-peptide –ve as no endogenous insulin production.

T Insulin replacement, patient education, regular follow-up.

C DKA, DM retinopathy, DM nephropathy, DM neuropathy, PVD, cardiovascular disease, autonomic dysfunction (postural hypotension, gastroparesis).

Pr Depends on good control. Likely to limit life expectancy by 10–20 years.

Type 2 diabetes

P Relative insulin deficit and resistance to insulin action.

A Genetics + environment (high density food intake, obesity, lack of exercise, chronic pancreatitis, Cushing's). Peak incidence 50 years.

S High BMI, central obesity, acanthosis.

Sx May be asymptomatic initially, recurrent infections, polyuria, polydipsia, weight loss (less marked compared to type 1), HONK.

I Plasma glucose, serum ketones, blood gas for PH and bicarbonate, electrolytes.

T *Lifestyle measures:* diet, exercise, smoking cessation, patient education.

Medical control: sulphonylureas, biguanides, glitazones, GLP-1 analogues, and DPP-4 inhibitors, using a stepwise approach. See Box 5.1.

Surveillance: regular follow-up and HbA_{1c} to monitor glycaemic control (levels relate to glucose levels over previous eight weeks) and complications.

- Biguanides
  - Metformin: 1st line in obese patients BMI >25. Improves sensitivity to insulin, does not cause hypoglycaemia. SEs: nausea, lactic acidosis (monitor renal function).
- Sulphonylureas
  - Gliclazide: 1st line in non-obese patients. Stimulates insulin release. SEs: hypoglycaemia.
- Thiazolidinediones
  - Rosiglitazone: improves sensitivity to insulin. SEs: weight gain, fluid retention, deranged LFTs.
- Glucosidase inhibitors
  - Acarbose: prevents intestinal sugar absorption. SEs: flatulence.

Box 5.1: Oral antiglycaemics

C Cardiovascular disease, DM retinopathy, DM nephropathy, DM neuropathy, peripheral vascular disease.

Pr Can be life limiting due to four-fold increase in cardiovascular disease, 10–20 year reduction in life expectancy.

HONK (Hyperosmolar non-ketotic coma)

P Hyperosmolar hyperglycaemia with dehydration and haemoconcentration. Counter-regulatory hormone excess with relative insulin deficit (able to switch off ketogenesis but not to control hyperglycaemia).

A Elderly with intercurrent infections, intake of drinks with high sugar content, myocardial infarction, drugs (eg steroids, thiazide diuretics).

S Dehydration, confusion, coma, polyuria, slurred speech, signs of stroke.

Sx Lethargy, confusion, altered consciousness, neurological symptoms.

I Lab glucose (usually>40mmol/L), serum electrolytes, serum osmolality (>350 mosmols).

Calculated osmolality = 2 × (Na + K) + urea + glucose

T IVI (8–10 litre deficit to be corrected slowly as risk of cerebral oedema), insulin (3–5 units/hour to reduce glucose ~ 5mmol/L/hour), thromboprophylaxis.

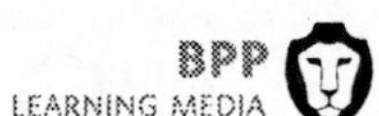

C Venous thromboembolism, permanent neurological sequelae.

Pr Mortality up to 50% especially in elderly.

DKA (diabetic ketoacidosis)

P Insulinopaenia causing diversion of metabolism to use alternate fuel. Also see pathology of diabetes above.

Remember D = diabetes, K = ketones, A = acidosis.

A First presentation of T1DM or in pre-existing diabetes from insulin omission / failed therapy or intercurrent infection.

S Dehydration 'pear drop' smell on breath, tachypnoea (Kussmaul's breathing), drowsiness, coma (~10% of cases), hypotension.

Sx Polyuria, polydipsia, weight loss, nausea, vomiting, lethargy, abdominal pain, headache.

I Glucose >11mmol/L (rarely euglycaemia), raised ketones (urine ≥3+ or serum ≥3mmol/L (near patient testing), blood PH ≤7.3, venous HCO_3 ≤15. Infection screen, CT head if prolonged low GCS, FBC (nb: can have leucocytosis without infection), U&Es, LFTs.

T DKA protocol (fixed rate IV insulin at 0.1 units/kg/hr, IV fluids 4–6 litres/24 hours with first two litres over three hours, potassium monitoring and replacement, and treatment of any intercurrent infections.

Resolution criteria: Venous PH >7.35, HCO_3 >18, and serum ketones <0.3mmol/L).

C Mortality 2–5% (up to 50% in elderly). More commonly causes increased morbidity.

Pr As above, usually good if recognised and treated appropriately.

Hypoglycaemia

P Mismatch in glucose supply, glucose utilisation, and circulating insulin. Blood glucose <4mmol/L.

A Poor oral intake, missed / delayed meal, drugs (insulin, sulfonylureas), ethanol ingestion (delayed effect), diabetic gastroparesis, Addison's disease, post exercise in insulin or SU treated subjects.

S Sx *Autonomic*: anxiety, sweating, hunger pangs, palpitations, tachycardia, tremor, pallor.

Neuroglycopaenic: inco-ordination, aggression, drowsiness, slurred speech, confusion, coma.

I Lab glucose, serum insulin and c-peptide (in non-diabetes patients), SST, pituitary profile, 72-hour fast (hypoglycaemia survey).

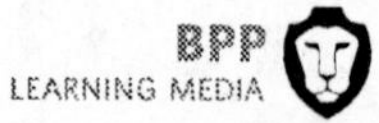

T Conscious patient: 20–30g of quick acting carbohydrate (eg six dextrose tabs, 100ml Lucozade, 150ml fruit juice). Unconscious: Glucagon 1mg IM or SC, 50–100ml 20% dextrose IV. Follow up with slow release carbohydrate, repeat glucose levels, and education to recognise and avoid further episodes.

C Injury, neurological (cognitive deficit, stroke etc), coma, death.

Pr Usually good unless prolonged severe or recurrent hypoglycaemia.

Thyroid

Thyrotoxicosis

P Increased T3 and/or T4 (usually both) due to excess production causing increased basal metabolic rate and multiple end-organ effects.

A Primary: autonomous thyroid in multinodular goitre or autoimmune hyperthyroidism (Graves' disease).

Secondary: due to thyrotroph pituitary tumour, thyroiditis from drugs (eg amiodarone), infections, post-partum, radiation.

S Fine tremor, tachycardia, warm moist skin, palmar erythema, hair loss, muscle wasting / weakness, brisk reflexes, signs of congestive cardiac failure.

Graves' disease: may have neck swelling and eye signs, proximal myopathy, pre-tibial myxoedema, thyroid acropachy.

Eye signs: exophthalmos, proptosis, ophthalmoplegia.

Sx Anxiety, hyperactivity, sweating, heat intolerance, palpitations, weakness, weight loss (although *increased* intake), increased stool frequency, pruritus, oligo / amenorrhoea.

I *Bloods:* thyroid function tests (TFTs): ↑ T_4, ↑ T_3, ↓ TSH, antithyroid peroxidase (TPO) antibodies, TSH receptor (TRAb) antibodies (Graves' disease).

Imaging: ultrasound thyroid, thyroid uptake scan.

T *Medical:* symptomatic treatment with beta blockers (eg propranolol 40mg TDS), antithyroid drugs (carbimazole 20–40mg/d or PTU 50-400mg/d).

Radiation: radioiodine therapy.

Surgery: thyroidectomy.

C Atrial fibrillation, heart failure, osteoporosis.

Pr Usually good. Can cause exacerbation of pre-existing heart failure or arrhythmias.

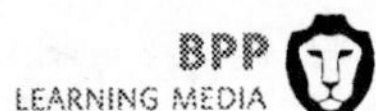

Hypothyroid

P Relative or absolute lack of thyroid hormones or resistance to thyroid hormone action.

A Endemic (iodine deficiency), autoimmune (Hashimoto's thyroiditis), congenital, drugs (eg lithium, amiodarone), thyroiditis (atrophic, post-partum), following thyroidectomy or radioiodine treatment, hypopituitarism.

S Dry skin, hoarse voice, hair loss, hypothermia, bradycardia, macroglossia, slowed reflexes, heart failure, serous effusions (eg pleural, pericardial).

Sx Lethargy, weight gain, cramps, constipation, cold intolerance, peri-orbital oedema, menorrhagia, ataxia, confusion (elderly), psychosis, depression.

I TFTs: $\downarrow T_4$, $\downarrow T_3$, $\uparrow$ TSH, thyroid antibodies, pituitary function, thyroid ultrasound.

T Replace with Thyroxine typically 100–150mcg/day in adults to normalise TSH or if due to central cause then T4 in the middle to upper part of normal range.

C Heart failure, ischaemic heart disease, delayed development and mental retardation (if congenital).

Pr Usually good.

Parathyroid

- *Parathormone (PTH):* from parathyroid glands increases serum calcium by mobilising calcium from bone, and increasing gut absorption
- *Vitamin D:* causes increased deposition of calcium in bone and increases absorption from gut and urine
- *Calcitonin:* causes reduced GI absorption, increased renal excretion, and decreased bone calcium resorption

Box 5.2: Calcium regulation

Hypercalcaemia

P Raised serum calcium.

A Hyperparathyroidism, malignancy (direct metastases to bone causing lysis or humoral hypercalcaemia due to circulating PTH like factors), iatrogenic (especially renal failure, elderly etc), vitamin D toxicity, milk-alkali syndrome, sarcoidosis, critical illness / immobility.

S Sx No specific signs, non-specific symptoms: polyuria, polydipsia, constipation, nausea, vomiting, depression, confusion, fatigue.

- Bones: bone pain and fractures
- Stones: renal stones
- Moans: depression
- Groans: abdominal pain

Box 5.3: Signs and symptoms of hypercalcaemia

I Bloods: calcium, albumin, PTH, vitamin D, phosphate, magnesium, creatinine, urine calcium excretion, serum ACE level (sarcoid), autoimmune profile.

Imaging: renal ultrasound, ultrasound neck, sestamibi of parathyroids, bone scan for metastases etc.

T Rehydration, treatment of underlying cause, IV bisphosphonates.

C Cardiac arrhythmias, renal failure, renal stones.

Pr Depends entirely on underlying aetiology.

Hypocalcaemia

P Low calcium.

A Hypoparathyroidism, osteomalacia (vitamin D deficiency / resistance), hypomagnesaemia, drugs (bisphosphonates, calcitonin, cisplatin), osteoblastic metastases, acute pancreatitis, hungry bone syndrome.

S Sx Tingling, cramps, Chvostek's sign (pre-auricular tap → twitching of corner or mouth), Trosseau's sign (carpo-pedal spasm with inflation of BP cuff), hyper-reflexia, seizures.

I Bloods: calcium, PTH, vitamin D, phosphate, magnesium, creatinine, urine calcium excretion, autoimmune profile, serum ACE level (sarcoid).

Imaging: renal ultrasound, ultrasound neck, sestamibi of parathyroids, bone scan for metastases etc.

T IV or oral calcium supplementation. Magnesium supplementation if low, treat underlying cause.

C Cardiac arrhythmias, complications from seizure.

Pr Depends entirely on underlying aetiology.

Hyperparathyroidism

P Excess production of parathyroid hormone from the parathyroid gland causing hypercalcaemia, calciuria, renal stones, nephrocalcinosis, hypertension, osteoporosis.

A Primary: parathyroid adenoma (85%), multiple gland hyperplasia (10–15%), parathyroid carcinoma (1–5%). Can be part of multiple endocrine neoplasia (MEN) syndromes.

Secondary: renal disease.

Tertiary: autonomous hyperplasia.

S Sx 50% asymptomatic. Related to high calcium (see above). Could be an incidental finding. Also features of chronic kidney disease.

I ↑ PTH, ↑ Ca^{2+}, if MEN suspected then may need full pituitary profile and serum calcitonin assay (medullary thyroid cancer).

T *Medical:* bone protection, hydration, cinacalcet to reduce serum calcium.

Surgical: parathyroidectomy particularly if adenoma or carcinoma.

C Related to high calcium. Complications from surgery include haemorrhage, incomplete excision, and recurrent laryngeal nerve injury.

Pr Usually good unless underlying malignancy or CKD.

Hypoparathyroidism

P a) Failure of development of parathyroid
b) Failure to secrete
c) Damage to the gland
d) Failure of PTH action

A a) DiGeorge syndrome
b) Hypomagnesaemia, calcium receptor mutation
c) Autoimmue, radiation, surgery (eg thyroid), infiltration
d) Pseudohypo-parathyroidism

S Sx Features of hypocalcaemia, see Box 5.2 *Calcium regulation.*

I See Box 5.2 *Calcium regulation.*

T Activated vitamin D and calcium supplements. Aim for low normal calcium.

C Renal stones and nephrocalcinosis from calcium supplementation.

Pr Usually good. Can be associated with mental retardation, cataracts, extrapyramidal symptoms.

Adrenal

Adrenal cortex

- Glucocorticoids eg cortisol: ↑ blood glucose, ↑ fat, carbohydrate and protein metabolism
- Mineralocorticoids eg aldosterone: ↑ Na and water retention, ↑ K excretion to ↑ BP
- Androgens

Adrenal medulla

- Catecholamine eg adrenaline and noradrenaline

Box 5.4: Adrenal hormones

Cushing's syndrome

P Cortisol excess from exogenous or endogenous source.

A See Box 5.5.

Exogenous

- Steroids: usually iatrogenic
- Pseudo-Cushing's: ETOH excess, depression

Endogenous

- ACTH Dependant (↑ ACTH)
  - Pituitary adenoma secreting ACTH
  - Ectopic ACTH secretion: eg small-cell lung cancer, carcinoid. Presents with hyperpigmentation, hypokalaemic alkalosis, weight loss
- ACTH independent (↓ ACTH due to –ve feedback)
  - Adrenal adenoma or carcinoma

Box 5.5: Causes of Cushing's syndrome

S Central obesity, easy bruising, proximal myopathy, thin shiny skin, painful purple striae, oedema, virilisation-excess hair, deep voice, coarse skin etc (suggests adrenal cause).

Sx Fluid retention, weight gain (weight loss in malignancy), tiredness, depression, headaches.

I FBC, U&Es (hypokalaemia), LFTs, 24-hour urine free, cortisols × 2, overnight dexamethasone suppression test, low dose dex suppression test +/– CRH testing, inferior petrosal sinus sampling (central:peripheral ACTH gradient of 4:1), pituitary MRI, CT chest-abdo-pelvis, localisation studies (MIBG, octreotide scan, PET scan etc). Nb all radiology ideally only after biochemical diagnosis.

T Gradual weaning of exogenous steroids, removal of pituitary tumour, excision of ectopic source, bilateral adrenalectomy (ACTH dependant when source not identified / eradicated). Also bone protection, treatment of BP, ↑ glucose if any.

C Relapse, osteoporosis, recurrent infections, metabolic complications, panhypopituitarism, Nelson's syndrome (aggressive corticotroph tumour post bilateral adrenalectomy in pituitary Cushing's).

Pr Depends on underlying cause. Good if can be cured. Adrenal carcinoma has a poor prognosis.

Conn's syndrome

P Excess aldosterone production from the adrenal cortex (primary).

A Adrenocortical adenoma (60%): F >> M, 3–5th decade. Idiopathic / hyperplasia (40%): M = F, 5–7th decade.

Adrenal Ca: older group, F > M.

S Those of moderate hypertension (not optimised despite at least three agents).

Sx Usually related to hypertension. Rarely myopathy, weakness, polyuria from severe hypokalaemia.

I Hypokalaemia (normal in many cases), elevated serum aldosterone (ng/dl), suppressed plasma renin, (ratio usually >30–50ng/ml/h used as screening test).

T *Medical:* aldosterone antagonists eg spironolactone or epleronone.

Surgical: if adenoma, adrenalectomy can cure ~ 75% of cases.

C All associated with poorly treated hypertension.

Pr Usually depends on level of BP control.

Addison's disease

P Primary: glucocorticoid (cortisol) and mineralocorticoid (aldosterone) deficiency due to failure of adrenal glands. Secondary hypoadrenalism: ACTH deficiency as part of hypopituitarism.

Tertiary: withdrawal of exogenous steroids, hypothalamic tumours / infiltration.

A See Box 5.6.

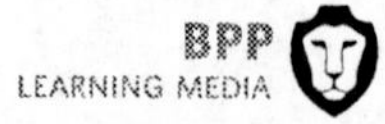

- Autoimmune (90%. Can be part of autoimmune polyglandular syndromes)
- Infections (TB, fungal, HIV related)
- CAH
- Infiltration (amyloid, sarcoid etc)
- Vascular (haemorrhage / infarction) – anticoagulants, meningococcal sepsis, antiphospholipid syndrome
- Iatrogenic: adrenalectomy, ketoconazole, metyrapone etc

Box 5.6: Causes of adrenal insufficiency

S Hyperpigmentation (palmar creases, buccal, scars etc), postural hypotension, muscle wasting, vitiligo.

Sx Fatigue, weight loss, nausea, poor appetite, dizziness.

I Bloods: ↓ Na, ↑ K, hypoglycaemia, ↑ Ca^{2+}, exclude anaemia, B_{12} ↓ (coeliac, pernicious anaemia), thyroid (hypofunction and autoimmunity), adrenal antibodies, Coeliac screen.

Short synacthen test: ACTH analogue.

Imaging: CXR (suspected malignancy, TB), CT adrenals (calcification in TB, infiltration etc), bone density (monitoring for osteoporosis).

T Hydrocortisone 10–20mg/day in div doses, fludrocortisone 0.05–0.2 mg/day. Double former when ill and give IV/IM if oral route compromised. Adrenal crisis → **S**alt (saline), **S**ugar (dextrose), **S**teroids, **S**upport, **S**earch (precipitant), **S**trategy.

C Adrenal crisis at presentation / intercurrent illness. Steroid over-replacement, other autoimmune conditions.

Pr Life expectancy reduced by 10–20 years. Steroid over-replacement → increased morbidity.

Phaeochromocytoma

P Catecholamine secreting tumours of the adrenal medulla

A M = F; commonly 3–4th decade. Can be sporadic (unilateral < 10cm) or familial autosomal dominant: MEN 2, Chr 10, RET protoncogene mutation; Von Hippel-Lindau tumour suppressor gene Chr 3; Neurofibromatosis NF1 gene, Chr 17.

- 10% extra-adrenal
- 10% bilateral
- 10% familial (eg MEN, Von Hippel-Lindau)
- 10% malignant

Box 5.7: 10% rule in phaechromocytoma

S Labile hypertension, postural hypotension, features of cardiac failure.

Sx Typical spells: sweating, flushing, pallor, pyrexia, headache, palpitations.

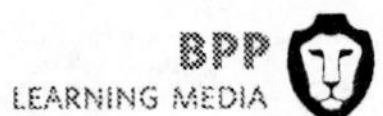

I Elevated 24-hour catecholamines, calcium (MEN), serum calcitonin (medullary thyroid carcinoma), fundoscopy for retinal angiomas (VHL), MRI/CT adrenals, radionuclide imaging (MIBG or PET avid lesions).

T *Medical:* alpha blockade with phenoxybenzamine (irreversible blockade) followed by beta-blockade for reflex tachycardia. *Surgery:* adrenalectomy +/- adjuvant treatment with peptide radionuclide therapies.

C Pressor crisis, end organ damage from hypertension, operative mortality <2%.

Pr HTN curative in ~ 75% with surgery. Five-year survival ~44% for metastatic disease.

Congenital adrenal hyperplasia

P 21-hydroxylase deficiency → diversion of steroid biosynthesis → androgenic by-products.

Adrenocortical insufficiency → raised ACTH → adrenal hyperplasia.

A Point mutation (adults) in CYP21 gene. Gene deletion or subversion causes more severe disorder (infancy) with salt wasting and virilisation.

S Sx Hirsutism, acne, oligomenorrhoea, subfertility in 50% women. Asymptomatic in males.

I ↑ serum 17-OH progesterone (9 AM >15nmol/L in follicular phase of menstruation). Normal <5 nmol/L, 5–15>needs SST with 17-OHP levels. ↑ plasma testosterone.

↑androstenedione. Sub-optimal cortisol post SST.

T Prednisolone 2.5mg or dexamethasone 0.5mg ON (↓17-OHP~ 2 × norm). Cyproterone and OCP to treat hirsutism/hyperandrogenism. Fludrocortisone.

C Rarely salt wasting, psychological burden, subfertility, morbidity from steroid overreplacement. Infants of mothers – screening with 17-OHP levels. Can have adrenal crisis and 'sick day rules' similar to Addison's.

Pr Usually good with appropriate treatment and support.

Pituitary

Pituitary tumours

P Monoclonal tumours with tumour activity depending on cell type >> corticotrophs: Cushing's, comatotrophs: ↑ GH, thyrotrophs: ↑ TSH, gonadotrophs: FSH/LH secretion. Many non-functioning, few co-secrete. Hormonal ↑, local pressure effects (eg optic chiasm), and Rx related effects → hyper/hypofunctioning.

A Tumorigenic mechanisms unclear. Mutations in oncogenes eg *Gsα* (~40% of GH-secreting tumours), *Ras* (aggressive tumours).

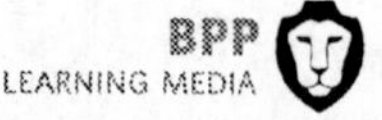

S Related to specific hormone excess or deficiency. Local effects can cause bitemporal hemianopia, CSF rhinorrhoea, signs of raised ICP (esp. if haemorrhage).

Sx Headache, fatigue, myalgia, double vision, nasal congestion, etc.

I Pituitary profile. Likely to need *dynamic endocrine testing*. Humphrey's field test, MRI pituitary.

T Transsphenoidal surgery (resection of smaller tumours, debulking big tumours, sight preservation).

Medical: dopamine agonists (eg cabergoline, somatostatin analogues), radiotherapy for larger tumours.

C Apoplexy (bleed into pre-existing tumour), hypopituitarism, specific hormone axes are dealt with in respective topics.

Pr Good where tumour fully resected and no hormone pathology. Also depends on tumour type and effects. Most tumours are very slow growing.

Hypopituitarism

P Loss of pituitary function due to lack of development, damage from natural pathology or treatment for same. Can develop insidiously over many years.

A Congenital, neoplastic (pituitary (non-functioning adenoma most common), extrapituitary), vascular (haemorrhage, infarction), inflammation (eg Wegener's, neurosarcoid), infiltration, infection (TB, syphilis), post-irradiation, traumatic brain injury.

S See specific hormone deficiencies eg hypothyroidism, congenital adrenal hyperplasia.

Sx See specific hormone deficiencies eg hypothyroidism, congenital adrenal hyperplasia.

I Pituitary profile. Likely to need *dynamic endocrine testing*. MRI pituitary, Humphrey's field test.

T Replacement of secondary axes (ie thyroid, adrenal, gonadal etc). Growth hormone replacement until full growth potential / peak bone mass attained on entering adulthood and then dependant on AGHDA-Qol scoring.

C Poor quality of life, sub-fertility, increased cardiovascular morbidity and mortality, osteoporosis.

Pr Depends on underlying cause, life expectancy may be shortened by several years, increased morbidity (multifactorial).

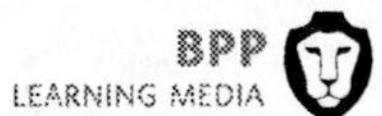

Acromegaly

P Prolonged excessive growth hormone production.

A Somatotroph adenoma (99% cases), GHRH secretion – hypothalamic tumours, ectopic secretion (carcinoid or other neuroendocrine tumours). M = F.

S Prognathism, frontal bossing, enlarged nose, deep voice, macroglossia, coarse skin texture, enlargement of hands and feet, nerve entrapment, multiple skins tags.

Sx Excess sweating (majority), headaches, change in shoe / ring size, joint pains, sleep apnoea, symptoms of diabetes.

I Fasting growth hormone and IGF-1 levels, full pituitary profile, OGTT with GH series (GH fails to suppress with glucose loading), MRI pituitary, skin thickness, photographs from the past.

T Trans-sphenoidal surgery followed by medical therapy (somatostatin analogues) +/– radiotherapy. Treatment of metabolic parameters.

C Cardiovascular disease and heart failure, carpal tunnel syndrome, sleep apnoea, osteoarthritis, diabetes (20%), colonic polyps and cancer, hypopituitarism.

Pr Double expected mortality in untreated patients.

Hyperprolactinaemia

P Excess prolactin production either from a micro / macro prolactinoma or any cause of pituitary stalk disruption.

A Prolactinoma (most common), macroadenoma compressing stalk, empty sella, craniopharyngioma, infiltration, radiation, drugs (DA therapy, neuroleptics, anti-depressants etc), physiological, metabolic.

S **Sx** Reduced / absent menstruation (F), galactorrhoea, breast tenderness, headaches, visual defects, lack of libido, sub-fertility.

I Serum prolactin, pituitary function, visual fields, MRI pituitary.

T Stop drugs causing raised prolactin, dopamine agonist therapy with bromocriptine or cabergoline to normalise prolactin (particularly tumour related).

C Microadenomas can resolve on two to five years Rx or post-menopause in the majority. The rest receive lifelong treatment. Some tumours can be aggressive / erode the skull.

Pr Usually good prognosis.

Diabetes insipidus

P Deficiency of anti-diuretic hormone causing free water loss. Can be central DI (due to stalk compression or damage) or nephrogenic DI (receptor insensitivity). Can be transient (eg post cranial surgery, trauma).

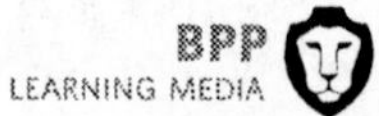

A Central tumour, infiltration, infection, trauma, congenital.

Nephrogenic drugs (eg lithium, demeclocycline, colchicine), familial (X-linked AVP receptor gene).

S Dehydration, polyuria.

Sx Excessive thirst (unless hypothalamic damage), polyuria, weight loss.

I Paired serum (increased) and urine osmolality (inappropriately dilute) after overnight water deprivation. DASHE Water dep test. MRI pituitary.

T Mild DI usually managed by free fluid intake. Central DI can be treated with desmopressin. Nephrogenic DI – stop offending medications.

C Neurological sequelae (rapid correction of Na), ↓ Na (over Rx).

Pr Depends on underlying cause. Mild to moderate disease can be treated effectively; severe DI with hypothalamic damage (loss of thirst) can be difficult.

Syndrome of inappropriate ADH (SIADH)

P Inappropriate anti-diuretic hormone secretion leading to excess total body water and relative hyponatraemia. Euvolaemic, hyposmolar, with normal adrenal and thyroid function, and renal function.

A
- Idiopathic (by exclusion)
- Respiratory
- CNS
- Drugs
- Malignancy

S Related to low sodium.

Sx Fatigue, confusion, falls, seizures, inappropriate thirst.

I Paired osmolalities, urine sodium, SST, TFT.

T Fluid restriction to 750–1,000ml, demeclocycline,

C Related to low sodium.

Pr Usually good for idiopathic or drug related causes.

Other endocrine conditions

Carcinoid tumour

P Tumour of enterochromaffin cells of neural crest secreting 5-hydroxytriptamine (serotonin, 5-HT).

Location: appendix (45%), ileum (30%), rectum (20%) also bronchi, ovary / testis (5%).

80% tumours >2cm metastasise.

A Commonest neuroendocrine tumour. Peak age >30 years.

S Sx Flushing, abdo pain, diarrhoea, wheeze, right-sided heart valve disease, peripheral oedema.

I Urine: 24-hour collection for 5-hyroxyindoleacetic acid (5-HIAA) a metabolite of 5-HT

Imaging: CT / MRI / MIBG scan to locate tumour.

T Medical: ocreotide (blocks tumour mediators and reduces peripheral effects), 5-HT antagonists.

Surgical: resection of tumour +/- chemotherapy.

C Heart failure, liver mets.

Pr Slow growing tumour. 95% five-year survival for local disease.

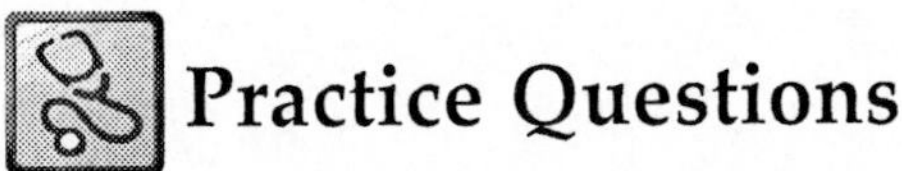

Practice Questions

Single Best Answers

1. Select the hormone-action pairing that is false

   A Calcitonin – lowers blood calcium level
   B Insulin – promotes gluconeogenesis and glycogen synthesis
   C TSH – stimulates production and release of thyroid hormones
   D Parathyroid hormone – lowers blood vitamin D level
   E Somatostatin – inhibits release of glucagon

2. Select the cell type which is mismatched with the organ.

   A Islets of Langerhans – pancreas
   B Somatotrophs – anterior pituitary
   C Chief cells – parathyroid
   D Papillary cells – adrenals

3. Most hormones are

   A Glycoproteins
   B Polypeptides
   C Steroids
   D Carbohydrates
   E Polymers

4. Surgical treatment is not usually considered as first line treatment for which of the following pituitary conditions?

   A Acromegaly
   B Thyrotroph adenoma
   C Cushing's disease
   D Non-functioning pituitary adenoma

5. All of the following are true with regards to primary hyperparathyroidism except

   A The parathyroid glands are usually palpable in the neck
   B It is the commonest cause of outpatient hypercalcaemia
   C Malignancy and primary hyperparathyroidism account for the majority of hypercalcaemia
   D Unilateral adenoma accounts for ~85% of cases
   E A sestamibi scan may help delineate the abnormality

6. All are true in primary hyperaldosteronism except

   A Hypertension needing multiple drugs is the commonest feature
   B Only unilateral adenoma (Conn's syndrome) can be surgically treated
   C Serum potassium can be normal in a number of cases
   D Dehydration and hypernatraemia is typical

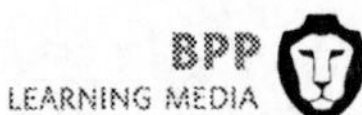

7. Congenital adrenal hyperplasia – all are true except

   A Autosomal recessive inheritance
   B Some cases may have salt losing nephropathy
   C Causes ambiguous genitalia in females
   D Can be diagnosed and treated prenatally with dexamethasone given to the mother
   E Can cause Cushing's syndrome

8. Select the part of the brain responsible for temperature regulation, satiety, and thirst.

   A Pons
   B Cerebellum
   C Pituitary
   D Hypothalamus
   E Corpus callosum

9. Hyperglycaemia can lead to all of the following except

   A Acidosis
   B Hypernatraemia
   C Polyuria
   D Increased glucagon
   E Blurred vision

10. All of the following can result in hypoglycaemia except

   A Delay in meals
   B Miscalculation of insulin dose
   C Renal failure
   D Metformin monotherapy
   E Hypoadrenalism

Extended Matching Questions

Match the following scenarios to their diagnosis.

A Diabetes insipidus
B Prolactinoma
C Sheehan's syndrome
D Pituitary apoplexy
E Pituitary adenoma
F Cavernous sinus thrombosis

1. A 32-year-old female two months post-partum is unable to breastfeed due to failure to lactate and feels fatigued with weight gain of 10 pounds. Delivery was complicated by significant blood loss and low blood pressure. Bloods show an LH <0.5, FSH 0.8, Oestradiol 102, fT4 9.0, TSH 0.6.

2. A 40-year-old male presents with sudden onset severe headache, diplopia, blurred vision. He has photophobia, left ptosis, eye is down and out. His random cortisol is 58 nmol/L and fT4 10.2, TSH 1.0.

3. A 46-year-old male has been in a road traffic accident with head injuries. He is on ITU for a period of observation and is noticed to be polyuric 5 litres/day or dilute urine with serum sodium 152, and serum osmolality 300.

4. A 44-year-old female presents with history of fatigue, weight gain, dizziness, and frontal headaches for three months. She has been bumping into objects accidentally. Her vision shows a bi-temporal field loss on confrontation and is confirmed by Humphrey's visual field test.

5. A 39-year-old female presents with secondary amenorrhoea, lack of libido, breast tenderness and headaches. Her prolactin is 4,500 nmol/L.

Match the following diagnoses to their presentation.

A. Grave's disease
B. Addison's disease
C. Hypogonadotrophic hypogonadism (Kallman's syndrome)
D. Primary hyperparathyroidism
E. Primary hypothyroidism

6. A 25-year-old male presents with fatigue, dizziness, weight loss. He has postural hypotension, buccal pigmentation, and has a sodium 128, potassium 5.6, and low cortisol.

7. A 26-year-old female presents with fatigue and weight gain. She has a family history of goiter with free T4 6.8, TSH 18, anti-TPO antibodies<10.

8. A 24-year-old male presents with poor development of secondary sexual characteristics, testosterone 4nmol/L, and FSH 2.5, LH 1.9. He has also got loss of smell.

9. A 29-year-old female presents with palpitations, tremor, weight loss and increased irritation, redness etc to both eyes. There is evidence of lid lag and mild proptosis.

10. A 65-year-old female complains of fatigue, aches and pains, constipation. She has a history of renal stones.

Match the following complications / side effects to treatments for endocrine problems.

A Carbimazole
B Spironolactone
C Thyroidectomy
D Cranial radiotherapy
E Desmopressin
F Bilateral adrenalectomy
G Sulfonylurea (eg gliclazide)

11. Hypocalcaemia

12. Hypoglycaemia

13. Nelson's syndrome

14. Neutropaenia

15. Hypnatraemia

16. Gynaecomastia

17. Hypopituitarism

Match the following syndromes to their descriptions.

A Waterhouse-Friedrichson syndrome
B Nelson's syndrome
C Multiple endocrine neoplasia type 1
D Multiple endocrine neoplasia 2a
E Polyglandular autoimmune syndrome type 1
F Cushing's disease
G Hyperosmolar Hyperglycaemic syndrome

18. Cortisol excess from an ACTH secreting pituitary tumour.

19. Hypothyroidism, hypoadrenalism, mucocutaneous candidiasis.

20. Bilateral adrenal haemorrhage due to meningococcal sepsis.

21. Medullary thyroid cancer, parathyroid hyperplasia, phaeochromocytoma.

22. Dehydration, confusion, very high blood glucose levels, modest or absent ketones.

23. Enlargement of a corticotroph adenoma causing ACTH excess and hyperpigmentation following bilateral adrenalectomy.

24. Parathyroid hyperplasia, pituitary adenoma, insulinoma.

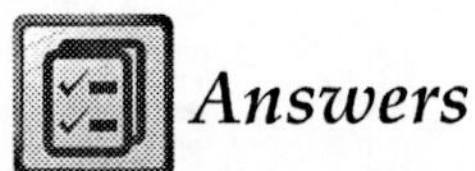

Answers

SBAs		EMQs	
1	D	1	C
2	D	2	F
3	B	3	A
4	D	4	E
5	A	5	B
6	D	6	B
7	C	7	E
8	D	8	C
9	B	9	A
10	D	10	D
		11	C
		12	G
		13	F
		14	A
		15	E
		16	B
		17	D
		18	F
		19	E
		20	A
		21	D
		22	G
		23	B
		24	C

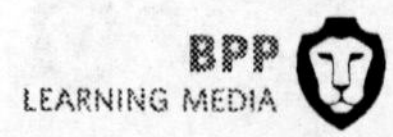

Chapter 6

Neurology

Dr Madhu Ramamoorthi

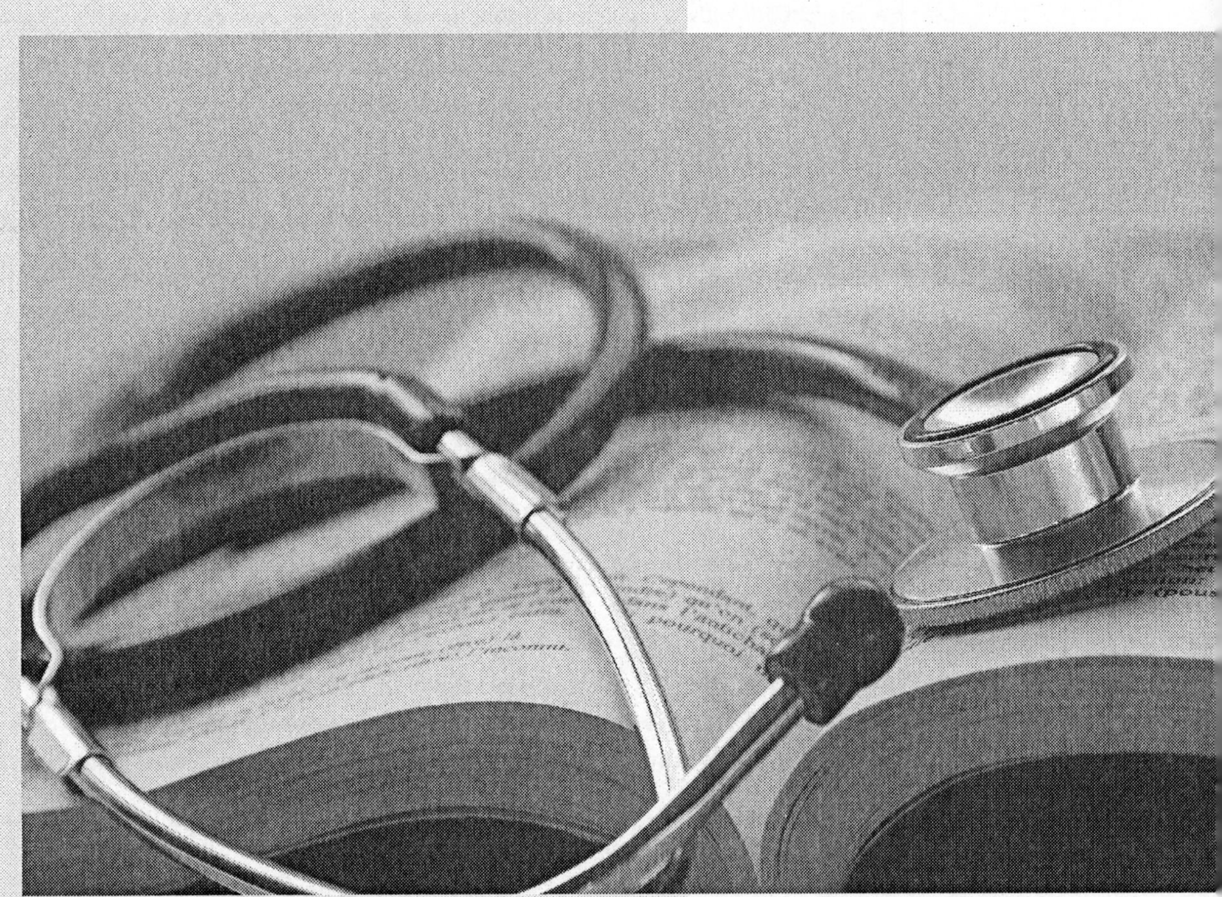

Headache

Migraine

P Pathogenesis unknown.

Classical migraine: migraine with visual aura.

Common migraine: migraine without visual aura.

Hemiplegic migraine: sporadic or familial – associated with calcium / sodium channel mutations.

A Mechanism of migraine remains unclear. Possibly genetic as tends to be more common in patients with family history.

Triggers: food such as chocolate, cheese etc, exercise, menses, hunger, lack of sleep, stress.

S Sx See Box 6.1.

Typical migraine attack consists of sequence of phases:

- Prodromal phase: non specific symptoms such as difficult concentration, irritability, hunger, excessive yawning, tiredness etc
- Aura phase: visual symptoms such as scintillations, zigzag lines, scotomas; somatosensory symptoms such as parasthesia, dysphasia and hemiparesis
- Headache: mostly unilateral throbbing or pulsating associated with photophobia, phonophobia and nausea.

Box 6.1: Signs and symptoms of migraine

I Nil as clinical diagnosis. Consider brain imaging in atypical migraine or in the presence of red flags (age > 50, sudden severe headache, focal neurological signs, fever etc).

T Acute: aspirin, paracetamol, NSAIDs (with antiemetics such as domperidone or metoclopramide), triptans.

Prophylactic: beta blockers, pizotifen, antiepileptic drugs such as topiramate and sodium valproate, amitryptilline and methysergide.

Idiopathic intracranial hypertension

P As the name suggests, this condition is caused by an idiopathic increase in intracranial pressure with no evidence of an underlying structural brain pathology.

A This condition is commonly encountered in obese women of child bearing age group.

Sx Headache worse with coughing, sneezing, bending down, visual obscurations, pulsatile tinnitus and papilledema. 6th nerve palsy may also be seen (false localising sign).

I MRI brain with contrast to exclude structural brain lesions such as tumour, venous sinus thrombosis etc.

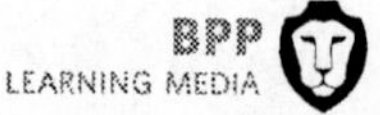

Lumbar puncture shows an elevated CSF opening pressure (usually >25cmH_2O) with normal constituents.

Humphrey's visual field test should be done to look for any field defects.

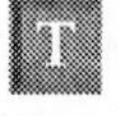

Weight loss is an effective treatment that reduces intracranial pressure and improves symptoms.

Therapeutic lumbar punctures to reduce CSF pressures could be performed at intervals in symptomatic patients.

Drugs such as acetozolamide (carbonic anhydrase inhibitor) and chlorthalidone (diuretic) help to some extent.

In patients with threatened vision surgical options such as optic nerve fenestration, lumbo-peritoneal shunt procedure should be considered.

Stroke

Transient ischemic attack (TIA)

P TIAs are transient, brief episodes of focal brain, spinal cord or retinal ischemia with clinical symptoms usually lasting less than 24 hours and without evidence of acute infarction on CT.

A Risk factors: see *Stroke* below.

Sx These depend on the areas of brain involved and can present as brief episodes of visual loss, speech disturbance, hemiparesis or sensory symptoms.

I CT or MRI brain, carotid doppler, ECG, ECHO and 24-hour cardiac tape.

T Address modifiable risk factors, antiplatelets (aspirin, clopidogrel), antihypertensives and statins.

C 15% strokes preceded by TIA.

Pr ABCD2 score (A – age, B – blood pressure, C – clinical symptoms D – duration of symptoms and diabetes) is used to predict the risk of stroke following a TIA.

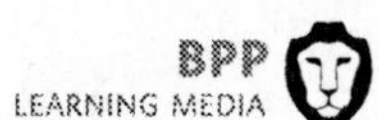

Ischaemic stroke

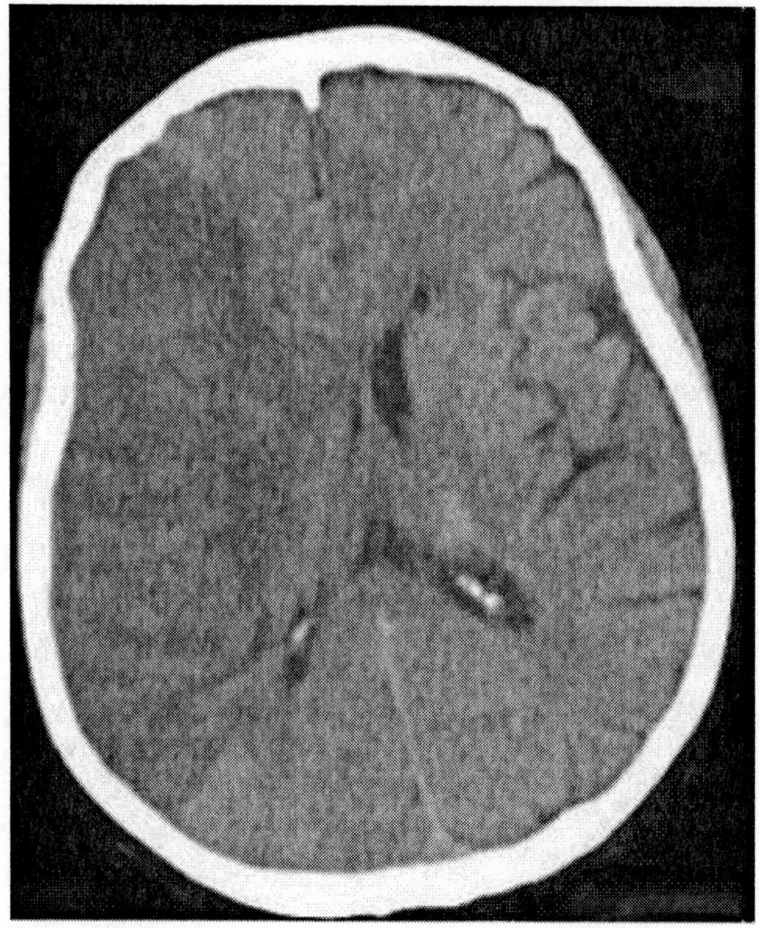

Figure 6.1: Right middle cerebral artery infarct. (Reproduced with permission from SW Deanery.)

P Acute occlusion of intracranial blood supply leading to hypoxia and infarction. 80–90% of strokes are ischaemic, 10–20% are haemorrhagic.

Total anterior circulation infarct (TACI):

- Eg entire middle cerebral artery territory occluded
- Highest mortality (60% 1 year)
- Contralateral hemiparesis
- Contralateral homonymous hemianopia
- Higher cortical dysfunction (dysphasia)

Partial anterior circulation infarct (PACI):

- Two of three features of TACI
- Deficit often incomplete but risk of recurrence

Posterior circulation infarct (POCI):

- Highest risk of recurrence
- Contralateral homonymous hemianopia

OR

- Cerebellar signs (DANISH: **D**ysdiadockokinesia, **A**taxia, **N**ystagmus, **I**ntention Tremor, **S**canning speech/dysarthria, **H**ypotonia/Hyporeflexia)

OR

- Brainstem signs (Horner's, conjugate gaze palsy)

Lacunar infarct (LACI):

- May be pure motor or pure sensory
- Four features are absent
  - No higher cortical dysfunction
  - No homonymous hemianopia
  - No drowsiness
  - No brainstem signs

Box 6.2: Classification of stroke

A Non-modifiable risk factors: age > 65, male gender, family history.

Modifiable risk factors: hypertension, diabetes, smoking, hypercholesterolemia, atrial fibrillation, obesity.

S Sx Dependent on area affected. See Box 6.2.

I Full blood count, fasting sugar, lipids, clotting, ECG, CT or MRI brain, carotid doppler.

Young patients < 60 years should have thrombophilia screen, homocysteine levels and bubble ECHO.

T Acute treatment: consider thrombolysis with recombinant-tissue plasminogen activator (rt-PA) in patients presenting within 4.5 hours of onset of symptoms.

Secondary prevention: antiplatelets (aspirin, clopidogrel), antihypertensives, statins.

Warfarin therapy in AF patients.

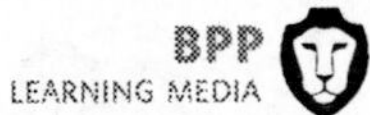

Address modifiable risk factors.

Carotid endarterectomy if significant >70% carotid artery stenosis.

Rehabilitation.

C Disability, sepsis, arrythmias, DVT, pressure sores, contractures, dysphagia, seizures, death.

Carotid and vertebral artery dissection

P Tear in the artery wall intima allowing blood between the inner and outer wall layers. This produces luminal stenosis, complete occlusion or clot embolism compromising blood supply to the brain.

Accounts for nearly a quarter of strokes in young patients.

A Spontaneous: associated with Ehlers-Danlos, Marfan's, fibromuscular dysplasia.

Traumatic: head injury, RTA, chiropractic manipulation.

Sx Ipsilateral headache, neck pain and Horner's syndrome, scalp tenderness, pulsatile tinnitus, cranial neuropathies and subarachnoid hemorrhage.

I CT or MR angiogram.

Formal cerebral angiography is the gold standard investigation.

T Aspirin or warfarin.

Angioplasty and stenting may be considered in a small percentage of patients with dissection presenting with recurrent thromboembolism.

Epilepsy

P Transient seizures due to abnormal excessive or synchronous neuronal activity in the brain.

- Partial seizures: focal in onset and originate in one hemisphere. Further classified as:
  - simple partial: consciousness is preserved
  - complex partial: where consciousness is impaired
- Generalised seizures begin in both hemispheres simultaneously

Box 6.3: Classification of epilepsy

A See Box 6.4.

- Structural: trauma, space occupying lesion, vascular malformation
- Metabolic alcohol withdrawl, high/low glucose, high/low sodium, low oxygen
- Infection: HIV, encephalitis, syphilis

Box 6.4: Causes of epilepsy

S Sx These depend on the cortical areas involved and are variable.

Absence seizures: 'petit mal' lapse of consciousness for <10 seconds while maintaining postural tone.

Tonic-clonic seizures: 'grand mal' loss of consciousness followed by stiffness of body / limbs (tonic phase) and jerky movements of the limbs (clonic phase). During the tonic phase, there may be associated tongue biting and urinary / faecal incontinence. This is followed by a postictal phase with drowsiness and confusion for several minutes.

Myoclonic seizure: sudden limb contractions then loss of consciousness.

Status epilepticus: defined as seizures lasting for more than 30 minutes or recurrent seizures without regain of consciousness in between. This can be convulsive or non-convulsive status.

I Bloods: exclude sepsis, electrolyte abnormalities, hypoglycemia.

MRI brain: exclude structural pathology.

EEG, ECG.

CSF analysis should be considered in suspected underlying encephalitis.

T Partial focal seizures: 1st line lamotrigine, carbamezepine. Generalised and unclassified seizures: 1st line sodium valproate.

Refractory epilepsy: vagal nerve stimulation, epilepsy surgery.

Status epilepticus: 1st line IV benzodiazepines, IV phenytoin / valproate, consider ICU admission for sedation with anesthetic agents (propofol, thiopentone) for resistant status epilepticus.

C Injury, refractory seizures, SUDEP (sudden unexplained death in epilepsy), side effects of AEDs (including teratogenicity in pregnancy).

Infection

Meningitis

P Infection of the meninges.

Viral disease is self-limiting, bacterial can be fatal.

A Neonates: strep. B, E. coli.

Adults: strep. pneumoniae, N. meningitidis.

Elderly: listeria.

Also viral infections and TB.

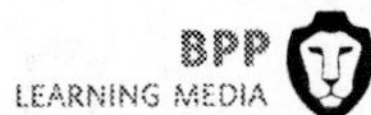

S Kernig's sign +ve, Brudzinski's sign +ve.

Sx Fever, chills, headache, photophobia, neck stiffness, vomiting and changes in mental state. Rash may be present, this is non-blanching and may be urticarial, maculopapular or petechial.

I CT or MRI brain, LP, grams stain, PCR, and blood cultures.

T Abx: IV ceftriaxone immediately in suspected cases without awaiting confirmatory tests. In adults, the addition of vancomycin and ampicillin should be considered especially in elderly and immunocompromised. A short four-day course of dexamethasone is recommended in pneumococcal meningitis patients along with antibiotic therapy.

Prevention: meningococcal and pneumococcal vaccine, chemoprophylaxis (ciprofloxacin, rifampicin) in close contacts.

C Acute: seizures, cerebral abcess, stroke, disseminated intravascular coagulation, gangrenous necrosis of limbs, coma, death.

Long term: (especially in pneumococcal meningitis) deafness, cognitive impairment and focal deficits.

Pr Prognosis is dependent on early diagnosis and commencement of antibiotic therapy. There is increased risk of both mortality around 10% and morbidity of around 30%.

Herpes simplex encephalitis

P Herpes Simplex Virus (HSV) is a DNA virus. Pathologically characterised by a necrotising microencephalitis associated with oedema, haemorrhage, and encephalomalacia.

A HSV-1 is associated with orofacial infection.

HSV-2 is associated with genital infections.

Herpes simplex encephalitis should be strongly suspected when there are focal features clinically or radiologically suggestive of temporal lobe or orbitofrontal cortex involvement. Majority of cases are caused by HSV-1 and is spread through droplets and casual contact with infected person.

S Sx Headache, fever, personality changes, alteration of consciousness, seizures, focal deficits such as dysphasia, hemiparesis, visual field defects.

I MRI brain: temporal / orbitofrontal lobe high signal changes.

CSF cell count shows lymphocytosis with elevated protein and normal glucose.

Viral PCR for HSV is usually positive.

EEG: may show focal changes in temporofrontal areas.

T IV acyclovir (10mg/kg tds) for 14–21 days. Antiepileptic drugs may be required.

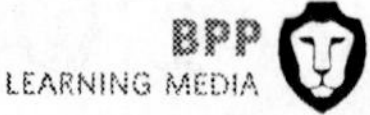

C Long-term neurological sequelae such as cognitive impairment and seizures.

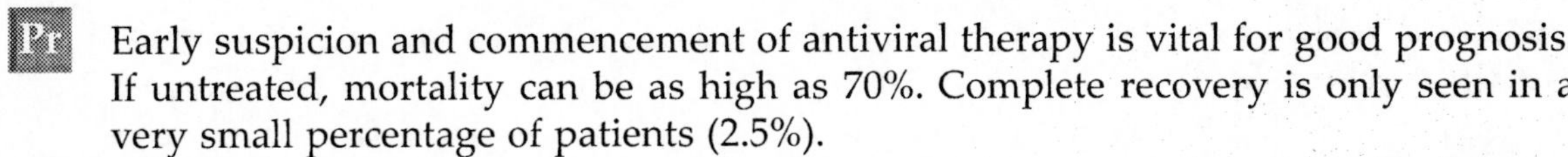

Pr Early suspicion and commencement of antiviral therapy is vital for good prognosis. If untreated, mortality can be as high as 70%. Complete recovery is only seen in a very small percentage of patients (2.5%).

Cruetzfeldt Jacob disease

P CJD belongs to family of human transmissible spongiform encephalopathy. This is a rare and fatal degenerative brain disease caused by an abnormal prion protein.

Incidence: one case per million per year.

A Sporadic: most common type. The cause is uncertain but is likely due to spontaneous mutation resulting in abnormal prion protein.

Genetic: autosomal dominant inheritance, commonest mutation being E200K mutation in PRNP gene on chromosome 20.

Iatrogenic: very rare. Transmission is through infected human growth hormone, corneal grafts, dural grafts, intracranial EEG electrodes.

New variant: this is the human form of bovine spongiform encephalopathy acquired by consumption of infected beef.

Sx Early stages: lethargy, headache, insomnia, poor appetite and depression. Symptoms gradually progress to include impaired memory, personality changes, inco-ordination, visual hallucinations, impaired speech / swallow, dementia, pyramidal / extrapyramidal / cerebellar signs, myoclonus, blindness, coma.

I MRI brain: may show changes in basal ganglia / thalamus and cortex.

CSF: positivity for 14-3-3 and S100 proteins, although not specific, is supportive of a diagnosis of CJD in the presence of strong clinical suspicion.

EEG: presence of biphasic / triphasic periodic sharp waves is also supportive.

Blood for genetics for PRNP mutations.

Tonsil biopsy.

Brain biopsy is the gold standard test, which shows spongiform changes with vacuolation, neuronal loss and gliosis. The definitive diagnosis is usually made at post mortem examination.

T No curative treatment available yet.

Pr Fatal. Symptoms relentlessly progress resulting in death. Sporadic CJD patients have a prognosis of about four to six months. This is slightly better in variant CJD patients with a prognosis of around one year.

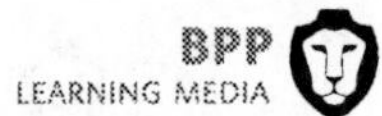

Demyelination

Multiple sclerosis

P Demyelinating inflammatory disease affecting the brain, spinal cord and optic nerve. Several sub-types:

- Commonest: relapsing-remitting type
- Others: primary progressive, secondary progressive, progressive relapsing, benign MS

A Unknown. Proposed mechanisms: autoimmune, genetic, viral (EBV related).

S Sx Depend on areas of inflammation: focal neurological signs both motor / sensory, visual symptoms (optic neuritis, internuclear ophthalmoplegia, extraocular muscle palsies), transverse myelitis, Lhermitte's sign (sensory symptoms on neck flexion), fatigue, spasticity, cognitive impairment, depression, constipation, bladder and sexual dysfunction.

I MRI brain / spine, CSF analysis for oligoclonal bands, visual evoked potentials.

T Acute relapses: short course of IV / PO methyl-prednisolone.

Severe relapsing remitting MS: disease-modifying drugs such as beta interferons, glatiramer acetate or monoclonal antibody such as natalizumab, alemtuzumab should be considered.

Symptom relief: spasticity (baclofen, tizanidine, benzodiazepines, botulinum toxin), fatigue (amantadine, modafinil), laxatives, antidepressants (SSRIs), bladder spasticity (oxybutinin), erectile dysfunction (sildanafil) and neuropathic pain (gabapentin, pregabalin, carbamezepine).

C About 50% of relapsing remitting MS patients after ten years and 90% by 25 years progress into secondary progressive phase. 10–15% of MS patients are progressive from onset.

Pr Average life expectancy in MS patients is lower by around ten years compared to general population.

Guillain-Barré syndrome

P Autoimmune mediated acute inflammatory demyelinating polyneuropathy resulting in ascending motor paralysis, sensory symptoms and loss of deep tendon reflexes.

A In most cases there is a history of preceding viral or diarrhoeal illness.

S Sx Ascending motor weakness usually starting in the lower limbs, parasthesia, areflexia, cranial nerve palsies, symptoms of dysautonomia such as fluctuating BP, temperature, heart rate.

Respiratory muscle weakness can occur in severe cases.

I Bloods: serology for viruses such as EBV, CMV, HIV. Atypical pneumonia screen.

Stool for campylobacter jejuni.

Anti ganglioside antibodies such as Anti GM1, Anti GD1a. Anti GQ1b is specific for Miller Fisher variant.

CSF shows albumino-cytologic dissociation (markedly increased CSF protein compared to low cell count).

Nerve conduction studies.

T Intravenous immunoglobulins.

Plasma exchange.

Cardiac monitoring (autonomic syptoms) and regular lung function tests.

ITU admission and ventilation for respiratory compromise.

Rehabilitation.

C Cardiac arrhythmias, respiratory arrest, LRTI.

Pr Majority of patients recover fully, 5–10% left with significant disability. Poor prognosis is associated with elderly, significant disability at two weeks, history of preceding diarrhoea and significant abnormality in nerve conduction studies. Recurrence of GBS is very rare.

Transverse myelitis

P Inflammatory demyelinating disease of the spinal cord with associated axonal loss with symptoms evolving over several hours–days.

A See Box 6.5.

- Idiopathic: commonest, nearly two-third of cases
- Infective: viral (several including CMV, EBV, HIV, adenovirus, coxsackie, HTLV-1, hepatitis C, HSV, VZV), bacterial (mycoplasma, Lymes, brucellosis, tuberculosis), parasitic
- Inflammatory: multiple sclerosis, and neuromyelitis optica should be considered especially in recurrent cases, acute disseminated encephalo myelitis (ADEM)
- Autoimmune: SLE, sarcoid, Sjögren's, Behçet's
- Neoplastic: glioma, lymphoma, secondary metastasis, paraneoplastic myelitis
- Metabolic: vitamin B12 deficiency, vitamin E deficiency, copper deficiency

Box 6.5: Causes of transverse myelitis

S Sx Depend on the level of inflammation in the cord. These include back pain, motor weakness (mainly in the legs, this may be flaccid weakness initially due to spinal shock and gradually progresses to spasticity) sensory level (commonly thoracic), parasthesia, sphincter dysfunction such as urinary retention, sometimes hyperesthesia at the dermatome above the sensory level.

I MRI spine, consider MRI brain, CSF analysis, blood tests for infection / autoimmune / connective tissue disorder screen, NMO IgG antibodies (in suspected cases of neuromyelitis optica).

T Treat underlying cause if found. IV methyl prednisolone, IV immunoglobulins, plasma exchange, long-term immunosuppression depending on underlying cause.

Symptom control with neuropathic painkillers (gabapentin, amitryptilline), muscle relaxants (baclofen, tizanidine, benzodiazepines), long-term urinary catheter.

Pr Roughly one-third will make full recovery, one-third will have some residual disability and one-third will have severe disability.

Dementia

Parkinson's disease

P Degeneration of dopaminergic neurons in substantia nigra.

A Risk factors: male, family history, smoking may be protective.

Sx Tetrad of: resting tremor, rigidity, bradykinesia and postural instability.

Motor symptoms: festinant-gait, small hand writing and masked facies.

Non-motor symptoms: depression, sleep disorders, sexual dysfunction, hallucinations, restless legs syndrome, constipation, dementia.

I The diagnosis is clinical, MRI brain and DaT scan (dopamine transporter scan) could be considered in atypical cases.

T Symptomatic treatment only.

Levodopa in combination with dopa decarboxylase inhibitors such as carbidopa and benserazide.

Adjuvant medication: dopamine agonists (ropinirole, pramipexole), monoamino oxidase-B inhibitors (selegiline, rasagiline) and catecholamine-O methyl transferase inhibitors (entacapone, tolcapone).

For advanced PD: consider apomorphine, and deep brain stimulation.

C Depression.

Pathology:

Syndromes where apart from parkinsonian features such as tremor, rigidity and bradykinesia, there are additional neurological signs, which distinguish them from an idiopathic Parkinson's disease. These generally progress more rapidly and have a poor response to levodopa therapy.

- **Progressive supranuclear palsy**: parkinsonism with vertical gaze palsy, frequent falls, axial rigidity and cognitive decline
- **Multi system atrophy**: parkinsonism with autonomic dysfunction such as orthostatic hypotension, dry mouth, erectile dysfunction etc and cerebellar signs such as ataxia
- **Cortico basal degeneration**: parkinsonism with parietal lobe signs such as apraxia and sensory symptoms, alien hand syndrome and cognitive decline

There are neither diagnostic tests nor curative treatment for Parkinson's plus syndromes. Symptomatic treatment with anti parkinson medications such as levodopa and cholinesterase inhibitors such as rivastigmine may offer little benefit. Supportive measures such as physiotherapy, occupational therapy, family and carer support help.

Box 6.6: Parkinson's plus syndromes

Alzheimer's disease

P Classically the presence of cerebral neuronal cell loss, senile plaques, neurofibrillary tangles and beta-amyloid deposition.

A This is the most common cause of dementia predominantly affecting memory. The age of onset is usually from 6th decade onwards.

Sx Short-term memory loss progressing gradually over a few years to involve other cognitive domains such as language and executive function.

Progressive personality changes: apathy, depression, wandering and emotional labililty.

Language deficits: word finding difficulty, problems with reading and writing.

Apraxia develops and patients need assistance with activities of daily living.

In the advanced stage, mobililty, speech, swallow and memory are severely affected. Patients may develop signs of rigidity, myoclonus and seizures in the late stages. Death is usually due to sepsis.

I MRI or CT brain in Alzheimer's patients may show mesial temporal lobe atrophy.

Bloods: B12, TSH, syphilis, HIV to look for reversible causes of dementia.

T No curative treatment.

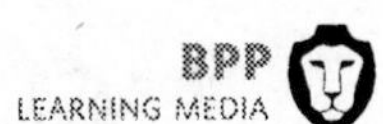

Central cholinesterase inhibitors such as donepezil, galantamine and rivatigmine may slow down disease progression for one to two years. Symptomatic treatment with antidepressants / neuroleptics should be considered.

With disease progression, multidisciplinary approach in the form of physiotherapy, occupational therapy, family and carer input and nursing home placement may be required.

Pr The average life expectancy from the time of diagnosis is around six to seven years.

Dementia with Lewy body (DLB)

P Lewy bodies (inclusion bodies containing alpha-synuclein and ubiquitin) found in the brain on post-mortem histology.

DLB is a neurodegenerative disorder characterised by parkinsonism, prominent visual hallucinations and dementia.

A The time of onset of cognitive symptoms is either concurrently or within one year of onset of parkinsonism. In contrast, Parkinson's disease with dementia is diagnosed in well-established Parkinson's disease patients who develop cognitive symptoms at least more than one year after onset of parkinsonism.

Sx Cognitive symptoms: impaired memory, apathy, executive dysfunction and visuospatial abilities.

Psychiatric symptoms: delusions, visual hallucinations and emotional lability.

Parkinsonian features of rigidity and bradykinesia but less of resting tremors.

Other prominent symptoms include frequent falls, transient episodes of depressed consciousness and autonomic symptoms such as dry skin, orthostatic hypotension, sexual dysfunction.

Symptoms suggestive of REM sleep disorder and restless legs syndrome may also be present.

I No diagnostic test available yet.

MRI/CT brain to exclude other causes of dementia such as tumours, subdural hematoma, normal pressure hydrocephalus.

DAT (dopamine transporter scan): reduced uptake of radioactive isotope in the basal ganglia.

T Dopaminergic therapy such as levodopa to help parkinsonism but response is usually poor.

Choline esterase inhibitors such as donepezil can be used to treat cognitive symptoms.

Atypical antipsychotics such as quetiapine can be used to treat psychiatric symptoms and hallucinations.

Avoid neuroleptic drugs such as haloperidol.

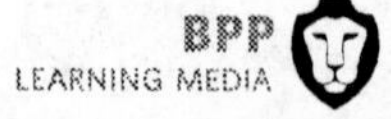

Pr Mean survival seven years from onset.

Huntington's disease (HD)

P Huntington's disease is an inherited progressive neurodegenerative disorder causing abnormal involuntary movements (chorea), psychotic symptoms and progressive cognitive decline and dementia.

A This is an autosomal dominant trinucleotide repeat disorder due to mutation in 'Huntingtin gene' on short arm of chromosome 4.

S Sx Usually begin around 4th decade of life.

Earliest symptoms: subtle personality changes, memory deficits, decreased executive skills and slowing of sacchadic eye movements.

Progressive symptoms: depression, anxiety, irritability, aggression, obsessive-compulsive behaviour and psychosis, choreiform movements, dystonia and balism, increased risk of falls, speech and swallow difficulties, progressive cognitive decline resulting in dementia.

I Blood tests for HD genetics, genetic counseling pre-testing for patient and family.

MRI brain may show atrophy of caudate lobe.

T There is no cure for HD yet, current treatment is symptomatic only.

Chorea: tetrabenazine.

Psychosis / depression: antipsychotics / SSRIs / benzodiazepines.

Dysphagia: modified diet, PEG feeding.

Multidisciplinary assessment including physiotherapy and speech and language therapy.

Pr Average survival after onset of symptoms is around 20 years. Pneumonia, cardiac disease and suicide are the common causes of death in HD patients.

Nerve disorders

Peripheral neuropathy

P Damage to nerves of the peripheral nervous system.

A Acquired: idiopathic, diabetes, alcohol, vitamin deficiencies (B12, folic acid), inflammatory, paraneoplastic, toxic.

Hereditary: commonest is Charcot-Marie-Tooth disease. Also HNPP (hereditary neuropathy with liability to pressure palsies).

S Sx Lower motor neuron symptoms and sensory symptoms of numbness, pins and needles.

Proprioceptive loss can cause gait difficulties.

I Basic neuropathy screen such as FBC, U&Es, LFTs, fasting blood glucose / oral glucose tolerance test, B12, folic acid, serum electrophoresis.

Extended neuropathy screen in atypical cases: autoimmune profile, ENA, ds-DNA, serum ACE levels, infection screen such as HIV, syphilis, Lyme disease, paraneoplastic antibodies.

T Treat underlying disease if found, symptomatic treatment with neuropathic pain killers such as amitryptilline, gabapentin, pregabalin, carbamezepine, duloxetine. Also TENS machine, topical capsaicin cream.

Bell's palsy

P Palsy of CN VII.

A This is the commonest cause of lower motor neuron facial palsy.

Idiopathic.

Other causes of LMN facial palsy include Ramsay Hunt syndrome, diabetes, sarcoidosis, Lyme disease, myasthenia gravis, Gullian-Barré syndrome.

I Clinical diagnosis.

T Not usually required but five- to seven-day course of oral prednisolone could be considered to hasten recovery.

Trigeminal neuralgia

P Unknown pathogenesis.

A Idiopathic, MS, vascular compression, tumours.

S Sx Painful disabling sensory symptoms in the distribution of the trigeminal nerve.

I MRI brain.

T Neuropathic pain killers such as carbamezepine, gabapentin, pregabalin, lamotrigine.

Severe cases: consider IV phenytoin, nerve injection with alcohol, glycerol could also be considered.

Surgical: microvascular decompression (if vascular loop compression of trigeminal nerve is present), partial rhizotomy of nerve.

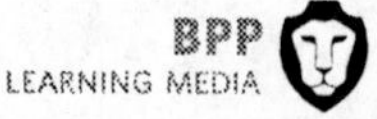

Neuromuscular disorders

Myasthenia gravis

P This is an autoimmune mediated neuromuscular disease characterised by fatigable muscle weakness resulting in various symptoms.

A Female:male 2:1, peak age 30 years.

S Sx Ptosis, opthalmoplegia, dysphagia, dysarthria, facial weakness, limb and respiratory muscle weakness. Weakness worse with exercise.

I Tensilon test: edrophonium, an intravenous acetylcholine esterase inhibitor may produce a transient improvement in certain symptoms.

Acetylcholine receptor antibodies: sensitivity of 85–90% in generalised myasthenia but may be negative in about 50% of ocular myasthenia.

Anti-MUSK (muscle specific kinase) antibodies: positive in about half of the patients who are negative for acetylcholine receptor antibodies.

CXR and CT thorax: presence of thymoma.

Repetitive nerve stimulation test showing a decrement of more than 10–15% of motor action potential with exercise is supportive of diagnosis.

Single fibre EMG (electromyography) is the most sensitive test (95%).

T Medical: corticosteroids, and acetyl choline esterase inhibitors are the mainstay treatment. IV immunoglobulins and plasma exchange are reserved for myasthenic crisis.

Patients with respiratory decompensation should be managed in ICU setting as they may require respiratory support such as non-invasive ventilation or intubation.

Steriod sparing drugs such as azathioprine, mycophenolate should be considered in those needing long-term steroid therapy.

Surgery: thymomas present in 10–15% of all myasthenic patients. Thymectomy is considered an effective therapy for these patients.

Lambert-Eaton myasthenic syndrome (LEMS)

P LEMS is an antibody mediated disorder causing muscle weakness, loss of reflexes and autonomic dysfunction. Antibodies interfere with calcium dependent acetylcholine release in the presynaptic junction of the nerve terminal. Both the muscle strength and reflexes improve post exercise, which is in contrast to MG.

A This is commonly a paraneoplastic phenomenon associated with small cell lung cancer but less frequently can also be non paraneoplastic.

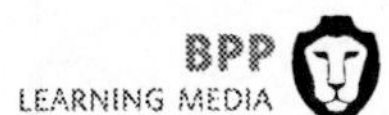

Sx Proximal muscle weakness, bulbar and eye muscle weakness are infrequent, reflexes are reduced but improve post exercise, ataxia.

Autonomic symptoms: orthostatic hypotension, impaired sweating, dry mouth, urinary incontinence.

I Blood test for voltage gated calcium channel antibodies.

Neoplastic screen: CXR, CT chest to look for lung cancer.

Nerve conduction studies / repetitive nerve stimulation / single fibre.

EMG: this show classical increment in compound muscle action potentials after few seconds of voluntary exercise of the tested muscle.

T Successful treatment of an underlying tumour if found, can significantly improve symptoms of LEMS.

Symptomatic treatment with acetylcholine esterase inhibitors like pyridostigmine.

Suppression / removal of autoantibodies with corticosteroids, intravenous immunoglobulin and plasma exchange can be effective.

Motor neuron disease (MND)

P This is caused by degeneration of motor neurons in the cortex, brainstem (corticobulbar tracts), cranial motor nuclei and anterior horn cells in the spinal cord resulting in various neurological symptoms.

- Amyotrophic lateral sclerosis
- Primary lateral sclerosis
- Progressive bulbar palsy
- Progressive muscle atrophy
- Flail limb variant

Box 6.7: Sub-types of MND

A Sporadic or familial (5–10%): SOD1, TDP43 mutations.

S Sx Upper motor neuron signs: spasticity, brisk reflexes, positive Babinski.

Lower motor neuron signs: fasciculations, muscle wasting and weakness.

Bulbar symptoms such as dysarthria, dysphagia, tongue fasciculations / atrophy, brisk jaw jerk are also frequently seen.

Sensory symptoms are minimal or absent.

I MRI brain and spine to exclude other diagnoses.

Nerve conduction studies / electromyography show signs of chronic denervation in the muscles.

T Riluzole (anti glutamate antagonist) only licensed treatment available.

Management is mainly symptomatic: non invasive ventilation, PEG feeding, medications to help symptoms of spasticity, sialorrhea and communication devices such as light writers.

Pr Average survival is usually between two to five years from onset.

Five-year survival is 25%.

Eye signs

All other eye muscles are innervated by CNIII except lateral rectus (CNVI) and superior oblique (CNIV): **LR6 SO4 AO3**.

Third nerve palsy

P Damage to occulomotor nerve.

A Medical: diabetes, demyelination, brainstem infarct.

Surgical: compression of CNIII eg posterior communicating artery aneurysm.

S Sx Ptosis, eye held 'down and out' by action of unaffected lateral rectus and superior oblique. Dilated pupil in surgical CNIII palsy due to compression of parasympathetic fibres.

Fourth nerve palsy

P Damage to trochlear nerve.

A Trauma (30%), raised ICP, congenital palsy.

S Sx Diplopia, eye is held slightly elevated and is unable to look down and in.

Sixth nerve palsy

P Damage to abducens nerve.

A Demyelination, raised ICP, vasculitis.

S Sx Horizontal diplopia, eye unable to abduct beyond midline.

Horner's syndrome

P Horner's syndrome is characterised by miosis, ptosis and anhydrosis and is caused by lesions in the oculosympathetic pathway.

A See Box 6.8.

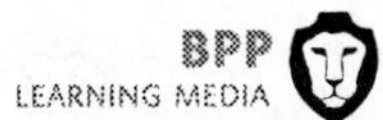

- Central causes: lesions involving hypothalamus, brain stem and cervical cord such as infarct, bleed and demyelination
- Preganglionic: cervicothoracic cord trauma, tumours or syrinx, lower brachial plexus injuries, apical lung tumours, cervical rib
- Postganglionic: migraine, cluster headache, internal carotid artery dissection, cavernous sinus pathologies

Box 6.8: Causes of Horner's syndrome

I Cocaine test (topical cocaine dilates normal eye but has no effect on Horner's eye) and apraclonidine test (topical alpha agonist which constricts normal eye and reverses Horner's eye) help confirm the diagnosis.

Depending on the localisation of the cause for Horner's imaging studies such as MRI brain / cervical cord, MR angiography, CT' chest should be considered.

T Symptoms of Horner's syndrome are usually mild and do not require any intervention. Surgical correction of ptosis could be considered in some cases. Identification and treatment of the underlying cause is important.

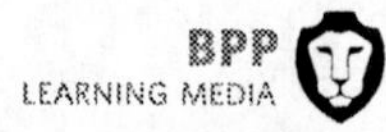

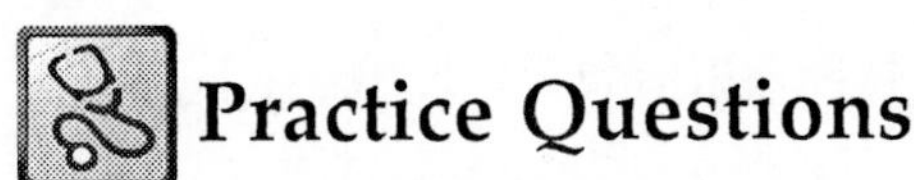

Practice Questions

Single Best Answers

1. Which of the following statements is false regarding weakness?

   A Proximal myopathy (weakness of the thighs) is a classical feature of thyrotoxicosis
   B Proximal myopathy (weakness of the thighs) is a side effect of glucocorticoid use
   C Leg weakness is a typical feature of Guillain-Barré syndrome
   D Ipsilateral leg weakness is a typical characteristic of middle cerebral artery stroke

2. An inferolateral gazing eye and ptosis is caused by:

   A Lesion of Cranial Nerve VII
   B Cavenous sinus mass
   C Brain stem infarct
   D Horner's syndrome

3. The following is true regarding pupillary reflexes:

   A Decreased with occipital lobe infarcts
   B May be spared in 3rd CN palsy
   C Beta blockers lead to constriction
   D The need for mydriatic is increased if the iris is very dark

4. Features of cerebellar syndrome include:

   A Hemianopia
   B Contralateral hemiplegia
   C Proximal myopathy
   D Nystagmus

5. Clinical features of Parkinson's disease include:

   A Proximal myopathy
   B Progressive distal sensory loss
   C Complete ptosis
   D Festinant gait

6. Ptosis, meiosis and anhydrosis is classical of which condition?

   A Horner's syndrome
   B Bell's palsy
   C MND
   D Brain stem infarct

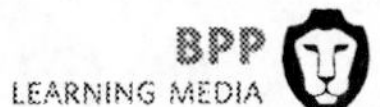

7. Kernig's and Brudzinski's signs are indicative of which condition?

   A Central pontine myelinolysis
   B Brown-Séquard syndrome
   C Meningitis
   D Vertebral artery dissection

8. The following is true regarding Guillain-Barré syndrome.

   A Presents as a distal muscle weakness
   B The majority of patients have permanent muscle paralysis
   C Autonomic and respiratory function should be closely monitored
   D Is always preceded by campylobacter infection

9. Which of the following is the most appropriate first line treatment for a generalised seizure?

   A Sodium valproate
   B Lamotrigine
   C Phenytoin
   D Carbamazepine

10. Proximal muscle weakness that progressively improves with exercise suggests which condition?

   A Myasthenia gravis
   B Lambert-Eaton syndrome
   C Miller-Fischer syndrome
   D Guillain-Barré syndrome

Extended Matching Questions

Causes of unilateral facial palsy

A Stroke
B Brainstem tumour
C Multiple sclerosis
D Acoustic neuroma
E Otitis media
F Cholestertoma
G Bell's palsy
H Ramsey-Hunt syndrome
I Parotid tumours
J Trauma
K Post-meningitis
L Sarcoidosis

Match the following scenarios with the most likely diagnosis.

1. A 30-year-old woman has developed ear pain and facial weakness. On otoscopy she has an inflamed, bulging tympanic membrane.

2. A 35-year-old woman has suddenly developed facial palsy. Six months before this, she had an episode of blurred vision and unsteadiness. On examination, she has mild ataxia and an afferent papillary defect.

3. A 70-year-old man has suddenly developed facial weakness, which was preceded by two days of severe left ear pain, vertigo and deafness. On examination, he has vesicles around his ear and on his soft palate.

4. A 50-year-old woman has developed complete palsy of the left side of the face including the forehead. She also has mild facial pain and watering of the eye on that side. Her sense of taste is impaired.

5. A 56-year-old woman with a history of atrial fibrillation develops sudden weakness of the right side of her face. She is still able to wrinkle both sides of her forehead and her smile is asymmetrical.

6. A 35-year-old man has developed a slowly progressive right-sided facial palsy with deafness and tinnitus. As well as facial asymmetry, he is unable to adduct his right eye. His father had been similarly affected.

Headaches

A Cervival spondylosis
B Stroke
C Bacterial meningitis
D Cerebral tumour
E Extradural haemorrhage
F Tension headache
G Encephalitis
H Subarachnoid haemorrhage
I Congenital heart disease
J Trigeminal neuralgia
K TIA
L Migraine

Match the following scenarios with the most likely diagnosis.

7. A 25-year-old, highly stressed Junior House Officer complains of a headache that has been persistent for weeks. She describes the pain as being 'like a tight band around her head'. Over the counter medication has been used to no avail.

8. A 40-year-old housewife complains of a repeated history of a unilateral throbbing headache lasting several hours for six months. The headache is associated with a disturbance of vision. She claims that eating cheese may trigger it.

9. A 19-year-old male first year university student complains of a rapidly developing headache and a stiff neck. He has been vomiting and his friends say that he cannot stand to be in bright rooms. Examination reveals a pyrexia of 37.5°C.

10. A 70-year-old man presents to his GP surgery with repeated episodes of left sided hemiparesis. A recent ECG reveals that he is in atrial fibrillation. His symptoms fully resolve within 24 hours.

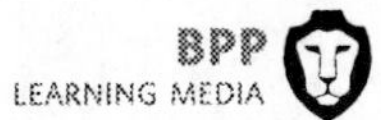

11. A 55-year-old known hypertensive male complains of a sudden devastating occipital headache. He says that he feels as though he had 'been kicked in the head' even though he has not experienced any trauma in the last few weeks. He is feeling drowsy and during the examination he loses consciousness.

Causes of confusion

A Alzheimer's disease
B Delerium tremens
C Postictal state
D Hypoxia
E Cerebrovascular accident
F Hypoglycaemia
G Hypothermia
H Encephalitis
I Urinary tract infection
J Intoxication
K Acute psychosis
L Hypothyroidism

Match the following scenarios with the most likely diagnosis.

12. A 30-year-old man has been picked up in the street by police. He was initially drowsy but is now agitated and aggressive. His trousers are wet with urine.

13. A 75-year-old woman has gradually become confused over three or four years. She forgets the names and birthdays of her family. She gets lost when she goes shopping alone. She sometimes leaves her cooker on all night.

14. A 20-year-old man is irritable and confused. He appears disturbed by loud noises. He is also complaining of a headache and has a pyrexia and mild neck stiffness.

15. A 30-year-old man two days post appendicectomy is now agitated and confused. He is sweaty with a marked tremor of his hands. He claims that his sleep was disturbed by insects in his bed.

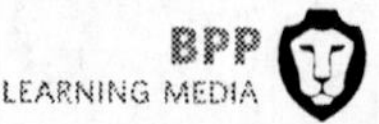

Answers

SBAs		EMQs	
1	D	1	E
2	C	2	C
3	B	3	H
4	D	4	G
5	D	5	A
6	A	6	B
7	C	7	F
8	C	8	L
9	A	9	C
10	B	10	K
		11	H
		12	J
		13	A
		14	H
		15	B

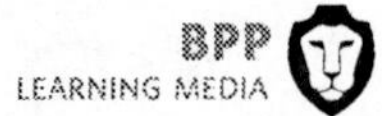

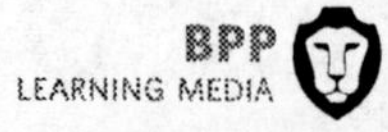

Chapter 7

Haematology

Dr Winifred French and
Dr David Veale

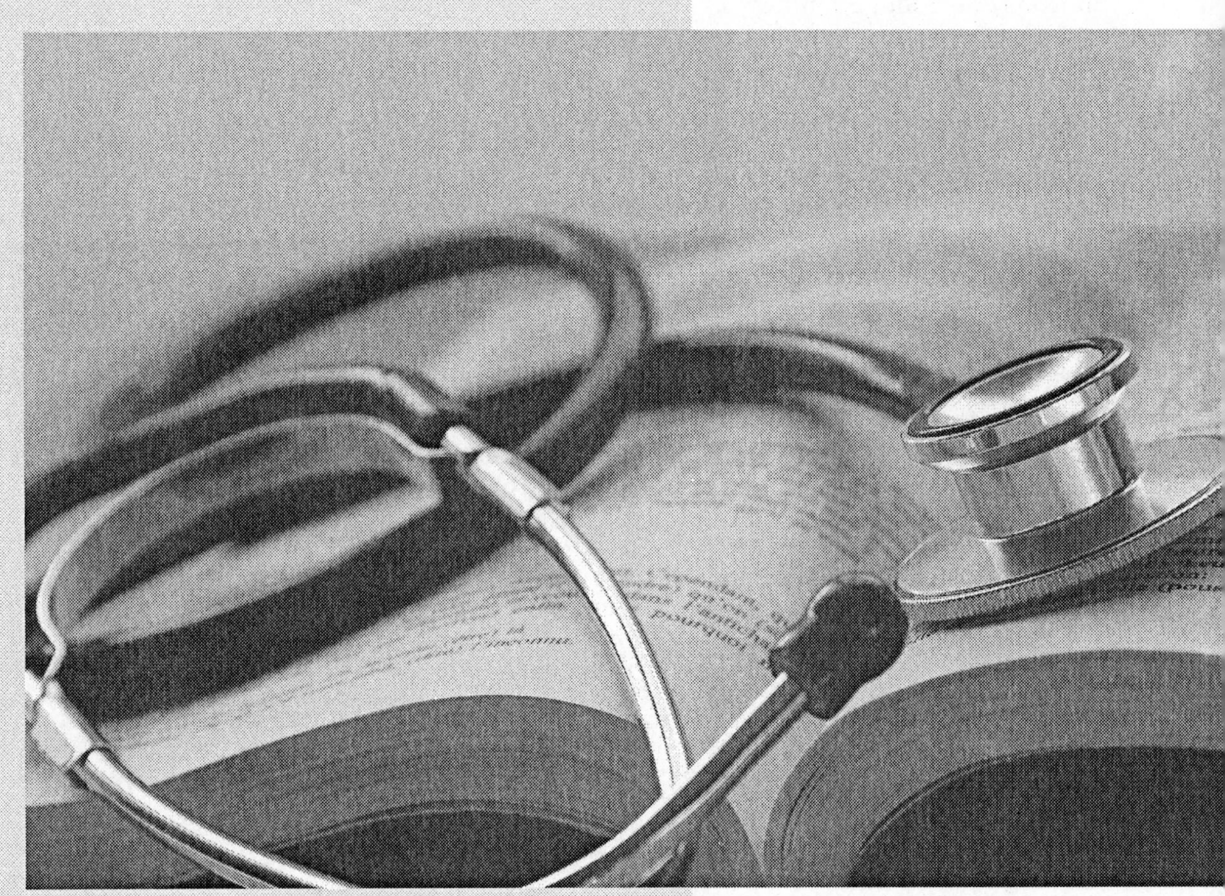

Anticoagulants

Coumarins

Definition and mode of action: are coumarin analogues; act by inhibiting the vitamin K dependent gamma carboxylation of coagulation factor precursors – factors II, VII, IX, X, protein C and protein S.

Most commonly used agent: Warfarin – an oral agent T1/2 >40 hours.

Uses: treatment and prevention of thrombosis. Slow onset of action and need for regular monitoring of levels by the INR.

Adverse effects: bleeding. Skin rashes and necrosis. Numerous drug interactions, leading to increased or decreased serum levels of coumarins.

Heparins

Unfractionated heparins (UFH)

Naturally occurring glycosaminoglycans. Act by inhibiting thrombin, factor Xa and factor II.

Administered intravenously or subcutaneously.

Uses: to treat or prevent thrombosis, rapid onset of action.

Short T1/2 – about 30 minutes.

Monitored by measuring the APTT (Activated Partial Thromboplastin Time).

Adverse effects: bleeding. Allergic reactions. Heparin induced thrombocytopenia (HIT). Osteopenia with long-term use.

Low molecular weight heparins (LMWH)

Are the products of depolymerization of unfractionated heparin.

Uses: to treat or prevent thrombosis.

Administered subcutaneously. No need for regular monitoring.

Adverse effects: Less risk of osteopenia, otherwise similar to UFH.

Antiplatelet agents

Action: inhibit the action of platelet at the sites of endothelial damage.

Uses: to treat or prevent arterial thrombosis eg. aspirin, clopidogrel, tirofibran.

Adverse effects: bleeding.

T1/2 and other side effects vary between agents.

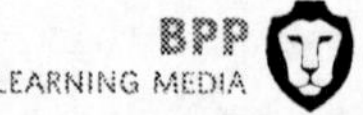

Anaemia

Haemoglobin less than expected for age, sex and physiological state.

Commonly <13.5g/dL in men and <11.5g/dL in women.

Symptoms: pallor, SoB, malaise.

Microcytic (MCV <76)	Normocytic (MCV 76–96)	Macrocytic (MCV >96)
• Iron deficiency anaemia • Thalassaemias • Lead poisoning • Sickle cell anaemia	• Acute blood loss • Anaemia of chronic disease • Marrow infiltration • Haemolysis • Hypothyroid	• B12/Folate deficiency • Alcohol axcess • Liver disease • Myelodysplasia • Hypothyroid

Table 7.1: Classification of anaemia

Microcytic anaemia

Iron deficiency anaemia

P Chronic iron deficiency leads to iron deficient red cells and tissue hypoxia. Total body Iron = 4g (3g in Hb, 1g in cells). Iron is absorbed in the duodenum, transported in blood via transferrin and stored as ferritin.

A Blood loss: most common, dietary deficiency, malabsorption.

S Often none, pallor, fatigue, CHF, kolonychia, angular stomatitis.

Sx Usually none, fatigue, features of underlying cause of blood loss.

I ↓ Hb, ↓ Serum ferritin, ↓ serum iron, ↓ transferrin saturation, ↑ total iron binding capacity (TIBC), endoscopy (OGD/colonoscopy).

T Oral ferrous sulphate, treat underlying cause, dietary advice.

Rarely red cell transfusion is required.

C Usually none, lethargy.

Pr Good.

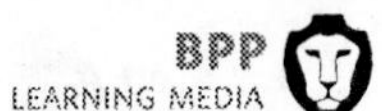

Thalassaemia

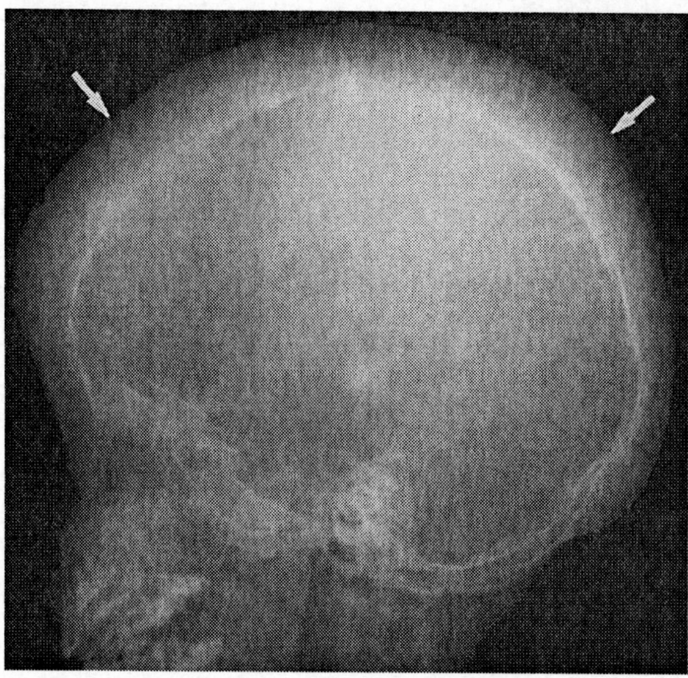

Figure 7.1: 'Hair-on-end' appearance on skull XR in a child with β thalassaemia major. Due to expansion of the diploic space secondary to extramedullary haemopoiesis. (Reproduced with permission from SW Deanery.)

P Imbalance in the production of one or more globin chains. Increased or reduced chains, leading to chronic haemolysis.

α thalassaemia: impaired production of α-chains leading to excess β-chains. HBA1 and HBA2 genes involved.

β thalassaemia: impaired production of β-chains leading to excess β-chains.

A Autosomal recessive inherited genetic defect.

Most common inherited haematological disorder, commonest in middle east and Asia.

S Sx *β thalassaemia trait (heterozygotes)*: none or mild anaemia. *β thalassaemia major (homozygotes):* failure to thrive, stunted growth, skeletal hypertrophy due to extramedullary haemopoiesis (frontal skull bossing, 'chipmunk facies' due to overgrowth of maxilla, 'hair-on-end' skull), hydramnios in pregnancy, severe anaemia, splenomegaly.

Number of alleles affected/genotype	Symptoms
• One (- α/ α α): *Silent carrier*	Asymptomatic
• Two (--/ α α): *α Thalassaemia trait*	Asymptomatic or mild anaemia
• Three (--/- α): *Haemoglobin H disease*	Microcytic anaemia, jaundice, gallstone, hepatosplenomegaly
• Four (- -/ - -): *Bart's hydrops*	Hydrops fetalis, foetus unable to survive leading to still birth

Table 7.2: α **thalassaemia alleles affected and symptoms**

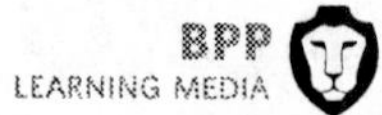

I FBC, blood film, haemoglobin electrophoresis, genetic studies.

T Folic acid, red cell transfusion, desferioxamine (iron chelation), splenectomy, bone marrow transplant, prenatal genetic counseling.

C Haemosiderosis from repeated transfusions, recurrent infections, early death.

Pr Variable depending on genes inherited and available supportive treatment.

Sickle cell anaemia

P Polymerisation of hemoglobin S, which sickles when O_2 and pH are low in small vessels in organs. Anaemia results from splenic destruction of red cells.

A Homozygous inheritance of the Bs gene results in sickle cell anaemia. Heterozygosity for the gene gives rise to various types of Sickle cell disease.

S Sx

HbAS (sickle cell trait)	HbSS (homozygous)
• Only sickle under severe hypoxic conditions eg aircrafts. Otherwise asymptomatic • Protects against falciparum malaria	• Haemolytic anaemia • Sickle cell vasoocclusive crisis: bone pain, dehydration, worse in cold, infection • Aplastic crisis • Splenic sequestration • Gallstones (due to haemolysis) • Avascular necrosis • Hand dactylitis • Retinal damage, priapism, leg ulcers

Box 7.1: Signs and symptoms of sickle cell disease

I Blood film: marked variation in red cell size; varying amounts of sickle cell.

Sickle cell test (HbS insoluble in phosphate buffers).

Hb electrophoresis: HbS 80–90%. Hb F may be raised.

T Prevent / minimise triggers for hypoxaemia and acidosis eg infection, dehydration, hypoxia. Folic acid. Prophylactic antibiotics. Prompt treatment of infections. Red cell transfusion / exchange transfusion. Hydroxycarbamide to increase Hb F. Bone marrow transplant. Genetic counseling.

C Infarcted organs: bone, spleen, kidneys, CNS, pulmonary hypertension. Proliferative retinopathy. Developmental and psychosocial problems.

Pr Variable depending on combination of genes inherited and available supportive treatment.

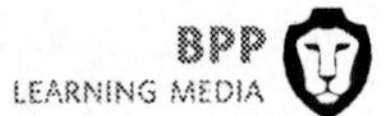

Normocytic anaemia

Haemolysis

P Shortened red cell life span (normally 120 days), secondary to increased destruction.

A See Box 7.2.

Congenital

- *Membrane:* hereditary spherocytosis
- *Enzyme:* G6PD deficiency, pyruvate kinase deficiency
- *Hb defect:* sickle cell, thalassaemia

Acquired

- *Immune:* autoimmune haemolytic anaemia (AIHA), incompatible transfusion
- *Mechanical:* microangiopathic haemolytic anaemia (MAHA), prosthetic heart valves
- *Infection:* malaria
- *Drugs:* dapsone, amyl nitrate

Box 7.2: Causes of haemolysis

S Few, pallor, jaundice, features of underlying condition.

Sx Fatigue, shortness of breath, haemoglobinuria.

I Bloods: ↑ reticulocytes, ↑ unconjugated bilirubin, ↑ lactate dehydrogenase, ↓ serum haptoglobin.

Blood film: reticulocytosis, spherocytes, bite cells, schistocytes (red cell fragments).

Direct Coombs test, urinary haemosiderin.

T Treat cause of haemolysis, folic acid, steroids / immunosuppression. Blood product support.

C Depends on underlying cause.

Pr Generally good.

Hereditary spherocytosis

P Abnormal red cell membrane resulting in spherocytes, with increased osmotic fragility.

A Autosomal dominant inheritance.

S There may be none, mild jaundice during an infection, splenomegaly.

Sx Often none, lethargy, abdominal pain.

I Family history usually positive, FBC, reticulocyte count, blood film (spherocytes ++), uncongugated bilirubin, LDH EMA test, abdominal USS.

T Folic acid, blood transfusion only if severely anaemic.

Splenectomy (not often required), cholecystectomy.

C Cholecystits.

Pr Good.

G6PD deficiency

P Defective enzyme causes red cell membrane to be damaged by oxidative stress, usually infections or drugs. Abnormal cells are destroyed in the spleen.

A X- linked inheritance.

S None, in steady state, pallor, neonatal jaundice, jaundice on exposure to oxidants or infection.

Sx None, fatigue, abdominal pain, discoloured urine.

I Bloods: FBC (reticulocytosis), uncongugated bilirubin, LDH, haptoglobin, urinary urobilionogen.

Blood film: spherocyres, irregularly contracted red cells, red cell fragments, Heinz bodies.

T Avoid all drugs associated with oxidative haemolysis, red cell transfusion, IV fluids, exchange transfusion for affected neonates, folic acid.

C Cholecystitis.

Pr Good.

Aplastic anaemia

P Bone marrow aplasia.

A Most cases idiopathic.

Other causes: hereditary eg Fanconi syndrome, post viral eg hepatitis A, B, C, drug induced eg carbamazepine, busulpan, exposure to high dose irradiation.

S Sx Chronic pancytopenia, bleeding, respiratory and soft tissue infections, lethargy.

I FBC, blood film, reticulocyte count.

Bone marrow aspirate and trephine biopsy, flow cytometry, cytogenetics.

T Careful observation only, in mild cases. Blood product support, immunosuppressive therapy, androgens, bone marrow transplant.

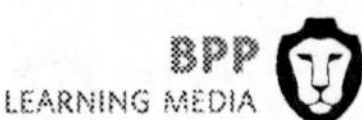

C Progression to more severe disease. Progression to acute leukaemia. Development of paroxsymal nocturnal haemoglobinuria.

Pr Potential for cure with bone marrow transplant. Immunosuppression may give good results.

Macrocytic anaemia

Vitamin B12 deficiency

P B12 is required for DNA synthesis.

A Lack of gastric intrinsic acid for binding with dietary B12 or failure of absorption in terminal ileum. less often dietary deficiency (body stores last two to three years).

S Often none, pallor, CHF, peripheral neuropathy, confusion, SACD.

Sx Of anaemia, neuropathy, bowel disease.

I FBC, serum B12 (and folate).

Blood film: oval macrocytosis, hypersegmented neutrophils.

Bone marrow biopsy, serum ferritin, LDH, homocysteine levels, Autoantibody screen (for gastric parietal and intrinsic factor antibodies), Schilling test.

T Intramuscular hydroxycobolamin replacement and long-term maintenance plus folic acid, oral B12, if clear dietary deficiency. Antibiotics for bacterial overgrowth in blind-loop syndrome. Supportive measures for CHF.

C Neurological damage may be permanent.

Pr Good.

Folate deficiency

P Folate required for DNA synthesis.

A Dietary deficiency / malabsorption, increased utilisation in rapid turnover eg haemolyticanaemias, pregnancy, anti-folate drugs eg, methotrexate.

S Sx As for B12 deficiency.

I As for B12 deficiency, except autoantibody screen and Schilling test.

T Replace folic acid only after any B12 deficiency has been corrected. Maintain folic acid in chronic haemolytic syndromes.

Pr Good.

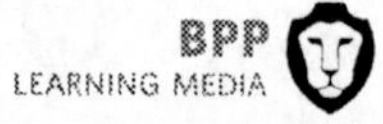

Anaemia of chronic disease

P Disordered iron metabolism.

A Inflammatory factors, cytokines, hormones, associated with chronic inflammatory or malignant disorders, prevent available iron from being adequately utilised.

S Sx Features of anaemia and the underlying condition.

I Iron studies, EPO levels, hepcidin levels, bone marrow biopsy.

T Treat the underlying condition.

C Due to the underlying condition.

Pr Depends on the underlying condition.

Coagulation disorders

Common pathway:

- Factor X & V

Extrinsic pathway:

- Factor VII & TF (Tissue Factor)

Intrinsic pathway:

- Factor VIII, IX & XI

PT measures common and extrinsic pathway
APTT measures common and intrinsic pathway

Box 7.3: Coagulation pathways

Haemophilia A and B

P Haemophilia A: low levels of factor VIII.

Haemophilia B: low levels of factor IX.

A X linked genetic defect in the responsible genes (male only disease, females are carriers).

S Sx Haemarthrosis, spontaneous bleeds into muscles and soft tissue, haematuria, GI bleed.

I Clotting screen: ↑ APTT, normal PT, normal vWF, ↓ factor VIII (Haemophilia A), ↓ factor IX (Haemophilia B).

T Factor VIII and IX replacement, desmopression increases factor VIII.

C Chronic arthropathies, contraction of Hepatitis A, B, C, HIV. Risk of variant CJD.

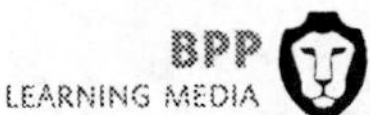

Pr Good with prophylactic and replacement recombinant factor therapy. Fatal hemorrhage in the absence of factor replacement.

Von Willebrand disease

P Low or abnormal vWF resulting in low levels of factor VIII and disorders of platelet function.

A Autosomal dominant inheritance.

S Sx Intermittent mucocutaneous bleeding, easy bruising, menorrhagia, epistaxis.

I Clotting screen: ↑ APTT, normal PT, ↓ vWF levels and function. ↓ factor VIII, ↑ bleeding time.

T Desmopressin (can increase vWF levels), vWF rich factor VIII, vWF concentrate, tranexamic acid, FFP.

C From bleeding or factor replacement.

Pr Usually very good.

Autoimmune thrombocytopaenic purpura

P Antibody mediated destruction of megakaryocytes and platelets.

A Unknown, often preceded by a viral infection in children.

S Sx Epistaxis, menorrhagia, bruising, gingival bleeding.

I FBC: ↓ PLTs, blood film.

Clotting screen: normal.

Bone marrow biopsy: normal / increased megakaryocytes.

T If PLTs <30 × 10^9/L: steriods or immunosuppression.

Splenectomy.

C Life-threatening bleeding, risk of life threatening infections post splenectomy or immunosuppression.

Pr Good.

Disseminated intravascular coagulation (DIC)

P Activation of the haemostatic system within the intravascular system resulting in widespread deposition of fibrin, activation of platelets and consumption of coagulation factors.

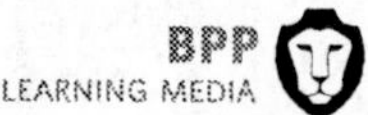

A See Box 7.4.

- Tissue damage and burns
- Malignancy
- Complications of pregnancy
- Infection
- Immunological reactions
- Toxins
- Liver disease

Box 7.4: Causes of DIC

S Sx Bleeding (major symptom), thrombosis, features of the underlying condition. Patients are usually very ill.

I FBC, blood film.

Clotting screen: ↑ PT, ↑ APPT, ↑ thrombin time, ↓↓ fibrinogen, ↑ fibrinogen degradation products (FDP), ↑ D-dimer.

T Treat underlying cause, blood products if bleeding (FFP, PLTs,).

Pr High mortality: greater than 80% in severe cases.

Deep vein thrombosis (DVT)

P Formation of a clot in a deep vein, usually of the lower extremities or pelvis.

A Several factors increase risk: age, known thrombophilia, malignancy, high BMI, previous DVT, pregnancy, oestrogens, immobility, severe illness, recent surgery.

Virchow's Triad: venous stasis, hypercoagulation, vascular injury.

S Sx Pain, swelling, erythema, warmth, pitting oedema.

Homan's sign: increased pain on dorsiflexion in calf DVT (risk of dislodging thrombus).

I Clinical assessment of risk, ↑ D-dimer (also raised in infection, only useful if no other cause), doppler ultrasound scan, venogram.

T Low molecular weight heparin (LMWH), oral anticoagulant, support stockings, investigation of underlying cause, IVC filter.

C Pulmonary embolism (PE), extension of thrombus, post thrombotic syndrome, recurrence of DVT.

Pr Good if promptly and adequately treated. Risk of recurrence.

Thrombophilia

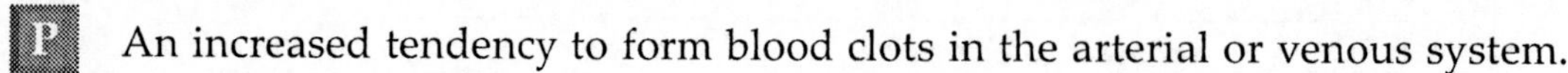

P An increased tendency to form blood clots in the arterial or venous system.

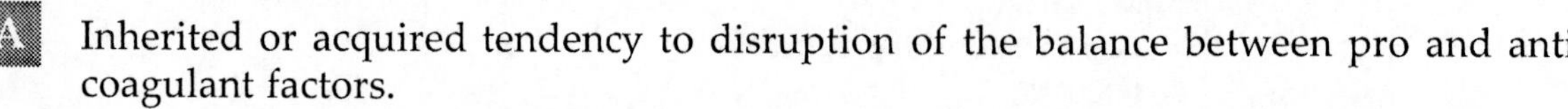

A Inherited or acquired tendency to disruption of the balance between pro and anti coagulant factors.

Primary

- Reduced coagulant factors:
  - Protein C deficiency
  - Protein S deficiency
  - Antithrombin III deficiency
- Reduced effectiveness of anticoagulant clotting factors:
  - Factor V Leiden (commonest hereditable thrombophilia)

Secondary

- Immobility
- Recent surgery
- Malignancy
- Smoking
- Pregnancy
- Antiphospholipid syndrome
- Oestrogens (OCP)

Box 7.5: Causes of thrombophilia

S Sx Asymptomatic or features of thrombosis, PE/DVT, recurrent thromboembolism or miscarriage, thrombosis in atypical sites, FH of thrombosis.

I FBC, clotting screen, lupus anticoagulant, anticardiolipin antibodies, assays for antithrombin, protein C and protein S, PCR for factor V Leiden.

T Treatment of any thrombosis. Prophylactic measures in individuals and family members at high risk of thrombosis.

C Variaible risk of thrombosis and its complications.

Pr Variable.

Myeloproliferative disorders

Polycythaemia vera (PV)

P Neoplastic clonal disorder of bone marrow stem cells causing excessive production of erythrocytes (often with neutrophils and platelets too).

Differential diagnoses include causes of secondary polycythaemia: smoking (hypoxia), alcohol excess, kidney disease (eg polycystic kidneys), EPO-producing tumours (eg bronchial carcinoma), drugs.

A 95% is caused by mutation of JAK-2 (product of the mutated gene drives cell growth and differentiation).

Median age 60 years.

S Plethoric complexion, hepatosplenomegaly, thrombosis (arterial more commonly than venous), hypertension.

Sx Often asymptomatic, headache, drowsiness, symptoms of thrombosis, pruritis, haemorrhage.

I Bloods: FBC, U&Es, LFTs, JAK-2 mutation analysis.

If JAK-2 is positive, no further investigation required.

If JAK-2 negative: serum erythropoeitin, bone marrow aspirate and trephine biopsy, ABG, CXR, red cell mass and plasma volume.

T No cure, venesection, low doses of chemotherapy eg hydroxycarbamide long-term, radioactive phosphorous, aspirin.

C Transformation of PV to myelofibrosis, AML.

Pr Median survival approximately 14 years if treated.

Essential thrombocythaemia

P Persistent thrombocytosis (>450 × 10^9/l) which is not reactive or due to another myeloproliferative neoplasm or myelodysplasia.

A Unknown 50% have JAK-2 mutation. Not associated with radiation, drugs, chemicals.

S Sx Often asymptomatic, thrombosis (arterial more than venous, eg CVE, MI, hepatic vein thrombus), headache, light-headedness, haemorrhage (as platelets are functionally abnormal and cannot produce clots), erythromelalgia (burning sensation and erythema in hands and feet caused by microthrombi). Splenomegaly less common than in PV.

I Bloods: platelets persistently >450, Hb usually normal, may have microcytic anaemia due to chronic bleeding, WCC normal.

Blood film: giant platelets and platelet clumps.

JAK-2 mutation analysis (present in 50%).

Bone marrow aspirate and trephine biopsy.

T Lifestyle changes to reduce clot risk, treat thrombotic risks.

Treat according to risk of thrombosis and haemorrhage.

- Low risk (young, no PMH of either, platelets <1,500, no cardiovascular risks): aspirin if not contraindicated
- High risk: aspirin (unless thrombocytosis >1,000), chemotherapy eg hydroxycarbamide

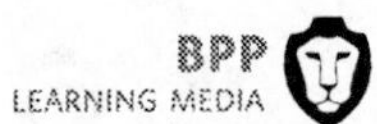

C Risk of transformation to myelofibrosis or AML (less likely than in PV).

Pr Life expectancy near normal.

Myelofibrosis

P Proliferation of haemopoeitic stem cells with bone marrow fibrosis. Fibrosis is caused by release of growth factors by abnormal megakaryocytes (platelet precursors), which stimulate fibroblasts.

A Rare, median age 65 years. Most are primary. Commonest secondary causes are PV, then ET. Rarely caused by chemotherapy, radiotherapy, myelodysplasia, carcinoma.

S 20% asymptomatic at diagnosis, majority have splenomegaly (moderate to massive) +/- hepatomegaly, gout, portal hypertension and ascites.

Sx Weight loss, sweats / fever, fatigue, abdominal discomfort, marrow failure.

I Bloods: usually normochromic normocytic anaemia.

Blood film: teardrop poikilocytes, giant platelets.

JAK-2 mutation analysis often positive.

Bone marrow aspirate and trephine: often unsuccessful (fibrosis prevents release of cells) 'dry tap', trephine shows variable cellularity and increased fibrosis.

T Incurable, watch and wait if asymptomatic, blood product support palliation, consider splenic radiotherapy or splenectomy if spleen painful or massive.

Drugs: thalidomide, androgens, corticosteroids.

Allogeneic stem cell transplant if fit enough (chance of cure).

C Haemorrhage, transformation to AML, infection, thrombosis, progressive cachexia.

Pr Poor, median survival three to five years.

Leukaemia

Acute myeloid leukaemia

P AML is a malignant proliferation of haematopoetic (blood making) precursor blast cells of non-lymphoid lineage.

A AML usually develops without a clear precipitant. Commonest leukaemia in adults.

More frequent with increasing age: median onset 64 years.

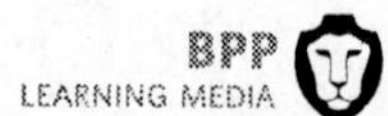

De novo AML (most cases): aetiology unclear Secondary AML • Preceding haematological disease (myelodysplasia, myeloproliferative neoplasm) • Previous chemotherapy (especially alkylating agents) • Benzene exposure • Ionising radiation • Congenital chromosomal abnormalities eg Fanconi's anaemia, Down's syndrome

Table 7.3: Causes of AML

S Sx Anaemia, infection, bruising and bleeding.

Gum hypertrophy (caused by infiltration with blasts) or skin infiltration (fleshy nodules), signs of leucostasis (hypoxia, retinal haemorrhage, confusion), lymphadenopathy infrequently.

I Bloods: ↓ Hb, platelets and neutrophils, blood film (pancytopaenia with circulating blast cells), U&Es, LFTs, B12, folate, ferritin, coagulation screen, blood group, antibody screen and direct Coombs test, infectious mononucleosis screen if young, blood cultures.

Bone marrow aspirate +/- biopsy including cytogenetics (check for aberrant mutation(s) in abnormal clone) and immunophenotyping.

T Depends on age, patient wishes and performance status. Neutropaenic infection prophylaxis. Intensive chemotherapy if fit enough (usually three to four cycles, each requiring four weeks of inpatient stay). Palliative measures if less fit.

May use low dose chemotherapy, blood product support, allogeneic stem cell transplant if high risk of relapse when in remission after induction chemotherapy or for relapsed disease.

C Chemotherapy induced: life threatening infection, bleeding, organ damage (renal, cardiac, liver toxicity), hair loss, GI toxicity, infertility.

Supporting drug induced: antibiotics, antifungals, antivirals damaging kidneys, hearing, liver.

Pr Variable depending on: age (<50 favourable), cytogenetic abnormalities, molecular genetic abnormalities, presenting blast count (<25 unfavourable), AML classification, preceding myelodysplasia (poor prognosis).

Acute lymphoblastic leukaemia

P ALL is a malignant proliferation of haematopoetic (blood making) precursor blast cells of lymphoid lineage.

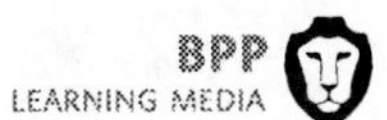

A Unknown.

Predisposing factors: ionising radiation, congenital chromosomal abnormality (Down's, Klinefelter's and Fanconi syndromes).

Commonest leukaemia in children. Median age 3.5 years. Rare in adults.

S Sx Anaemia, infection, haemorrhage, failure to thrive, CNS involved more commonly than in AML, hepatosplenomegaly, bone or joint pain, SVC obstruction. Lymphadenopathy more common than AML.

I Bloods: ↓ Hb, platelets and neutrophils usually low, WCC often high, may be very high.

Blood film (pancytopaenia with circulating blast cells), U&Es, LFTs, B12, folate, ferritin, coagulation screen, blood group, antibody screen and direct Coombs test, blood cultures.

Bone marrow aspirate +/- biopsy including cytogenetics and immunophenotyping.

CXR: mediastinal mass if T-lineage ALL.

Lumbar puncture.

T Counselling of child + parents, blood product support, treat infection +/- septic shock, prophylaxis for neutropaenic infections, central venous catheter insertion, chemotherapy, radiotherapy if indicated, allogeneic stem cell transplant if indicated.

C Chemotherapy induced: life threatening infection, bleeding, organ damage (renal, cardiac, liver toxicity), hair loss, GI toxicity, infertility, growth retardation, avascular necrosis (steroids).

Supporting drug induced: antibiotics, antifungals, antivirals damaging kidneys, hearing, liver.

Radiotherapy induced: accelerated coronary artery disease, reduced IQ, growth retardation.

Pr Childhood ALL >80% cure, adults poorer as higher relapse rates, dependent on age, cytogenetic abnormalities (eg Philadelphia chromosome), presence of CNS disease, high WCC at diagnosis, long time to complete remission after starting chemotherapy.

Chronic myeloid leukaemia

P Malignant tumour of the pleuripotent stem cell which produces excessive numbers of granulocytes (neutrophils and myelocytes), eosinophils and basophils.

Characterised by the presence of the Philadelphia chromosome (translocation between chromosomes 9 and 22, resulting in bcr-abl gene that produces tyrosine kinase).

A Unknown. Rarely caused by ionising irradiation. Incidence increases with age.

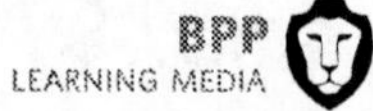

S Sx Usually insidious onset, 30% asymptomatic, fever, weight loss, anaemia, sweating, local (pressure) symptoms of massive splenomegaly, bruising, bleeding, gout, hyperviscosity and leukostasis (deafness and pulmonary infiltrates).

I Bloods: WCC often >100 (neutrophils, myelocytes, basophils, eosinophils), anaemia, platelets can be low, high or normal, LDH, urate.

Bone marrow aspirate: chronic phase if blasts <10%, 10–20% in accelerated phase, >20% in acute leukaemia (transformed from CML), molecular genetics.

Bone marrow trephine (rule out fibrosis).

T Tyrosine kinase inhibitors eg imatinib.

Consider allogeneic stem cell transplant in young patients with HLA matched sibling donor.

C Modest increased infection risk, progression to accelerated phase, acute leukaemia or myelofibrosis.

Pr Improving with advent of tyrosine kinase inhibitors, 84% survival at five years post-diagnosis.

Dependent on age, spleen size, platelet count, % of blasts in blood at diagnosis.

Chronic lymphocytic leukaemia

P Progressive proliferation and accumulation of mature (usually) B-lymphocytes found in blood, bone marrow, lymph nodes liver and spleen.

A Unknown. Small proportion familial. No link with radiation, chemicals, drugs.

Commonest leukaemia in adults. Increasing incidence with age.

S Sx Often asymptomatic, marrow failure (infection, anaemia, bleeding), autoimmune haemolytic anaemia or thrombocytopaenia. Lymphadenopathy can be bulky.

'B' symptoms in advanced disease (sweats, weight loss, anorexia, malaise).

I Bloods: lymphocytosis >5, usually >20, anaemia +/- low platelets, blood film.

Immunophenotyping (differentiates CLL from lymphomas or acute leukaemias).

Immunoglobulins (often low).

Bone marrow aspirate and trephine: infiltration of lymphocytes +/- reduced normal haematopoeisis, send for cytogenetics to help with prognosis.

Lymph node biopsy rarely needed.

T Usually 'watch and wait'.

Start chemotherapy if patient is fit, and:

- Rapidly increasing WCC or
- B symptoms
- Marrow failure
- Autoimmune anaemia or low platelets
- Massive splenomegaly or lymphadenopathy

Allogeneic stem cell transplant if young and fit.

Blood product support.

C Depends on choice of chemotherapy: gut toxicity, infections, anaemia, bleeding, hair loss, marrow failure, dysplasia caused by chemotherapy, secondary malignancy.

P Incurable unless transplanted.

Median survival varies between 1 year and >13 years depending on staging (according to presence of marrow failure, lymphadenopathy, splenomegaly and hepatomegaly).

Lymphoma

Hodgkin's lymphoma

P Clonal proliferation of abnormal B-lymphocytes (Reed-Sternberg cells) with reactive proliferation of other T- and B-lymphocytes.

A Often no cause found, may follow EBV infection, increased incidence if HIV positive, increased risk in first degree relatives of affected individuals. Usually affects young adults / adolescents.

S Usually painless rubbery lymphadenopathy, often cervical, occasionally hepato- or splenomegaly. Rarely bulky mediastinal nodes cause SVC obstruction or bronchial obstruction, pleural effusion, infection, eg shingles.

Sx 'B' symptoms common (weight loss, anorexia, sweats, fever, fatigue), pruritis, painful lymph nodes on drinking alcohol.

I Bloods: normochromic, normocytic anaemia, may have thrombocytopaenia, increased WCC, LFTs may be deranged if liver involved.

CT chest, abdo, pelvis (+ neck if involved).

Consider CT:PET scan (helpful in assessing response to treatment, as sometimes patients have residual scar tissue in a previously active node).

Lymph node biopsy.

Bone marrow aspirate and trephine for staging.

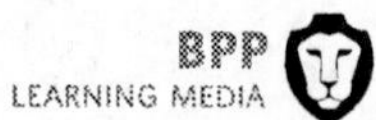

- Stage I: confined to single LN
- Stage II: Two or more LN groups confined to one side of the diaphragm
- Stage III: Two or more LN groups on both sides of the diaphragm
- Stage IV: involvement of extralymphatic sites (eg bone marrow)

A = Absence of systemic symptoms
B = Presence of systemic symptoms

Box 7.6: Ann Arbor staging for Hodgkin's lymphoma

T Counselling regarding disease, treatment and fertility, consider sperm banking in males or oocyte harvesting in females if facilities are available.

Chemotherapy (curative), consider adjuvant radiotherapy to localised residual disease.

Autologous (self) stem cell transplant in relapsed disease.

Allogeneic stem cell transplant in refractory / multiply relapsed disease.

C Early: infection, bone marrow failure, organ damage.

Late: reduced fertility, premature menopause, secondary malignancy, particularly after mediastinal radiotherapy, lung fibrosis (after radiotherapy), lung / thyroid toxicity.

Pr Variable depending on stage, FBC, albumin, gender, and age of the patient eg:

- Stage I/II (ie early), good risk, classical HL five-year overall survival 95%
- Stage III/IV (advanced), poor risk classical HL five year OS 59%

Non-Hodgkin's lymphoma

P Abnormal proliferation of B- or T-lymphocytes.

Multiple histological subtypes with very variable clinical courses

- B- or T- cell lymphomas
- High-grade (aggressive but potentially curable) or low grade (more indolent but incurable with chemotherapy) lymphomas

A Increasing incidence worldwide, geographic variation in prevalence of subtypes around the world.

Can be associated with: (see Box 7.7)

- Inherited immunodeficiency (eg ataxia telangiectasia)
- Acquired immunodeficiency (eg HIV, immunosuppressive drugs post transplant or in IBD etc)
- Infection:
  - HTLV-1 (Human T lyphotrophic virus) in a T lymphoma
  - EBV in Burkitt lymphoma
  - H. pylori in MALT lymphoma
- Family history
- Dye / chemical exposure

Box 7.7: Associations of NHL

S Usually non-tender lymphadenopathy, vary according to affected site, any organ can be affected.

Sx Can be asymptomatic, particularly in low grade, early stage disease, 'B' symptoms (fever, weight loss, anorexia, sweats), marrow failure (anaemia, haemorrhage, infections), local symptoms eg bowel obstruction.

I FBC: marrow failure, high WCC, U&Es, LFTs, calcium, urate, LDH, immunoglobulins.

CT chest, abdo, pelvis (+ neck / brain if involved).

Bone marrow aspirate and trephine.

Biopsy of other affected lymph node, organ or other tissue.

Lumbar puncture +/- MRI if worried about CNS involvement.

T Very variable depending on subtype and patient.

- 'Watch and wait' if early stage low grade disease
- Antibiotics (H. pylori eradication can cure MALT lymphoma)
- Powerful combination chemotherapy for very high grade lymphoma
- Monoclonal antibodies (recognise lymphoma surface structures eg CD20 on B lymphocytes, and destroy those cells only)
- Radiotherapy
- Autologous or allogeneic stem cell transplants for relapsed disease

C Dependent on treatment choice, can be life-threatening eg sepsis, organ failure.

Pr Dependent on: age, stage, presence of disease outside lymph nodes, performance status (ie presence of co-morbidities), high LDH.

Myeloma

P Clonal proliferation of plasma cells (type of B lymphocyte). 1% of all cancers. Median onset 66 years. They usually produce monoclonal immunoglobulins (paraprotein) or part of an immunoglobulin (light chains). Excess osteoclastic activity.

A Usually unclear. Weak association with radiation, benzene, pesticide and farm working. Few familial clusters reported.

S **Sx** Often asymptomatic, bone pain (often back) caused by lytic lesions and pathological fractures, hypercalcaemia, marrow failure, hyperviscosity (blurred vision, bleeding, headaches). Spinal cord compression rarely.

I Blood film: normochromic normocytic anaemia, thrombocytopaenia, rouleaux.

Bloods: ESR high, U&Es, calcium, LFTs, serum free light chains.

Immunoglobins: all low apart from high abnormal paraprotein.

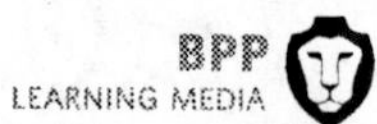

Protein electrophoresis: characterises paraprotein.

Urine: Bence Jones protein (light chains found in the urine).

X-rays of all long bones, skull, spine and pelvis (skeletal survey) +/- MRI.

Bone marrow aspirate +/- trephine biopsy including cytogenetics.

T Treatable, not curable.

Supportive treatment: bisphosphonates to reduce fracture risk, bone pain, calcium, local radiotherapy to painful bone lesions, blood transfusion if needed, hydration in hypercalcaemia, orthopaedic surgery to fractures, or critical bone lesions.

If fit, treat with combination chemotherapy (outpatient) then autologous (self) stem cell transplant.

Aim of chemotherapy is to allow extended period of time before disease (inevitably) relapses.

2nd, 3rd etc line combination chemotherapy on relapse if still fit enough.

C Chemotherapy side effects: infection, anaemia, bleeding, hair loss, GI toxicity, organ damage.

Pr Depends on lots of variables: age, performance status (are they fit for chemo?), severity of disease at diagnosis (very high calcium / paraprotein, low Hb, advanced bone disease, high LDH / β2Microglobulin). Improving with new drugs. Median survival approximately five years (very variable).

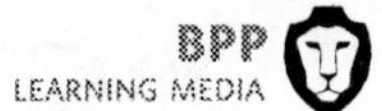

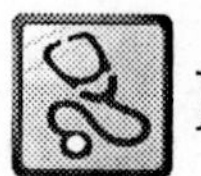

Practice Questions

Single Best Answers

1. Anaemia of chronic disease is associated with:

   A Cytokines and inflammatory factors
   B An aplastic marrow
   C Haemolytic anaemias
   D G6PD deficiency

2. Folate deficiency:

   A Occurs years after dietary deficiency
   B Is investigated using the Schilling test
   C May be caused by very rapid cell turnover
   D Can de differentiated from B12 deficiency by a blood film

3. A four-year-old child is suspected of having acute lymphoblastic leukaemia on blood tests taken by her GP. Which of the following symptoms or signs would support this diagnosis?

   A Splenomegaly
   B Lymphadenopathy
   C Weight loss
   D All of the above

4. Chronic lymphocytic leukaemia is a disease characterised by abnormal proliferation of:

   A Haematopoetic (blood making) precursor blast cells of lymphoid lineage
   B Plasma cells
   C Mature (usually) B-lymphocytes
   D Haematopoetic precursor blast cells of myeloid lineage

5. Which of the following is not a cause of secondary polycythaemia?

   A Chronic hypoxia
   B Polycystic kidneys
   C Erythropoeitin-secreting bronchial carcinoma
   D Polycythaemia vera

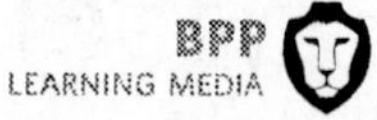

Extended Matching Questions

Haemolytic anaemias

A Frontal bossing
B Leg ulcers
C EMA test
D G6PD deficiency

Match the below scenarios with the co-existing symptoms above.

1. Three family members with spherocytes on their blood films and stunted growth.

2. A young man with pallor and discoloured urine on the second day of a new prescription.

3. A young lady with recurrent painful crises.

Anticoagulants

A Vitamin K antagonist
B LMWH
C UFH

Match the following scenarios with the most appropriate option above.

4. Given as a drip following cardiac surgery.

5. Tablet requiring regular blood tests.

A Diabetes mellitus
B Unsuccessful bone marrow aspirate ('dry tap')
C Down's syndrome
D Polycythaemia Vera
E Mediastinal mass on CXR
F Congenital hypothyroidism
G Mild splenomegaly on abdominal ultrasound
H Essential thrombocythaemia
I White cell count of 324×10^6/l (predominately neutrophils and myelocytes with increased basophils and eosinophils)
J Primary myelofibrosis

Match the following scenarios with the most appropriate option above.

6. Presence of this condition predisposes to development of Acute Lymphoblastic Leukaemia.

7. This investigation finding is suggestive of myelofibrosis.

8. The JAK-2 mutation is present in 95% of patients with this condition.

9. The life-expectancy of someone diagnosed with this condition and treated as per guidelines is equivalent to the general population.

10. This investigation finding is suggestive of chronic myeloid leukaemia.

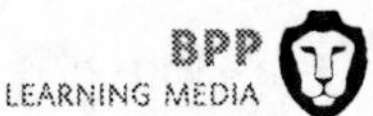

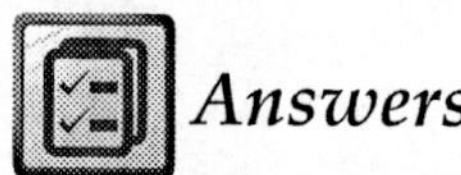

Answers

SBAs		EMQs	
1	A	1	C
2	C	2	D
3	D	3	B
4	C	4	C
5	D	5	A
6		6	C
7		7	B
8		8	D
9		9	H
10		10	I

Chapter 8

Rheumatology

Dr Mahdi Abusalameh and
Mr Alexander Young

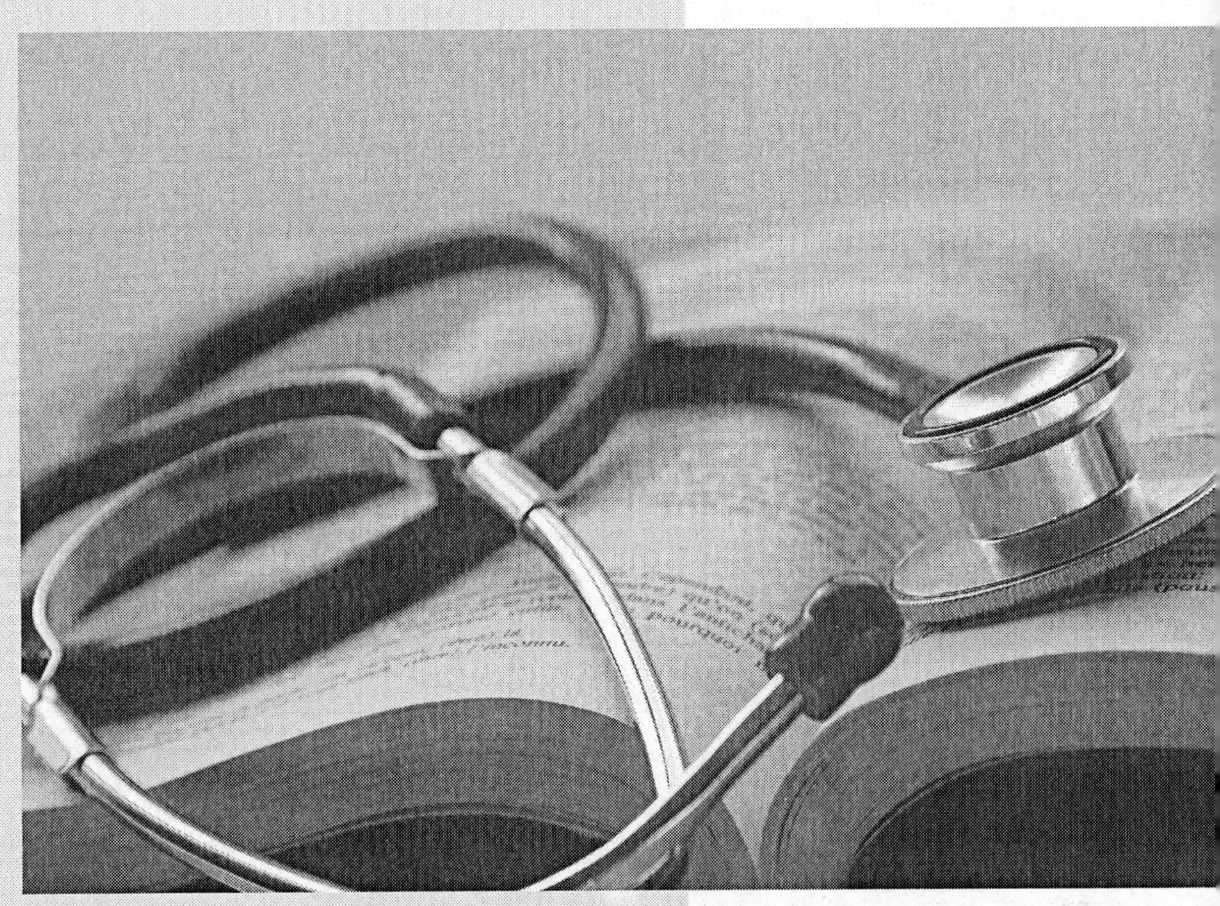

Terminology

- **ANA**: antinuclear antibody
- **ANCA**: anti-neutrophil cytoplasmic antibodies
- **AntiCCP**: anti-citrullinated protein antibodies
- **DEXA scan**: dual-energy X-ray absorptiometry scan
- **DIP**: distal interphalangeal joint
- **DMARDS**: disease-modifying antirheumatic drugs
- **EMG**: electromyography
- **HLA**: human leukocyte antigen
- **IL**: interleukin
- **MCP**: metacarpophalangeal joint
- **Monoarthritis**: one joint
- **MTP**: metatarsophalangeal joint
- **NCS**: nerve conduction study
- **Oligoarthritis**: two to four joints
- **PIP**: proximal interphalangeal joint
- **Polyarthritis**: more than five joints
- **RF**: rheumatoid factor
- **TNF**: tumour necrosis factors

Arthritis

Rheumatoid arthritis

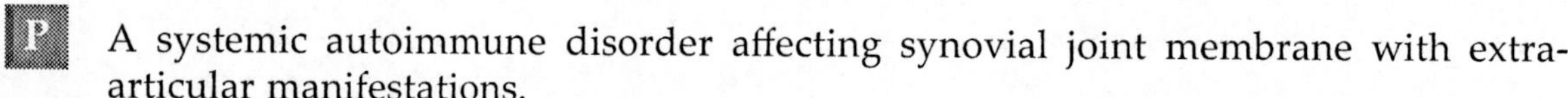

P A systemic autoimmune disorder affecting synovial joint membrane with extra-articular manifestations.

A Genetic, environmental, hormonal, immunologic, and infectious factors may play significant roles.

HLA-DR4 found in 60% of RA patients.

T and B lymphocytes play a role in RA pathogenesis, where T cells activate macrophages leading to the production of the proinflammatory cytokines (TNF-alpha and IL-1).

B cells secret antibodies ie RF, anti-CCP.

S Persistent symmetrical polyarthritis. The most commonly affected joints in decreasing order are: MCP, wrist, PIP, knee, MTP, shoulder, ankle, cervical spine, hip, elbow, temporomandibular joint. Atlanto-axial subluxation (following erosion of odontoid peg).

Rheumatoid nodules (elbow and lungs), lymphadenopathy.

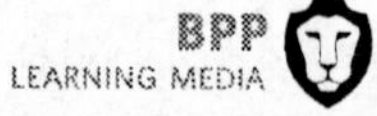

- Swan neck deformity: hyperextension at PIP, flexion at DIP due to damage of volar plate
- Boutonniere deformity: ('button-hole'= buttons through extensor tendon slip) flexion at PIP, hyperextension at DIP due to damage to central slip of extensor tendon
- Z-Thumb deformity: hyperextension at PIP with fixed flexion and subluxation of MCP
- Ulna deviation of fingers

Box 8.1: Hand involvement in rheumatoid arthritis

Sx *Joints:* inflammation with swelling, tenderness, warmth and decreased range of motion (ROM) and inactivity stiffness (worse in morning, improved with movement).

Extra-articular manifestations: generalised malaise, fatigue, rheumatoid nodules, pericaditis or pericardial effusion, vasculitis, pulmonary fibrosis. (See Box 8.3.)

Require 4 of 7 'RH RISES'

- **R**heumatoid factor (+ve 70%)
- **H**and joint involvement
- **R**heumatoid nodules
- **I**nvolvement of 3 or more joints
- **S**tiffness (early morning)
- **E**rosions on XR
- **S**ymmetrical arthritis

Box 8.2: Diagnostic criteria for rheumatoid arthritis

I Bloods: ↑ ESR, ↑ CRP; FBC: anaemia of chronic disease, thrombocytosis, leukocytosis; RF, anti-CCP is more sensitive and specific.

XR of the areas involved looking for erosions.

MRI / US scan to assess certain small joints as well as periarticular soft tissues ie tendons.

Joint aspiration: synovial fluid ↑ WCC, ↑ Protein.

T *Non-pharmacological therapies:* exercise, diet, massage, counselling, stress reduction, physiotherapy.

Pharmacological therapies:

NSAIDs: reduce swelling and pain, however, they do not slow disease progression.

Steroids: commonly used in patients with RA to bridge the time until DMARDs are effective.

DMARDs: see Table 8.1.

Bilogical therapy: TNF inhibitors eg adalimimab and immunomodulators eg rituximab. Used in adults with highly active disease that failed to respond to ×2 DMARDS.

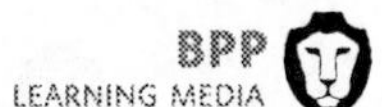

Surgery: synovectomy, tenosynovectomy, tendon realignment, reconstructive surgery or arthroplasty, and arthrodesis.

Name	Side effects
Hydroxychloroquine (HCQ)	Visual disturbance, psoriasis
Sulfasalazine (SSZ)	Agranulocytosis
Methotrexate (MTX)	Teratogenic, hepatotoxic, ↓ folate
Azathioprine (AZP)	Bone marrow suppression, teratogenic
Gold salts	Thromobocytopenia, proteinuria
Penicillamine	Aplastic anaemia, SLE, glomerulonephritis

Table 8.1: DMARDS for rheumatoid arthritis

C Extra-articular in 20%. See Box 8.3.

- CVS: endocarditis, myocarditis, pericarditis
- Eyes: episcleritis, scleritis, keratoconjunctivitis
- Neurology: peripheral neuropathy
- Respiratory: nodules, pleural effusion, fibrosing alveolitis
- Caplan's syndrome: RA in coal miners with pneumoconiosis (due to coal particles)
- Felty's syndrome: RhF +ve, splenomegaly, neutropenia
- Still's disease: juvenile arthritis, fever, rash

Box 8.3: Extra-articular manifestations of rheumatoid disease

Pr Systemic involvement is poor pronostic factor.

Septic arthritis

P Joints can be invaded by pathogens (most commonly bacteria) via different routes. Most commonly via bloodstream or direct inoculation in trauma.

A Previously damaged or prosthetic joints and those associated with the presence of inflammatory arthritis conditions are more susceptible.

Bacteria: staphylococcus aureus (most common pathogen), streptococcal species, such as s. viridans, s. pneumoniae.

Neisseria gonorrhoeae most common in young sexually active adults.

H. influenza most common in infants.

Other pathogens include borrelia burgdorferi that causes Lyme disease.

Sx Fever, joint pain, erythema, warmth and decreased range of movement are the main symptoms.

Can involve any joint: knee (50% of cases), followed by the hip, shoulder, ankle, and wrists. Hip commonest in infants.

I Bloods: ↑ WCC, ↑ CRP, uric acid (exclude gout).

XR: helpful in excluding osteomyelitis or signs of crystal arthropathy ie calcifications.

Joint aspiration: synovial fluid cloudy, ↑ WCC, M,C&S Blood cultures.

T IV antibiotics (after joint aspiration), analgesia, referral to orthopaedics if prosthetic joint (see Chapter 20).

C 50% have significant sequelae of decreased range of motion or chronic pain after infection. Also dysfunctional joints, osteomyelitis, and sepsis.

Pr Predictors of poor outcome in suppurative arthritis include the following:

- Age older than 60 years
- Infection of the hip or shoulder joints
- Underlying rheumatoid arthritis
- Positive findings on synovial fluid cultures after seven days of appropriate therapy
- Delay of seven days or longer in instituting therapy

The mortality rate depends primarily on the causative organism. N. gonorrhoeae septic arthritis carries an extremely low mortality rate, whereas that of s. aureus can approach 50%.

Spondyloarthritides

The spondyloarthropathies are a group of related disorders that includes ankylosing spondylitis, reactive arthritis, psoriatic arthritis, spondyloarthropathy associated with inflammatory bowel disease and undifferentiated spondyloarthropathy. They are linked by common genetics (human leukocyte antigen *HLA-B27*).

Ankylosing spondylitis

P The primary pathology is enthesitis with chronic inflammation, including cytokines particularly tumour necrosis factor-α (TNF-α) leading to fibrosis and ossification at sites of enthesitis.

A The cause of AS is unknown, but a combination of genetic and environmental factors leads to the clinical disease. The strong association of AS with *HLA-B27* (95%) is direct evidence of the importance of genetic predisposition.

Sx See Box 8.4.

- Low back pain and stiffness
- Onset of symptoms in those younger than 40 years
- Presence of symptoms for more than three months
- Symptoms worse in the morning or with inactivity
- Improvement of symptoms with exercise
- Peripheral enthesitis (pain at tendon insertion) with Achilles tendon insertion commonest
- Joint involvement most commonly in the hips and shoulders
- Iritis

Box 8.4: Features of AS

S Tenderness of the SI or a limited spinal ROM. While at late stages of the disease some patients may have a deformity of the spine, most commonly with a loss of lumbar lordosis and accentuated thoracic kyphosis.

Schober's test is the most popular test for limited spinal ROM but not specific for AS.

I Blood test: HLA-B27 in 90%, ↑ ESR, ↑ CRP, Normocytic anaemia. XR: sacroilitis, syndesmophyte formation, vertebral fusion (bamboo spine), marginal erosion.

T Long-term NSAIDs, DMARDs and biologics second line treatment.

Reactive arthritis (Reiter's syndrome)

P A seronegative oligoarthritis that develops two to six weeks after an infection, usually genitourinary or gastrointestinal infection.

Nomenclature has moved away from German physician Hans Reiter since his prosecution as a war criminal.

A Peak age 15–25, males > females. Associated with HLA-B27.

S Joint swelling, dactylitis, circinate balantitis, keratoderma blennorrrhagica (papules on penis, palms and feet).

Sx *Classic triad:* **U**rethritis, **C**onjunctivitis, and **A**rthritis plus malaise and fever. Low-back pain and heel pain is common because of enthesopathies at the Achilles tendon.

I ↑ ESR, ↑ CRP, ↑ WCC, RhF –ve, urine and vaginal / urethral swab for chlamydia, stool culture.

Early radiography is usually normal.

Joint aspiration to rule out crystals or septic arthritis.

T Rest, NSAIDs, intra-articular or oral steriods are an alternative, antibiotics to treat the underlying infection. DMARDs are of limited use and the benefit is uncertain.

C One-third have recurrent symptoms.

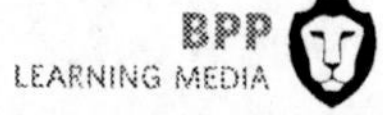

Psoriatic arthritis

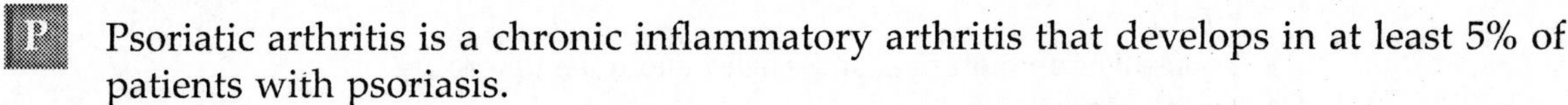

P Psoriatic arthritis is a chronic inflammatory arthritis that develops in at least 5% of patients with psoriasis.

A seronegative oligoarthritis found in patients with psoriasis, with characteristic differentiating features of distal joint involvement.

A Unknown, but genetic influences, environmental and immunologic factors are thought to contribute towards the development of the disease.

S Psoriatic rash on extensor surfaces, nail pitting or onycholysis, dactylitis with 'sausage digit' (35% of patients), enthesitis.

Sx See Box 8.5.

Five patterns of arthritis

- Asymmetrical oligoarticular arthritis (50 %)
- Symmetrical polyarthritis similar to RA (25 %)
- Distal interphalangeal arthropathy (5–10 %)
- Arthritis mutilans, which is destruction and shortening of small digits. (1–5 %)
- Spondylitis with or without sacroiliitis (5 %) with a male predominance

Box 8.5: Patterns of psoriatic arthritis

I Bloods: ↑ ESR, ↑ CRP, RhF –ve, ANA –ve.

XR: asymmetrical erosive changes in the small joints of the hands and feet, fluffy 'pencil in cup' periosteal bone formation (phalanges), asymmetric sacroillitis.

CT/MRI: periarticular involvement i.e enthesitis which is inflammation of tendon insertions.

T Arthritis and skin should be treated simultaneously.

NSAIDs, DMARDs (hydroxychloroquine) as well as biologic agents like anti-TNF medications.

Intra-articular injection of entheses or single inflamed joints with corticosteroids may be particularly effective in some patients.

Enteropathic arthropathies

P Inflammation of the GI tract may increase permeability, resulting in absorption of arthrogenic antigenic material, including bacterial antigens. These antigens may then localise in musculoskeletal tissues causing an inflammatory response.

S **Sx** See Box 8.6.

- Axial and peripheral arthritis: more common in Crohn's than ulcerative colitis
- Enthesitis: common sites are achilles and tibial tuberosity
- Extra-articular:
  - Intestinal: abdominal pain, weight loss, diarrhoea
  - Skin: erythema nodosum
  - Oral: aphthous ulcers
  - Ocular: uveitis

Box 8.6: Symptoms of enteropathic arthropathies

I FBC: iron deficiency anemia, leukocytosis, and thrombocytosis, ↑ ESR, ↑ CRP, HLA-B27 gene is found in only 30–70% of those with IBD-associated AS.

XR sacroilitis (arthritis is usually nonerosive), MRI.

T Steroids, DMARDs.

Crystal arthropathies

Recurrent episodes of joint inflammation caused by the formation of crystals within the joint space and deposition of crystals in soft tissue. If untreated, they can lead to joint destruction and renal damage.

Gout and pseudogout

P **Gout**: arthropathy caused by monosodium urate monohydrate (MSU) crystals. Uric acid is an end-stage product of purine metabolism removed by kidneys.

Pseudogout: arthropathy caused by calcium pyrophosphate (CPP) crystals.

A **Gout** *(hyperuricemia):* thiazide diuretics, ↑ dietary purine intake (alcohol, red meat), renal failure, lead, inherited enzyme deficiency, dehydration, low-dose aspirin.

Pseudogout: primary or secondary to hyperparathyroidism, haemochromatosis, hypothyroidism, hypophosphataemia, Wilson's disease.

S Sx *Acute:* monoarthritis, painful, swollen, hot, erythematous joint for 7–14 days.

Pain and inflammation in the metatarsal-phalangeal joint of the great toe (podagra) is highly suggestive of acute gout. However, ankle, wrist, and knee are commonly affected.

In pseudogout, the most common sites are shoulders, knees and wrists.

Chronic: Gout tophi on hands, pinna, polyarthritis.

I **Gout**:

Bloods: ↑ uric acid levels.

Joint aspirate: gout crystals are needle-shaped and strongly negatively birefringent on microscopy.

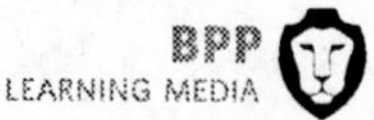

XR: cortical erosions, marginal sclerosis.

Pseudogout:

Joint aspirate: CPP crystals are rod-shaped and are positively birefringent on microscopy.

XR: chondrocalcinosis.

T *Acute:* NSAIDs or colchicine, while corticosteroids are used if renal function is impaired.

Prophylaxis in gout: allopurinol or febuxostat (xanthine oxidase inhibitors) aiming to reduce uric acid levels (do not use in acute attack).

Diet advice in gout: high-purine foods and alcohol should be avoided, or consumed only in moderation.

C Degenerative arthritis, uric acid nephropathy and renal stones, nerve or spinal cord impingement, increased susceptibility to infection.

Vasculitis

Wegener's granulomatosis

P Systemic vasculitis characterised by necrotising granuloma in the upper respiratory tract and necrotising glomerulonephritis in kidneys.

A Affects small-to medium-sized vessels, cANCA mediated.

S Pulmonary nodules ('coin' lesions) and infiltrates, purpura, oral ulceration and strawberry gingivitis, scleritis and conjunctivitis, progressive glomerulonephritis.

Sx Rhinitis and epistaxis (often first sign), perforated nasal septum, malaise, arthralgia (60%), hearing loss, pulmonary haemorrhage and haemoptysis, cough, haematuria.

I Bloods: ↑ WCC, ↑ PLTs, cANCA.

Urine: proteinuria, haematuria, red cell casts.

CXR: fluctuating lung shadows, pleural effusion, nodules, cavitation.

Biopsy: histology shows granulomatous change.

T Corticosteroids, immunosupression.

C Renal failure, destruction of nasal septum, hearing loss.

Pr Majority respond well, 20–40% suffer flare-ups.

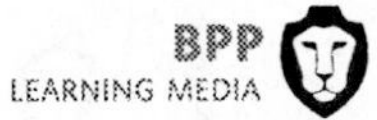

Giant cell arteritis (temporal arteritis)

P Systemic vasculitis affecting medium and large arteries.

Pathogenesis involves a chronic inflammatory process, predominantly of large arteries, resulting in the elaboration of various cytokines.

A Giant cell arteritis is commonly associated with polymyalgia rheumatica (PMR). Mostly aged >50 years, female > male.

S Sx See Box 8.7.

The presence of ≥3 citeria is highly diagnostic:

- Age 50 years or older
- Newly onset localized headache
- Temporal artery tenderness or decreased temporal artery pulse
- ESR of at least 50 mm/h
- Abnormal artery biopsy specimen characterised by mononuclear infiltration or granulomatous inflammation
- Proximal myopathy (typically shoulders, associated with PMR)

Constitutional symptoms, eg, fatigue, weight loss, and fever (50% of patients with giant cell arteritis have features of polymyalgia rheumatica and jaw claudication).

Pay attention to decreased vision secondary to arteritis as the most common serious consequence.

Box 8.7: Features of GCA

I ↑ ESR.

Temporal artery biopsy: should be obtained within 10 days of starting treatment in suspected cases. Histology shows inflammatory infiltrate (mononuclear cells) involving the entire vessel wall (panarteritis).

T High doses corticosteroids (40–60mg prednisolone) is the treatment of choice, and should not be delayed in suspected cases waiting for biopsy.

Maintain high-dose steroid therapy only long enough for symptoms to resolve and then taper to a maintenance dosage of prednisone over several months.

C Blindness, aortitis, aortic dissection / aneurysm.

Pr Relapse of giant cell arteritis (GCA) is common (25–60%).

Polymyalgia rheumatica (PMR)

P Syndrome of pain and stiffness, usually in neck, shoulders and hips. Associated with the HLA-DR4 and giant cell arteritis (15%).

A Older patients. The cause is unknown but there is suggestion of environmental factor–possibly a virus causes immune activation in genetically predisposed patients.

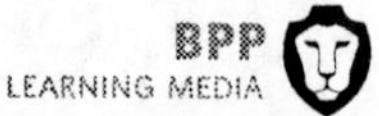

S Sx See Box 8.8.

Diagnostic criteria	Systemic symptoms
• Age 50 years or older at onset • Bilateral aching and morning stiffness for at least one month and involving at least two of three areas: neck, shoulders or arms, hips or thighs • ESR 40mm/h or greater • Prompt response of symptoms to corticosteroids (15mg/day)	• Low-grade fever and weight loss • Malaise, fatigue, and depression • Difficulty completing daily life activities • Morning stiffness for more than one hour. • Muscle stiffness after prolonged inactivity

Box 8.8: Diagnostic criteria and systemic symptoms of PMR

I ANA, RF, and CK are usually normal, while FBC reveals mild normocytic, normochromic anemia in almost 50% of cases.

↑ ESR is the most sensitive test for PMR

T Corticosteroids are the treatment of choice, where a low dose (15–20mg/day) is usually needed.

Pr With prompt diagnosis and adequate therapy, patients have an excellent prognosis. The average length of disease is three years.

Polyarteritis nodosa (PAN)

P Inflammatory vasculitis in small- and medium-sized arteries occur mainly at bifurcations and branch points. Aneurysms develop in the weakened vessel, carrying a subsequent risk for rupture and hemorrhage.

'Nodosa' are small aneurysms produced by fibrotic healing.

A Young men. The cause is unknown, but viral infections such as HIV, CMV, HBV are associated with PAN, explained by an immune complex-induced inflammation.

S ↑ BP, fever, livedo reticularis, mononeuritis multiplex (due to affect on vasa nervorum).

Sx Fever, malaise, anorexia and weight loss, myalgia and arthralgia. PAN is an acute multisystem disease, which can affect:

- *CVS:* pericarditis, myocardial infarction and congestive heart failure
- *CNS and PNS:* seizures, motor, sensory, or mixed sensorimotor polyneuropathy
- *Gastrointestinal:* abdominal pain, nausea and vomiting and rarly bowel infarction and perforation, hepatic infarction, or pancreatic infarction
- *Ophthalmologic:* retinal vasculitis, retinal detachment
- *Renal:* renal failure
- *Skin:* rash, purpura, nodules, cutaneous infarcts, and Raynaud phenomenon

I Bloods: ↑ ESR, ↑ CRP, FBC: neutrophilia, ANCA, viral serology, blood cultures.

Urine dip.

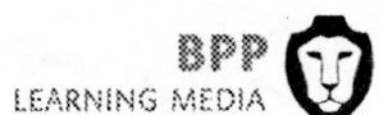

Imaging: CXR, angiography looking for aneurysms and stenosis.

EMG and NCS for peripheral neuropathy.

T Corticosteroids are the main treatment; cyclophosphamide; anti-viral therapy of hepatitis-related PAN.

C Renal effects are main cause of death, then cardiac. See Box 8.9.

- Cutaneous ulcerations
- Extremity gangrene
- Organ infarction
- Aneurysm rupture (intra-organ bleeding)
- Stroke
- Heart failure
- Myocardial infarction
- Pericarditis
- Renal failure
- Gastrointestinal (GI) bleeding
- Peripheral neuropathy

Box 8.9: Complications of PAN

Pr Better in patients with cutaneous PAN without systemic or visceral involvement.

Other eponymous vasculitidies

Kawasaki disease

P Affects medium-sized vessels, skin, mucous membrane and lymph nodes. Potentially fatal effect on coronary arteries in children.

A Commonest between six months to four years, peak incidence at 12 months. More common in Japanese patients, often following viral infection.

S 'Strawberry tongue', perineal rash, erythema / desquamation of palms, cervical lymphadenopathy, Beau's lines (transverse grooves across nails).

Sx High, prolonged fever (>5 days) not responsive to paracetamol (first sign), bilateral conjunctivitis, sore mouth, arthralgia, systemic upset.

I Clinical diagnosis.

↑ ESR, ↑ CRP, ECG + ECHO for cardiac complications.

T Immunoglobulin (IVIG) within first ten days lowers risk of coronary aneurysms.

Aspirin until six weeks or longer if abnormal ECHO to reduce risk of thrombosis.

Surgical treatment of coronary aneuryms if required.

C Coronary artery aneurysms (25% untreated cases).

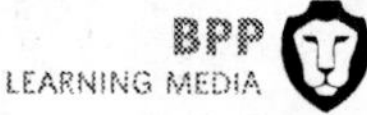

Pr Good with early treatment.

Churg-Strauss disease

P Also known as allergic granulomatosis. Affects small- to medium-sized vessels. Necrotising granuloma affecting vessels of lungs (begins as sever asthma), GI tract and peripheral nerves.

A Associated with pANCA.

S **Sx** Three distinct stages

1. Sinusitis and onset of allergies
2. Onset of acute asthma
3. Systemic involvement: skin purpura, GI upset, peripheral neuropathy

I Bloods: ↑ eosinophils, pANCA

Eosinophillic lung deposits.

T Steroids, immunosupression.

Takayasu's arteritis

P Chronic, progressive disease affecting large vessels including the aorta and branches.

A Peak in young to middle-aged asian women, 15–30 years.

S Loss of pulses, bruits, tender over palpable arteries.

Sx Claudication pain, systemically unwell.

I Bloods: anaemia, ↑ ESR, ↑ CRP.

T Steroids, immunosupression, angioplasty.

C Renal artery stenosis, hypertension.

Behçet's disease

P Inflammation of small-sized venules producing characteristic ulceration of skin, eyes and mucosa.

A HLA B51, commoner in Turkish / Iranian males.

S **Sx** *Major:* aphthous ulcers, skin lesions (papulo-pustules), uveitis / iritis, genital ulceration, pathergy reaction (papule >2mm 48 hours after skin needle-prick).

Minor: arthralgia, thrombophlebitis, epididymitis, malaise, GI ulceration.

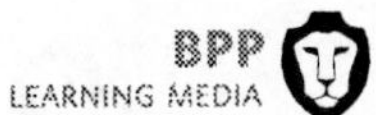

I ↑ ESR, ↑ CRP; papule swabs sterile.

T Steroids, ciclosporin, immunosuppressants.

C Optic atrophy, visual impairment.

Henoch-schonlein purpura

P Small vessel vasculitis characterised by deposition of IgA in skin and kidneys.

A Commoner in young males, often preceded by URTI.

S Sx *Classic triad:* purpura on legs and buttocks (100%), arthralgia (80%), abdominal pain (60%).

Also GI hameorrhage (often due to intussusception), haematuria.

I Bloods: ↑ ESR, ↑ CRP, ↑ PLTs (differentiates from ITP), ↑ U&Es, ↑ IgA (in 50%).

Skin biopsy: IgA and C3 in blood vessel wall.

T Spontaneous recovery within four weeks, analgesia for arthralgia.

C Long-term complications are secondary to renal involvement. Follow-up is required for one year to monitor renal function and blood pressure.

Pr Excellent.

Connective tissue disease

Systemic lupus erythematosus (SLE)

P A chronic inflammatory multisystem disease that follows a relapsing and remitting course, and characterised by an autoantibody response to nuclear and cytoplasmic antigens.

A Unknown, racial, hormonal, drug-induced and environmental factors. Peak in Afro-Caribbean women 25–35 years.

Associted with epilepsy, digital infarcts, alopecia and pleurisy.

Sx Arthralgia, fever, malaise.

S Malar 'butterly' rash ('lupine'), discoid rash, episcleritis, optic neuritis, retinal infarcts, Raynaud's phenomenon, Sjögren's syndrome, mucosal ulceration, symmetrical arthritis.

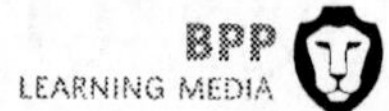

Require 4 out of the following 11 criteria 'SOAP BRAIN MD'

- **S**erositis: pleurisy or pericarditis
- **O**ral ulcers: usually painless.
- **A**rthritis: nonerosive, ≥2 peripheral joints
- **P**hotosensitivity: unusual skin reaction to light exposure.
- **B**lood disorders: ↓ neutrophils, ↓ PLTs, ↓ lymphocytes, hemolytic anemia
- **R**enal involvement: proteinuria or cellular casts
- **A**ntinuclear antibodies (ANAs): +ve in 90%
- **I**mmunologic phenomena: dsDNA or anti-Smith (Sm) antibodies or antiphospholipid antibodies / lupus anticoagulant
- **N**eurologic disorder: seizures or psychosis in the absence of other causes
- **M**alar rash: erythema over the cheeks and nasal bridge
- **D**iscoid rash: erythematous raised-rimmed lesions

Box 8.10: Diagnostic criteria for SLE

I Auto-antibody tests: ANA, anti-dsDNA, anti-sm (most specific antibody for SLE), anticardiolipin (IgG/IgM antibodies), anti-Ro/La, lupus anticoagulant, anti-histone (drug-induced lupus ANA antibodies are often of this type).

Bloods: ↑ ESR and CRP, direct Coombs' test +ve (haemolytic anaemia), ↓ complement levels ie C3/C4.

Renal biopsy: lupus nephritis.

T Depends on the organ involved.

NSAIDs for arthritis, corticosteriods, immunosuppressant (cyclophosphamide, azathioprine).

C *CVS:* pericarditis, myocarditis, endocarditis (Libman-Sacks).

CNS: stroke, fits, psychosis.

Renal: 50% develop lupus nephritis (50% require transplant).

Resp: ARDS, pleural effusion.

Systemic sclerosis (systemic scleroderma)

P Systemic connective tissue disease causing fibrosis and vascular damage to the skin and internal organs.

Excessive collagen deposition as a result immunologic system disturbances and vascular changes.

A Associated with malignancy, sub-type of scleroderma, affected organs and systems include the skin, lungs, heart, digestive system, kidneys, muscles, joints, and nervous system.

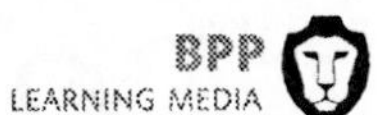

S Two major forms:

- *Limited cutaneous*: systemic symptoms occur late, skin of extremities affected early. CREST syndrome (see Box 8.11) ANA +ve 70%.
- *Diffuse cutaneous:* rapidly progressing, early systemic involvement, Scl-70 +ve 30%.

CREST syndrome
• **C**alcinosis • **R**aynaud's syndrome • **E**sophageal dysmotility • **S**clerodactyly • **T**elangiectasia

Box 8.11: Features of limited cutaneous systemic sclerosis

Sx Pruritus, Raynaud's phenomenon in 90% (pain in the affected digits, blanching, cyanosis, and hyperemia can follow), dysphagia, nausea, vomiting, weight loss, abdominal cramps, bloating, diarrhoea, shortness of breath, dry cough, palpitations, arthralgia, myalgia, weakness in 80% of patients.

One major and two minor criteria for diagnosis	
Major features:	Minor features:
• Centrally located skin sclerosis that affects the arms, face, and / or neck.	• Sclerodactyly (thickening and tightness of the skin of the fingers or toes) • Erosions • Atrophy of the fingertips • Bilateral lung fibrosis

Box 8.12: Diagnostic criteria for systemic sclerosis

I Bloods: ↑ or → ESR , ↑ MCV, ↓ PLTs, +ve ANA 90%, +ve ACA (limited > diffuse), Scl-70 +ve (diffuse > limited), haemolytic anemia, ↑ CK in patients with muscle involvement, ↑ U&Es in patients with kidney involvement.

CXR/CT Chest, ECHO, lung function tests.

T Depends on the organ affected:

- *Pruritus:* topical emollients
- *Raynaud phenomenon:* avoiding exposure to cold temperature, smoking cessation, calcium-channel blockers, vasodilating drugs, intravenous prostaglandins, prostacyclin analogs
- *Kidney:* ACE or angiotensin II inhibitor
- *GI*: PPI (eg, omeprazole) and H2 blockers to control reflux symptoms
- *Lungs:* calcium-channel blockers (eg, nifedipine), prostaglandins (eg, prostacyclin), and cyclophosphamide
- *Myositis:* corticosteroids

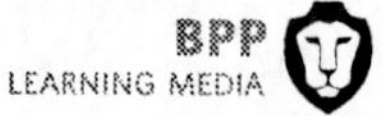

Sjögren's syndrome

P Systemic autoimmune disease that causes destruction of exoxrine glands.

A Primary or secondary in other autoimmune rheumatic disease (15% RA, 30% SLE), female:male 10:1.

S Xeroderma (dry skin), angular stomatitis, eye redness.

Schirmer's test (paper strips used to test tear production): poor tear production.

Sx Dry eyes, dry / sore mouth, mild polyarthritis, malaise.

I Bloods: ESR ↑, RhF +ve, anti-Ro/La.

Tissue biopsy.

T *Supportive:* artificial tears, mouthwash.

C Pancreatitis, interstitial nephritis, renal tubular acidosis, glomerulonephritis, B-cell lymphomas.

Polymyositis and dermatomyositis

P Polymyositis is an idiopathic inflammatory myopathy, which is an immune-mediated condition secondary to defective cellular immunity.

Dermatomyositis is muscle + skin involvement (Box 8.13).

A Primary or secondary to rheumatic disease or malignancy.

Sx Symmetrical, progressive proximal muscle weakness (difficulty standing from sitting, climbing stairs), dysphagia, myalgia, SoB.

- Heliotrope rash: lilac rash over upper eyelids
- Periorbital oedema
- Gottron's papules: red, scaly lesions on dorsum of hands
- Shawl sign: erythematous rash over back and shoulders

Box 8.13: Signs of dermatomyositis

I Bloods: ANA, Anti-Jo1 Ab, ↑ WCC, ↑ ESR, ↑ CRP, ↑ CK RhF +ve (50%).

Urine: myoglobinuria.

Electromyography (EMG) and muscle biopsy.

T Corticosteriods, immunosuppressive agents (methotrexate, azathioprine, cyclophosphamide), intravenous immunoglobulin (IVIG).

C Interstitial lung disease, aspiration pneumonia, heart block arrhythmias and malabsorption.

Pr Poor prognostic factors include advanced age, female, systemic disease, associated malignancy.

Fibromyalgia

P Fibromyalgia is a syndrome of persistent widespread pain, fatigue, disrupted sleep, and cognitive difficulties typically in young or middle-aged women.

A Multifactorial and includes both environmental and genetic factors. May be functional disorder.

It is a neurosensory disorder of central pain processing or a syndrome of central sensitivity.

S Sx Chronic widespread pain lasting more than three months, with associated fatigue, poor sleep, stiffness, cognitive difficulties, anxiety and / or depression.

Physical examination is usually normal except multiple tender points.

Criteria for diagnosis:

- Widespread pain in all four quadrants of the body
- Present for at least three months
- 11 out of 18 tender points

I Bloods: normal.

T Education: make sure patients understand the nature of the disease and that no cure exists.

Graded exercise over several sessions.

Relaxation techniques.

Pharmacological treatment includes tricyclic antidepressants, antidepressants, muscle relaxants, some anticonvulsants like gabapentin.

C Marked functional impairment, severe depression and anxiety.

Metabolic bone disease

Osteoporosis

P Low bone mass leading to increased fragility and fractures.

Bone undergoes a continual process of resorption and formation, bone loss results from an imbalance between the rates of those processes.

A *Primary:*

- Type I osteoporosis (postmenopausal osteoporosis) occurs in women aged 50–65 years
- Type II osteoporosis (age-associated or senile) occurs in women and men older than 70 years

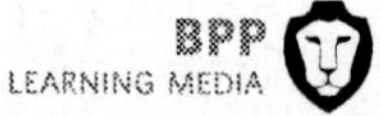

Secondary: endocrine (Cushing syndrome, adrenal insufficiency), corticosteroids, multiple myeloma, renal failure, alcoholism, reduced physical activity.

S Sx Osteoporosis is typically asymptomatic until a fracture occurs.

I Bloods: calcium, phosphate, ALP all normal.

XR: fractures, commonly wedge fractures in vertebrae.

DEXA scan: is test of choice to assess BMD (bone mineral density): T-Score compares bone density to peers.

- T-Score >–1 normal
- T-Score –1 to –1.5 osteopaenia
- T-Score < –2.5 osteoporosis

T No treatment can completely reverse established osteoporosis, so medical intervention aims to halt its progression.

Lifestyle: exercise, stop smoking, improved diet.

Pharmacological: calcium, vitamin D, bisphosphonates, oestrogen and calcitonin.

C Fractures.

Osteomalacia

P Defective bone mineralisation of new bone. Childhood form known as Rickets.

A Peaks in children and elderly. Due to Vitamin D deficiency: malnutrition, malabsorption, coeliac disease, hypophosphataemia, chronic renal failure, Fanconi syndrome, anti-convulsant therapy.

S Sx Proximal myopathy (waddling gait), bone pain, bone defomity (genu varum / valgum in children), hypocalcaemia, dental problems.

I Bloods: ↓ calcium, ↓ phosphate, ↓ 25-OH Vit D, ↑ ALP, ↑ PTH.

XR: pseudofractures / Looser's zones (radiolucent areas at right angles to cortex), protrusio acetabuli (disorder of hip joint).

T Vit D replacement, correct underlying pathology.

Paget's disease

P Chronic disorder of bone remodeling with excessive breakdown and formation of bone causing painful, misshapen bones and fractures with altered bone architecture.

A Elderly population, male > female.

S ↑ Head size, sabre tibia, warmth over affected area.

Sx Bone pain (commonly pelvis, femur, lumbar spine), hearing loss (due to compression of CNVIII).

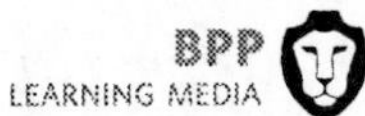

I Bloods: ↑ ALP, calcium and phosphate normal.

Urine: ↑ hydroxyproline (indicator of bone turnover).

XR: mixed osteolytic and sclerotic areas of bone affected.

T Bisphosphonates, calcitonin, surgery for fractures.

C Fractures, high-output cardiac failure, osteosarcoma, hypercalcaemia, immobility, hearing loss, loose teeth.

	ALP	Ca^{2+}	PO_4^-	PTH	Other
Osteoporosis	N	N	N	N	↓ bone mass
Osteomalacia	↑	↓	↓	↑	↓ mineralisation
Osteopetrosis	↑	N	N	N	↓ osteoclast activity (hard bone)
Paget's disease	↑	N	N	N	↑ remodelling

Table 8.2: Summary of blood tests in metabolic bone disease

Practice Questions

Single Best Answers

1. Which is the most appropriate treatment for acute gout?

   A Allopurinol
   B Oral prednisolone
   C NSAIDs such as ibuprofen
   D Furusemide

2. The following is a feature of SLE.

   A Appendicitis
   B Pityriasis rosea
   C Glomerulonephritis
   D Nose bleeds

3. Extra-articular features of RA include.

   A Retinopathy
   B Urethral stricture
   C Hepatomegaly
   D Lung nodules

4. The following is true regarding RA.

   A More common in women
   B RhF +ve in 95% of patients
   C The commonest affected joint is the hip
   D HLA-B27 carries a poor prognosis

5. The following is **not** a risk factor for developing osteoporosis.

   A Hyperthyroidism
   B Smoking
   C Cushing's syndrome
   D Oral contraceptive pill

6. The following test is helpful in diagnosing Paget's disease.

   A Calcitonin level
   B Urine hydroxyproline
   C Serum electrophoresis
   D Creatinine kinase

7. The following is true regarding ankylosing spondylitis.

   A Buttock pain is relieved by rest
   B Disease regresses with age
   C Iritis is a complication
   D Felty's syndrome is a complication

8. The following is due to accumulation of calcium pyrophosphate crystals.

   A Reiter's disease
   B Gout
   C Henoch-Schonlein purpura
   D Pseudogout

9. Calcium and phosphate levels are reduced in which of the following?

   A Paget's disease
   B Osteomalacia
   C Osteopetrosis
   D Osteoporosis

10. The classic triad of urethritis, conjunctivitis and arthritis is seen in which of the following?

   A Psoriatic arthritis
   B Sjörgen's disease
   C Dermatomyositis
   D Reiter's disease

Extended Matching Questions

Tests and disease

A ↑ ESR
B Anti-Sm
C Anti-Jo1 Ab
D pANCA
E cANCA

Match the following diseases with their serum markers.

1. Wegener's graulomatosis

2. SLE

3. Polymyositis / dermatomyositis

4. Churg-Strauss syndome

5. Giant cell arteritis

Match the following signs / symptoms with their disease.

A Dry eyes and skin
B Heliotrope rash
C CREST
D Sabre tibia
E Swan neck deformity

6. Paget's disease

7. Sjörgen's syndrome

8. Systemic sclerosis

9. Dermatomyositis

10. Rheumatoid arthritis

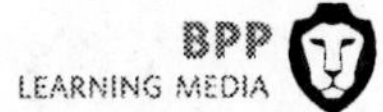

Answers

SBAs		EMQs	
1	C	1	E
2	C	2	B
3	D	3	C
4	A	4	D
5	D	5	A
6	B	6	D
7	C	7	A
8	D	8	C
9	B	9	B
10	D	10	E

Chapter 9

Infectious diseases

Dr Begoña Bovill

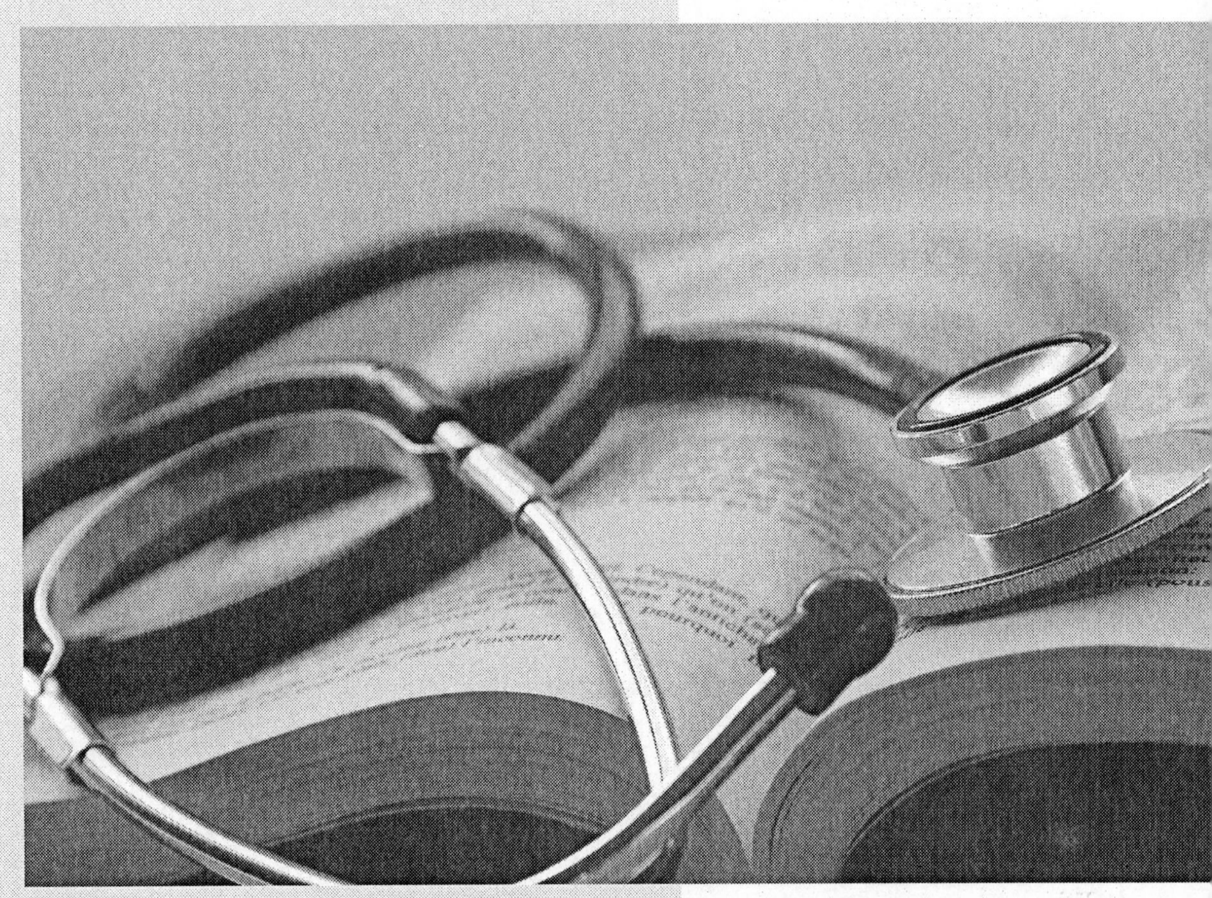

Immunisations

- DTaP: diphtheria, tetanus, pertussis
- Hib: haemophilus influenza type B
- MMR: measels, mumps, rubella
- BCG: Bacille Calmette-Guerin (TB vaccine)

Inactivated	Live attenuated	Toxoid	Polysaccharide conjugate	Protein subunit
Pertussis	BCG	Tetanus	Hib	Hep B
Rabies	MMR	Diphtheria	Meningococcal	
Influenza	Yellow Fever		Pneumococcal	
Hep A	Typhoid			
Cholera				
Polio				
Bubonic plague				

Table 9.1: Types of vaccine

Age	Immunisation
Neonates at risk	BCG
2 months	DTaP, Polio and Hib 1st dose Pneumococcal 1st dose
3 months	DTaP, Polio and Hib 2nd dose Meningococcal C 1st dose
4 months	DTaP, Pol, and Hib 3rd dose Men C 2nd dose Pneumococcal 2nd dose
12 months	Hib and Men C single booster dose
13 months	MMR Pneumococcal single booster dose
3–5 years	DTaP, Polio single booster dose MMR 2nd dose (different limb)
12–13 years	HPV (3 doses, 0, 2 and 6 months)
13–18 years	Diphtheria (low dose), Tetanus, Polio single booster dose

Table 9.2: Immunisation schedule

Global disease

Malaria

Disease found predominantly in tropical / subtropical areas. Protozoan parasitic infection transmitted by bite of female anopheline mosquito–bites at dusk.

All four species give rise to similar symptoms, but P. falciparum is responsible for most deaths and complications. P. ovale and P. vivax have dormant liver stages call hypnozoites, which can give rise to recurrent attacks over several months for up to five years.

> **Sexual phase**: occurs within female mosquito after ingesting blood containing male and female gametocytes.
>
> **Asexual phase in human**:
>
> - **Pre-erythrocytic stage (asymptomatic)**
>
>   Sporozoites from mosquito salivary glands enter human with bite, enter liver, and develop in hepatocytes as tissue schizonts. After ~11 days, merozoites burst out of the liver into bloodstream and invade erythrocytes.
>
> - **Erythrocytic phase**
>
>   Each **merozoite**, enters an RBC to become a **trophozoite.** It matures, and divides within the RBC turning into a **schizont.** The schizont ruptures, releasing merozoites into the bloodstream, each invading a fresh erythrocyte and continuing the cycle every 48 or 72 hours depending on species.
>
>   Red cell lysis releases toxins, which stimulate cytokines and give rise to the symptoms of malaria.

Box 9.1: Malaria life cycle

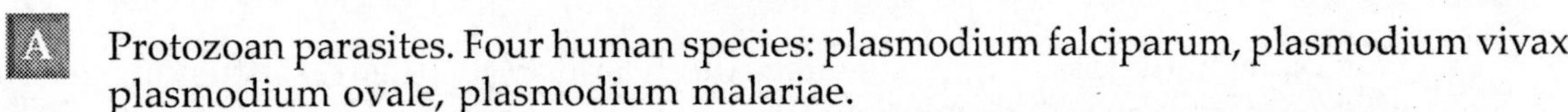

Protozoan parasites. Four human species: plasmodium falciparum, plasmodium vivax, plasmodium ovale, plasmodium malariae.

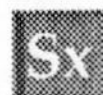

Uncomplicated malaria: chills and rigors 10–40 minutes (rapid temperature rise as schizonts burst), fever, intense headache and myalgias, headache and exhaustion persist till next paroxysm.

Complicated falciparum malaria (symptoms reflect pathology in affected organs):

- *Cerebral malaria* (WHO definition = grade 4 coma, but any of the below imply cerebral involvement)
  - Confusion, aggression
  - Focal neurological signs, fits
  - Retinal haemorrhage
  - Sequestration in CNS capillaries
- *Hypoglycaemia* (may cause cerebral signs)

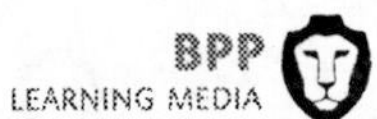

- *Diarrhoea (choleraic malaria)*
- *Pulmonary oedema / ARDS*
- *Spontaneous bleeding*
- *Severe anaemia and haemoglobinuria* (haemolysis)
- *Renal failure*

I FBC: anaemia, ↓ platelets, ↓ WBC, thick and thin blood films for malarial parasites, hypoglycaemia, U&Es, LFTs.

T *Uncomplicated malarias (vivax, ovale and malariae):* chloroquine, primaquine.

Falciparum malaria (seek expert advice always): Chloroquine resistance is almost universal for falciparum malaria, so if P. falciparum is suspected chloroquine should not be used.

Oral quinine 5–7 days as inpatient, follow with one week of doxycycline or malarone, ITU / HDU, IV quinine or artesunate, monitor fluids and hypoglycaemia.

C *Acute*: hypoglycaemia, pulmonary oedema, acute kidney injury, acidosis, secondary bacterial sepsis, cerebral malaria, algid malaria, splenic rupture (rare – vivax).

Chronic: quartan malarial nephropathy (p. malariae), hyper-reactive malaria splenomegaly, EBV associated lymphoma (Burkitt's).

Pr 2 million deaths / year globally – mostly due to plasmodium falciparum.

~10 deaths / year in UK ~ 2,000 cases.

Tuberculosis

P Caseating granulomatous disease.

Inhalation of infection through aerosol → alveoar macrophage engulfs bacterium, → local replication, → granuloma formation and enlargement of draining lymph nodes (the Ghon complex).

A Mycobacterium tuberculosis, mycobacterium bovis, M. africanum.

Sx Fevers, weight loss, night sweats, cough and SOB, pleural effusion, erythema nodosum, phlyctenular conjunctivitis, haematogenous spread (miliary tuberculosis), splenomegaly, hepatomegaly.

Pulmonary TB: Cough lasting >3 weeks unresponsive to antibiotics, creamy white sputum, haemoptysis, upper lobe cavitation / patchy consolidation and fibrosis.

Spinal TB: focal spinal pain +/- focal neurology, Gibbus deformity, Pott's disease, paraspinal abscess formation.

TB meningitis: subacute onset, headache, cranial nerve palsies, hydrocephalus, marked neck rigidity is uncommon, 40% have CXR signs of TB.

Genitourinary: haematuria, loin pain, sterile pyuria.

Cutaneous disease: lupus vulgaris (apple-jelly nodules).

Pericardial TB: constrictive pericarditis.

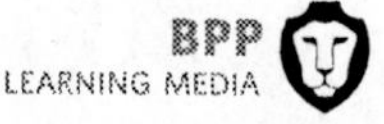

I CXR: miliary shadowing, hilar lymphadenopathy, pleural effusion, cavitating patchy consolidation in upper lobes, Ghon complex, signs of old healed TB.

Microbiology: direct microscopy for organism, sputum for acid-fast bacilli (AFB) using Ziehl-Neelsen (ZN) staining.

Immunological test: Mantoux (tuberculin skin test) or interferon gamma release assay.

Histology: tissue biopsy shows caseating granulomas with or without AFB on staining.

Inflammatory markers: CRP, ESR, plasma viscosity, WBC may be normal.

T Six months' antituberculous chemotherapy in fully sensitive uncomplicated TB.

12 months in TB meningitis, complicated bone and joint TB.

Longer duration if unable to use first line drugs (below).

Induction phase two months (RIPE):

- Rifampicin
- Isoniazid
- Pyrazinamide
- Ethambutol (ishihara test before prescribing)

Continuation phase four months (RI):

- Rifampicin
- Isoniazid

Pyridoxine 10–25mg daily protects against isoniazid related neuropathy.

Calcium and vit D supplementation.

Adjunctive steroids reduce sequelae in CNS TB and TB pericarditis.

C Cavitation in lungs leading to massive haemotysis.

Rasmussen's aneurysm: bronchial artery runs close to cavity and is eroded.

TB drug side effects:

- Hepatic (isoniazid, rifampicin and pyrazinamide)
- Rash
- Ocular toxicity (ethambutol – ishihara charts on commencing treatment)

Pr 1–2% recurrence after discontinuation of treatment. Poor adherence may lead to drug resistance.

AIDS (Acquired Immune Deficiency Syndrome)

P Human immunodeficiency virus (HIV), a retrovirus, infects CD4 lymphocytes and destroys them resulting in immunocompromise leading to opportunistic infections and tumours. When CD4 count is <200 cells/ml patient is said to have AIDS.

A Transmitted through sexual exposure, intravenous drug use, sharing needles. Perinatal infection through vaginal delivery.

Sx Seroconversion illness (two to ten weeks post-exposure): fever, headache, rash, sore throat, lymphadenopathy. First presenting symptoms often due to opportunistic infections.

I HIV test, CD4 count, viral load, contact tracing.

T *Combined highly active antiretroviral therapy* (HAART)

- ×2 nucleoside reverse transciptase inhibitors (NRTIs)
- *Plus* either non-nucleoside reverse transciptase inhibitors (NNRTI) or boosted protease inhibitor (PI)

Indications to start HAART:

- Symptomatic HIV
- CD4 count between 350–500, and certainly before it drops below 350. Before CD4 <200
- During pregnancy – reduces mother to child transmission from ~ 30% to < 1%
- Post-exposure prophylaxis (zidovudine reduces risk of seroconversion)

C Opportunistic infections, drug resistance, death.

P Without antiretroviral therapy progression to AIDS and death occurs within 7–10 years.

With antiretroviral therapy, life expectancy approaches that of a non-HIV infected person.

Opportunistic infections

Occur when CD4 count <200cells/ml blood.

Bacterial: Tuberculosis (4.5%): most lethal OI.

Mycobacterium avium complex.

Viral: CMV (3.7%): CMV etinitis in 45% AIDS.

HSV, HPV, HZV, oral hairy leukoplakia.

Fungal: Candidiasis (15%): Tx nystatin / amphotericin.

Aspergillosis, coccidiodomycosis, cryptococcal meningitis.

Protozoal: Pneumocystis carinii pneumonia (PCP) (43%): commonest life-threatening OI, low sats on minimal exertion. Tx co-trimoxazole (Septrin).

Toxoplasmosis (2.5%), cryptosporidiosis.

Malignancy: Kaposi's sarcoma due to human herpes virus-8 (10%): from capillary endothelial cells, purple papules on skin. Tx chemo / radiotherapy.

Lymphoma: EBV (2%), anal/cervical cancer: HPV

Neurological: HIV dementia, peripheral neuropathy.

Gastroenteritis

P Two main pathological processes are seen in acute gastroenteritis, Secretory diarrhoea: toxins interfere with the secretion or reabsorption of water and electrolytes from the small bowel.

Inflammatory diarrhoea: bowel wall inflammation secondary to bacterial invasion / toxin.

Both features may coexist with the same pathogen.

A See Table 9.3.

Causes of secretory diarrhoea	Causes of inflammatory diarrhoea
Viruses • Rotavirus • Norovirus • Coronavirus	Viruses • Rotavirus
Bacteria • E. coli • Vibrio cholera • Bacillus cereus (typically from uncooked rice dishes) • Campylobacter spp • Salmonella spp	Bacteria • E. coli • Shigella spp • Campylobacter spp • Yersinia spp • Clostridium difficile
Protozoa • Giardia intestinalis • Cryptosporidium parvum • Cyclospora cayetanensis	Protozoa • Entamoeba hystolitica • Balantidium coli

Table 9.3: Causes of diarrhoea

S Dehydration, fever, borborygmi, abdominal tenderness

I ↑ WCC in inflammatory diarrhoea, ↑ U&Es due to dehydration, stool cultures and microscopy.

Sx Anorexia, nausea and vomiting especially in first 24 hours, abdominal colic, diarrhoea, fever.

	Non-inflammatory diarrhoea	Inflammatory diarrhoea
Symptoms	Nausea Vomiting (pain and fever not prominent)	Abdominal pain Fever
Diarrhoea/ stool	Large volume Watery	Frequent Small volume Mucus Blood (dysentery)
Main site	Small intestine	Distal ileum and colon
Mechanism	Osmotic (non-absorbable solutes) Secretory Toxin-mediated Intestinal hurry	Invasion of enterocytes Mucosal cell death Inflammation

Table 9.4: Inflammatory versus non-inflammatory diarrhoea

T Rehydration: oral rehydration solution (ORS), IVI fluids, monitor fluid balance and stool chart.

ORS 1 litre solution contains:

20g glucose
3.5g NaCl
2.5g $NaHCO_3$
1.5g KCl

Box 9.2: Oral rehydration solution

C Complications of dehydration, bacteraemic spread.

P In developing countries diarrhoea is the fourth commonest cause of death – 2.5 million deaths/year mostly among infants.

Bacteria

Gram +ve	Gram –ve
Stain blue eg streptococcus, staph, listeria, enterococcus	Stain pink eg E. coli, salmonella, shigella

Box 9.3: Gram positive and gram negative bacteria

Clostridium difficile

P C. difficile is gram +ve anaerobe able to colonise the gut producing symptoms via two toxins: A (enterotoxin) and B (cytotoxin).

A Antibiotics, old age, hospital stay.

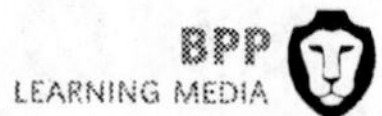

Sx Diarrhoea, abdominal pain, fever.

I Stool culture × 3, ↑ WCC.

T Isolation, barrier nursing, fluids, stool chart, metronidazole, vancomycin.

C Pseudomembranous colitis, sepsis, toxic megacolon.

Salmonella (non-typhoidal salmonellosis)

P Motile gram negative aerobic or facultative anaerobic rods. Acute superficial inflammation of large and small bowel. Secretory diarrhoea due to enteropathy with electrolyte and water transport defects.

A Over 2,000 species of salmonella. Associated with poultry, mammals, reptiles.

Sx No prodrome, 48 hours' vomiting and diarrhoea, abdominal cramps occur intermittently, symptoms usually resolve after two weeks.

I Blood cultures, stool culture.

T Rehydration, antibiotics for severe or invasive disease, or in immunocompromised: ciprofloxacin 500–750mg bd.

C Persistent faecal carriage (~1%), bacteraemia, vascular infections, reactive arthritis.

Pr Excellent, vascular complications carry high mortality.

Shigella

P Human-only, non-motile gram negative rods.

A Four shigella species (in descending order or severity): shigella dysenteriae, S. flexnerii, S. boydii, S. sonneii.

Incubation: one to seven days.

Sx Severe prodrome: headache fever and abdominal pain.

Diarrhoea, dehydration.

I Stool culture.

T Usually self-limiting. Antibiotics reduce the severity and time course of the disease by about two days and reduce infectivity.

C Rectal prolapse, HUS, seizures in small children, reactive arthritis.

Pr Excellent. Faecal carriage continues for three to four weeks, and abdominal symptoms may persist for four to five weeks.

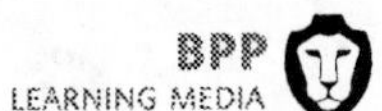

Campylobacter infection

P Campylobacter jejuni. Commonest cause of diarrhoea in UK.

A Associated with birds, poultry, pets, farm animals.

Incubation period: two to six days.

Sx Prodrome 24–36 hours: headache, abdominal pain. Nausea, vomiting, diarrhoea. Very high fever can be present. May mimic acute appendicitis.

I Stool culture × 3.

T Mainly supportive with ORS, IV fluids when required, antibiotics only for severe cases or immunocompromised.

C Guillain-Barré syndrome, transverse myelitis, reactive arthritis.

Pr Excellent.

Cholera

P Vibrio cholera, motile curved gram negative rod.

Secretory diarrhoea caused by toxin acting on enterocyte.

A Spread by faecal contamination of drinking water.

Incubation period: few hours to three days.

S Profound dehydration, electrolyte imbalance (reduced sodium, chloride and bicarbonate).

Sx Abrupt painless watery 'rice-water' diarrhoea (up to 30 litres a day).

I Blood gases: metabolic acidosis through loss of bicarb in stool, ↑ U&Es, stool culture.

T Accurate fluid balance, ORS, IVI fluids.

C Circulatory collapse, arrhythmias, death.

Pr Excellent with treatment and support. ORS has reduced mortality of severe cholera from 50% down to 1%.

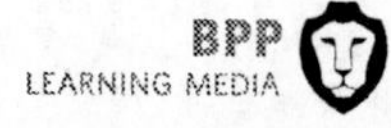

Tetanus

P Clostridium tetani: gram positive anaerobic spore-forming rod. Inoculation of organism or spore, potent exotoxin acts on synapse of motor nerves and blocks inhibitory neurone resulting in tetanic spasm.

A Seldom seen in developed countries with successful vaccination uptake and sanitary conditions.

Incubation: five to ten days.

Sx 24-hour prodrome: restlessness and malaise.

Hypertonicity: trismus (risus sardonicus) and neck muscle spasm, followed by spasm of truncal muscles. Lasts two to three months.

Reflex spasms: violent sustained muscle contraction while patient remains fully conscious. Lasts 7–21 days.

I Clinical diagnosis.

T Antitoxin: human tetanus immunoglobulin, benzylpenicillin IV, wound debridement, sedation, paralysis (tracheostomy and ventilation if any spasm post sedation).

C Aspiration pneumonia, exhaustion and death.

Pr Poor with short incubation period and onset of first spasm <24 hours.

Botulism

P Clostridium botulinum gram +ve rod produces heat-resistant neurotoxin leading to neuromuscular blockade.

A Improperly preserved food, also contaminated heroin in IVDU.

Sx Paralysis, nausea, diarrhoea, visual disturbance.

I Stool culture.

T IM Antitoxin, benzylpeniclin, HDU/ITU.

Pr Poor, 50% mortality.

Viruses

Chickenpox

P Varicella zoster virus. Usually mild infection in childhood.

A Droplet spread respiratory secretions, period of infectivity is one day before rash appears until last spot crusted, most infectious in first two days.

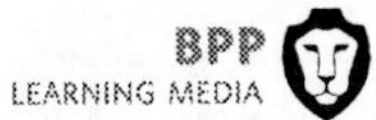

Sx Prodrome one to two days: headache, fever, malaise, sore throat, myalgia then vesicular rash (centripetal distribution).

I PCR for VZV secretions / vesicles.

T Calamine lotion, aciclovir for severe disease. **Never** give aspirin as may precipitate Reye's syndrome (encephalopathy and fatty degeneration of viscera).

C Pneumonitis, reactivation of latent virus gives rise to shingles, or herpes zoster infection.

Pr Complications and mortality increases with age.

Uncomplicated chickenpox prognosis is excellent.

Infectious mononucleosis (glandular fever)

P Epstein-Barr virus, enveloped DNA virus is transmitted via saliva and infects B lymphocytes, causing proliferation of mononuclear T-cells.

A Human infection with no animal reservoir.

Incubation: four to seven weeks.

S Fleeting macular rash and facial oedema, pharyngitis, generalised lymphadenopathy 100% of cases (especially posterior cervical chain), hepatosplenomagaly, jaundice (commonest cause of viral hepatitis in UK), petechial rash, rash with amoxicillin (90%).

Sx Childhood infection is usually asymptomatic. Fever, malaise, severe sore throat, myalgia, anorexia, abdominal pain, vomiting.

I FBC: ↑ WCC, thrombocytopenia, abnormal LFTs, positive heterophile antibody test: monospot / Paul-Bunnell test, viral PCR.

T Supportive. **Never** give amoxicillin due to rash.

C Lymphocytic meningitis, Guillain-Barré syndrome, autoimune haemolytic anaemia, splenic rupture, B cell lymphomas in immunocompromised.

Pr Excellent in infectious mononucleosis.

Mumps

P Paramyxovirus causing parotits ('mumbling' due to parotid gland infection).

A Droplet transmission. Preventable by MMR vaccine (15 months).

Sx Parotid swelling, fever, headache, orchitis.

I Clinical diagnosis.

T Supportive, analgesia.

C Meningitis, pancreatitis, orchitis, sub-fertility.

Measles

P Paramyxovirus.

A Droplet transmission. Preventable by MMR vaccine (15 months).

Sx 3Cs: cough, coryza, conjunctivitis and three-day fever.

Koplik spots: grey lesions on buccal mucosa.

Macularpapular rash: red / brown colour, head then rest of body.

I Clinical diagnosis.

T Supportive, analgesia.

C Pneumonia, gastroenteritis, panencephalitis.

Cytomegalovirus (CMV)

P Cytomegalovirus is a member of the herpesvirus family of DNA viruses.

A Shedding in secretions (saliva, urine, respiratory, genital and breastmilk). Crosses placenta giving rise to congenital infection, usually in primary maternal infection.

Incubation: 3–12 weeks.

S Lymphadenopathy is seen in 15% in contrast to EBV infection.

Sx Majority asymptomatic or fever three to five weeks, profuse sweats, lethargy.

I FBC: ↑ WCC, thrombocytopenia, deranged LFTs, CMV PCR. Histology: owl-eye nuclei (prominent nucleoli and intracytolpasmic inclusions).

T Supportive treatment.

Immunocompromised hosts or in complicated infection antivirals are available.

C Hepatitis, myocarditis, meningoencephalitis, thrombocytopenia, haemolytic anaemia, Guillain-Barré syndrome.

Pr Generally very good.

Poliomyelitis

P Enteroviral infection which has a predilection to affect the CNS/ PNS.

A Poliovirus (an enterovirus) is transmitted via faecal-oral route. Rare in communities where vaccine uptake is good, worldwide distribution.

Incubation 3–35 days.

Sx Most infections are asymptomatic.

Paralytic polio: presents as aseptic meningitis. After fever subsides secondary fever arises with onset of flaccid paralysis. Recovery is variable over next 12–18 months.

I Virus isolation from faeces, throat swab, CSF, antibody titre (rising titre to enterovirus).

T Isolation of patient, bedrest, ventilatory support if respiratory muscle involvement, care of pressure areas, physiotherapy for paralysed limbs, NG feeding for bulbar paralysis, vaccination of susceptible contacts.

C Paralysis, aspiration pneumonia.

Viral haemorrhagic fever (VHF)

P A group of viral infections which have broadly similar clinical features and are highly infectious in nosocomial settings and which carry significant mortality. Consider VHF in all travellers developing fever within three weeks of travel to endemic area.

T Isolation of patient, blood film to exclude malaria. Requires transfer of patient to high security infectious diseases unit and notification to appropriate authorities.

- Any fever and clinical features
- Travel history – onset <3 weeks from geographical exposure
- Exposure to sick person with unexplained fever +/- bleeding < 3 /52
- Exposure to animal reservoir (rodents, monkeys, bats, livestock)

Box 9.4: Risk assessment for VHF

Protozoa

Giardia intestinalis

P Giardia intestinalis (= lamblia / duodenale)

Commonest intestinal protozoanparasite. Produces small bowel overgrowth, malabsorption predominates.

A Worldwide distribution. Cysts can survive outside host for long periods in water facilitating spread, person to person spread.

Incubation: 3–21 days.

Sx Asymptomatic carriage.

Watery diarrhoea, steatorrhoea, abdominal discomfort, bloating, weight loss, fatigue, sulphurous belching, flatulence.

I Stools for OCP (giardia cysts, cryptosporidiosis, cyclosporiasis, and giardia), hairy string test (swallow capsule with string which unravels reaching duodenum. Giardia trophozoites cling onto string and can be seen on microscopy when string is pulled out), exclude coeliac disease and post infectious malabsorption.

T Tinidazole 2g two doses five days apart or metronidazole 400mg tds five days.

C Severe malabsorption with growth retardation.

Pr Generally good.

Toxoplasmosis

P Toxoplasma gondii, protozoan parasite. Definitive host: felines.

A Cysts excreted in cat faeces, which can cause infection through gardening, cat litter and grazing in herbivores.

S May be signs of old or active chorioretinitis on fundoscopy.

Painless lymphadenopathy.

Sx Primary infection: fever, lymphadenopathy, mild hepatitis.

Congenital infection: miscarriage, 60% triad of hydroccephalus, cerebral calcification and choroidoretinitis.

I Serology: toxoplsma dye test, IgM antibodies, viral PCR, histology.

T Supportive.

C Congenital infection, blindness, neurological sequelae.

Leishmaniasis

P Granulomatous inflammation caused by presence of protozoan parasite.

A Protozoan infection transmitted by sandfly, lutzomyia species in S America.

Sx Fever, weight loss, hepatosplenomegaly, leucopenia, cutaneous granulomatous lesion with raised border, ulceration and crusting.

I Leucopenia, PCR, culture of lymph from cutaneous lesion, histology, bone marrow biopsy.

T Sodium stibogluconate IV, liposomal amphotericin B – especially in HIV infection.

C Secondary bacterial infections, TB common sequel.

Enteric fever

Typhoid

P Salmonella typhi, salmonella paratyphi A, B and C, some non-typhoidal salmonella infections.

A Faeco-oral transmission via food / water.

Incubation period 10–20 days.

Sx *1st week:* fever, headache, dry cough, abdominal pain

2nd week: high fever, delirium, rose spots (between navel and nipples), foul 'pea soup' diarrhoea, bowel perforation, encephalitis.

3rd week: death or slow recovery.

I Blood culture, stool culture, WCC: low or normal, Widal test.

T Increasing prevalence of antibiotic resistance, ciprofloxacin 750mg BD, steroids for severe toxaemia.

C Intestinal haemorrhage, pneumonia, chronic carriage.

Pr Excellent with treatment. Death in 20% untreated.

Diptheria

P Corynebacterium diphtheria a gram positive rod.

A Spread by nose / throat of human carrier.

Incubation period: one to five days.

Sx Insidious onset: listlessness, fever, tachycardia and site-specific symptoms.

Faucial: (commonest) slow onset, fever, sore throat, nausea, vomiting, dysphagia.

Cutaneous: painful ulceration with offensive smell, may be superinfected with staphylococci or streptococci.

I Diagnosis should be clinical (and treatment started immediately) with lab confirmation, throat swab.

T Isolate patient, diphteria antitoxin, antibiotics (penicillin or erythromycin), bed rest, ECG monitoring, early tracheostomy and ventilation if signs of tracheal obstruction or respiratory muscle paralysis.

C Laryngeal obstruction, myocarditis, neuropathy.

Pr Overall mortality 5–10%, myocarditis – 50% mortality.

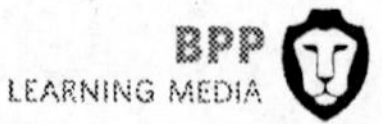

Spirochetes

Lyme disease

P Borrelia burgdorferi spirochaete.

A Transmitted by ticks, can be prevented by removal of tick within 24 hours, no human to human spread.

Sx Early localised infection (3–30 days): erythema migrans at site of tick bite, fever, headache, myalgia arthralgia.

Neurological manifestations: meningitis, cranial nerve palsies, periperal neuritis, painful radiculopathy especially cervical distribution.

Cardiac manifestations: heart block, arrhythmias.

Joint manifestations: arthralgia.

I ECG: arrhythmia / heart block.

Blood for antibodies to B. burgdorferi.

T Amoxicillin 500mg tds, doxycycline 100mg BD.

C Post-lyme syndromes: residual neurological sequelae and fatigue may persist for several months.

Pr Excellent. A few patients will have residual symptoms.

Leptospirosis / Weil's disease

P Leptospira species. L. interrogans icterohaemorrhagica causes most severe disease. Natural host: rat, dog and farm animals.

A Contact with water contaminated with rat urine eg sewer workers. Leptospires can survive in environment for months.

Incubation: 7–14 days.

Sx Fever, rigors, headache with photophobia (aseptic meingits, 'canicola fever'), conjunctival suffusion, marked myalgia, nausea, mild jaundice, mild renal impairment.

I FBC: neutrophilia, U&E: AKI, LFTs.

Urine: proteinuria and casts.

Serological tests: ELISA.

T Mainly supportive.

C Chronic eye infection.

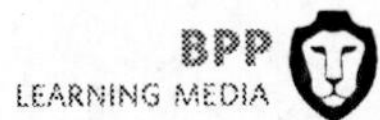

Sexually transmitted infections (STIs)

Chlamydia

P Due to chlamydia trachomatis.

A Most common STI in the UK.

Sx Women: asymptomatic or cystitis, lower abdo pain.

Men: asymptomatic or dysuria, discharge.

I Urine for chalamydia, PCR.

T Doxycycline, azithromycin, erythromycin.

C Peri-hepatits (Fitz-Hugh-Curtis syndrome).

Gonorrhoea

P Caused by neisseria gonorrhoea bacteria.

Incubation period 2–30 days, symptoms occur after 4–6 days.

A Sexual contact.

Sx Women: half are asymptommatic or have vaginal discharge.

Men: penile discharge.

I Microscopy of discharge.

T Cephalosporins.

C Septic arthritis.

Syphilis

P Due to treponema pallidum spirochaete.

A Sexual contact, pregnancy.

Sx See Box 9.5 below.

Primary syphyilis

- Chancre (painless, raised papule with ulcerated centre)
- Lymphadenopathy

Secondary syphilis (4–10 weeks after primary infection)

- Systemic mucocutaneous lesions
- Fever, malaise, headache, sore throat
- Lymphadenopathy

Tertiary syphilis (3–15 years after original infection)

- Gummatous (15%): formation of gumma (a form of granuloma) in liver, bone, skin and testes
- Cardiovascular syphlis (10%): syphlitic aortitis
- Neurosyphyllis (6.5%): infection involving CNS. Argyll-Robertson pupil, tabes dorsalis

Box 9.5: Symptoms of syphilis

I Bloods: VDRL (veneral disease research laboratory) and rapid plasma regain tests and TPHA (treponemal pallidum particle agglutination).

Microscopy: of chancre serous fluid.

T Penicillin.

C Progression to tertiary syphyllis as above.

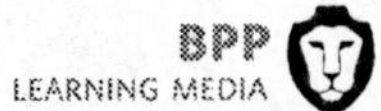

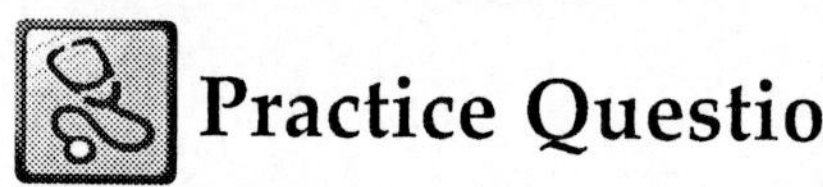

Practice Questions

Single Best Answers

1. Which of the following is true concerning HIV disease?

   A The most common mode of HIV infection is through heterosexual transmission
   B There is no risk of HIV transmission through oral sex
   C The median time from HIV infection to the development of AIDS is five to seven years
   D HIV can be detected in the blood at all stages

2. In HIV disease

   A Pneumocystitis carinii pneumonia is the commonest AIDS defining illness
   B CD8 cells are attacked
   C People with HIV infection have the same incidence of bacterial pneumonias as HIV negative people
   D Cytomegalovirus disease in HIV positive patients is primarily the result of reactivation of latent infection

3. Which of the following is not associated with infectious mononucleosis?

   A Jaundice
   B Thrombocytosis
   C Splenomegaly
   D Haemolysis

4. Which of the following is a live attenuated vaccines?

   A Influenza vaccine
   B Tetanus
   C BCG
   D Hepatitis B vaccine

5. Congenital cytomegalovirus (CMV) infection:

   A May be diagnosed by culture of urine
   B Is associated with congenital heart disease
   C Only occurs following a primary infection in pregnancy
   D Is diagnosed by detecting CMV IgG antibody in cord blood

6. Which of the following diseases is commonly spread by faecal or urinary contamination of water?

   A Plague
   B Syphilis
   C Leptospirosis
   D Diphtheria

7. Chickenpox is caused by which of the following?

   A Paramyxovirus
   B EBV
   C HSV
   D VZV

8. Trismus is a symptom of which type of infection?

   A Typhoid
   B Diphtheria
   C Tetanus
   D Botulism

9. Lyme disease may present with which of the following dermatological conditions?

   A Erythema nodosum
   B Erythema migrans
   C Pemphigoid
   D Erythema multiforme

10. Cerebral malaria is a complication of infection by which species?

   A Plasmodium falciparum
   B Plasmodium vivax
   C Plasmodium ovale
   D Plasmodium malariae

Extended Matching Questions

Match the following immunisations with their vaccine type.

A Live attenuated
B Inactivated
C Toxoid
D Protein subunit
E Polysaccharide conjugate

1. Diphtheria

2. Typhoid

3. Cholera

4. Hep B

5. Men C

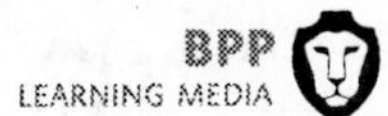

Match the following disease to the most appropriate investigation.

A Mantoux test
B Thick blood film
C Paul Bunnell test
D Widal test
E Owl eye nuclei on histology

6. Typhoid

7. TB

8. Infectious mononucleosis

9. CMV

10. Malaria

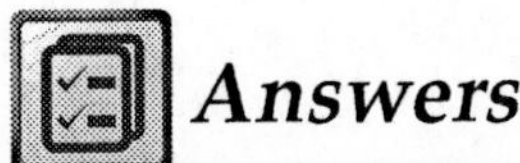

Answers

SBAs		EMQs	
1	A	1	C
2	A	2	A
3	B	3	B
4	B	4	D
5	C	5	E
6	C	6	D
7	D	7	A
8	C	8	C
9	B	9	E
10	A	10	B

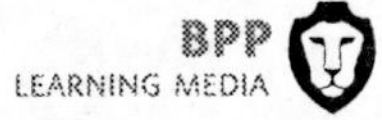

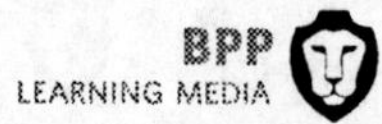

Chapter 10

Oncology and palliative care

Dr William Dougal

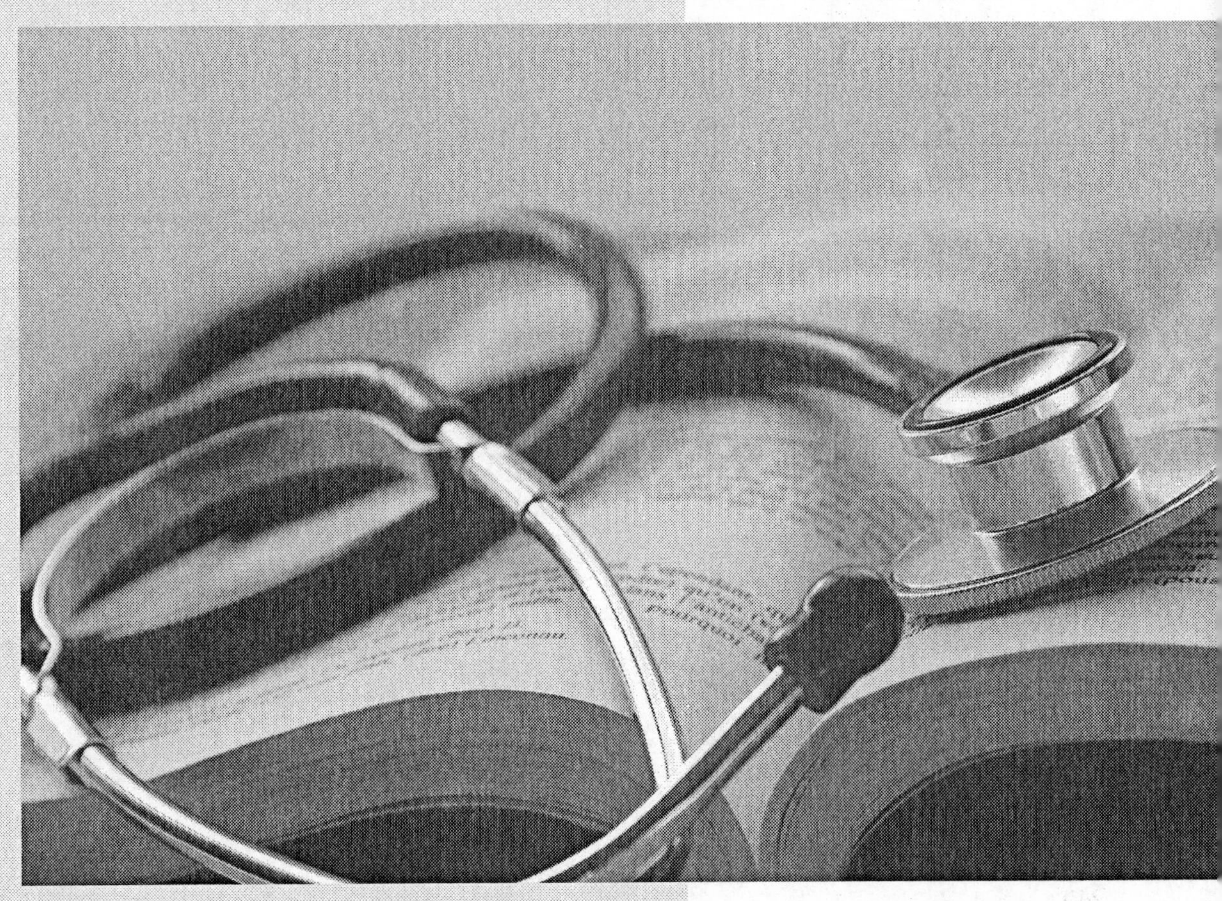

Terminology

- **Malignancy**: a tumour that invades and destroys the tissue in which it originates and can spread to other sites of the body
- **Metastasis**: the distant spread of a malignant tumour from its site of origin
- **Staging**: to classify a tumour by its size and the presence or absence of distal spread
- **Environmental risk factors**: risk factors from the environment
- **Genetic risk factors**: risk factors that are genetically determined
- **Curative / radical**: a treatment aimed to eradicate and cure the disease
- **Palliative**: a no curative treatment aimed at symptom control
- **Adjuvant**: chemo or radiotherapy after surgical treatment – aim is curative
- **Neo-adjuvant**: chemo or radiotherapy pre surgical treatment – aim is curative

Principles of oncology

Number	Male	Female
1	Prostate (23.9%)	Breast (30.9%)
2	Lung (14.7%)	Lung (11.6%)
3	Colorectal (14.2%)	Colorectal (11.6%)
4	Bladder (4.8%)	Uterus (5%)
5	NHL (4.1%)	Ovary (4.2%)
6	Malignant melanoma (3.6%)	Malignant melanoma (4%)
7	Oesophagus (3.5%)	NHL (3.6%)
8	Kidney (3.5%)	Pancreas (2.6%)
9	Stomach (3.2%)	Kidney (2.2%)
10	Leukaemia (2.9%)	Leukaemia (2.1%)
	Other sites (21.8%)	Other sites (22.1%)

Table 10.1: Top 10 malignancies male / female in the UK

Number	Male	Female
1	Lung (24%)	Lung (20.6%)
2	Prostate (12.7%)	Breast (15.7%)
3	Colorectal (10.5%)	Colorectal (9.9%)
4	Oesophagus (6.2%)	Ovary (5.8%)
5	Pancreas (4.7%)	Pancreas (5.6%)

Table 10.2: Top 5 cancer deaths male / female in the UK

Oncological therapies

Radiotherapy

Indications: neo-adjuvant, adjuvant or palliative.

Mode of administration: radiowaves.

Mechanism of action: ionising radiation producing free radicals that damage DNA. Kills cells with rapid turnover (ie cancerous cells), while normal cells have time to repair between doses.

Complications: early and late. Local side effects, therefore complications specific to site irradiated.

Early side effects (during / soon after Tx)	Late side effects (typically 6–12 weeks or longer after Tx)
Tiredness	Somnolence (CNS)
Skin reactions (range from erythema, desquamation and ulceration)	Pneumonitis (Lung Rx)
Mucositis (head and neck Rx)	Xerostomia, benign strictures and fistula formation (GI Rx)
Nausea and vomiting (abdominal or brain Rx)	Urinary frequency / fibrosed bladder and infertility (pelvic Rx)
Diarrhoea (abdo / pelvic Rx)	
Dysphagia (thoracic Rx)	
Cystitis (pelvic Rx)	

Table 10.3: Side effects of radiotherapy

Chemotherapy

Indications: neo-adjuvant, adjuvant or palliative.

Mode of administration: intravenous or oral.

Mechanism of action: cytotoxics that damage DNA. Kills cells with rapid turnover (ie cancerous cells).

Complications: nausea and vomiting. Alopecia. Neutropenia (typically day 7–14). Peripheral neuropathy. Transverse myelitis. Bone marrow suppression. Oral mucositis. Anorexia. Desquamation palms and soles.

Class of drug	Examples
Alkylating agents	Cyclophosphamide, Chorambucil
Antimetabolites	Methotrexate, 5-Fluorouracil
Vinca alkaloides	Vincristine, Vinblastine
Anti tumour antibiotics	Actinomycin, Doxorubicin
Others	Monoclonal antibodies, Epidermal Growth Factor Inhibitors (EGFR)

Table 10.4: Types of chemotherapeutic agents

Surgery

Indications: diagnostic, radical and palliative.

Complications: as with any surgery. Risk from GA. Risk of bleeding, infection and pain. Perforation with GI surgery. Post surgical complications such as DVT/PE, ACS etc.

Hormones

Indications: hormone responsive tumours, ie breast (Tamoxifen) or prostate (goserelin).

Mode of administration: oral, S/C

Mechanism of action: blocks or inhibits androgens.

Complications: Tamoxifen: menopausal symptoms, pro-thrombotic. Goserelin: similar to menopause in women.

Oncology emergencies

Neutropenic sepsis

P Sepsis occurring with neutrophils <1.0×10^9/l

A Bone marrow suppression induced by chemotherapy, rarely by huge dose radiotherapy.

S Neutrophils <1.0 × 10^9/l, temp ≥38°C.

Sx Can be asymptomatic, unwell, symptoms of infection in body system eg LRTI, UTI.

I Septic screen, FBC, U&Es, LFTs, CRP, clotting.

Blood cultures: from peripheral and central lines.

Urine: MC&S, stool culture, sputum, throat swab, line cultures. CXR.

T Follow local guidelines.

Immediate IV gentamicin and Tazocin 1st line, add vancomycin if MRSA suspected, add metronidazole if abdo cause suspected, add antifungal agent if not responding, remove central line if infected.

C Death.

Pr Prompt treatment improves prognosis. Antibiotics cover the patient while waiting for neutrophils to naturally recover.

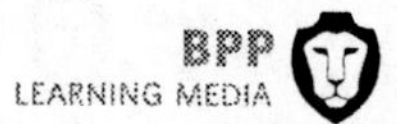

Hypercalcaemia of malignancy

P Increase of calcium release from bone.

A Primary tumours of bone, bone metastases, myeloma, tumours which secrete PTH related peptide and parathyroid tumours.

S Of hypercalcaemia.

Sx Of hypercalcaemia: lethargy, confusion, polydipsia, polyuria, constipation, nausea, weakness.

I Bloods: corrected calcium, U&Es (look for dehydration).

T Rehydration (3–4L IV saline over 24 hours), IV bisphosphonates (eg pamidronate), dose adjusted to level of calcium, control of underlying malignancy.

C Dehyration, arrythmias, renal stones.

Pr Depends on underlying malignancy.

Superior vena cava obstruction

P Obstruction of blood back to the right atrium via the SVC, (and tracheal compression).

A Any tumour causing compression of or in the SVC eg lung, lymphoma, thyroid, thrombus around a central line.

S Dyspnoea, orthopnoea, engorged veins, cyanosis.

Pemberton's test: lifting the arms over the head for one minute produces increased facial plethora, cyanosis, raised JVP and inspiratory stridor.

Sx Headache, swollen arm and face.

I CXR, CT, venography.

T Steroids: dexamethasone 4mg/6h PO, venoplasty and SVC stenting, radiotherapy or chemotherapy.

C Death. Complications from treatments.

Pr Depends on underlying malignancy, worse prognosis if tracheal compression.

Spinal cord compression

P Compression of the spinal cord.

A Extradural metastases, crush fracture, vertebral body tumour or direct extension of a tumour.

S Weakness, sensory level.

Sx Back pain with nerve root distribution (eg if T10 affected band of pain around abdomen at level of umbilicus), bladder and bowel dysfunction.

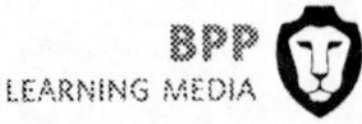

I Urgent MRI whole spine (within 24 hours).

T Steroids, dexamethasone 8–16mg IV, then 4mg/6h.

Radiotherapy or surgery.

C Paralysis.

Pr A high index of suspicion and prompt treatment improves prognosis. 30% may survive one year.

Raised intracranial pressure

P Increased pressure in a fixed container.

A Primary CNS tumour or metastases.

S Papilloedema, focal neurological deficit, seizures.

Sx Headache, nausea and vomiting.

I Urgent CT head.

T Steroids: dexamethasone 4mg/6h PO, radiotherapy or surgery.

C Seizures, stroke, herniation and 'coning'.

Pr Depends on underlying tumour.

Symptom control

WHO pain analgesia ladder:

3. ***Strong opioid*** *+- Non opioid +- Adjuvant*

2. ***Weak opioid*** *+- Non opioid +- Adjuvant*

1. ***Non opioid*** *+- Adjuvant*

Adjuvant: NSAIDs

Non opioid: paracetamol

Weak opioid: codeine, tramadol

Strong opioid: morphine, diamorphine, oxycodone, fentanyl, methadone, hydromorphone

Opiod	Relative potency	Equivalent daily dose (mg)
Oral codeine	×1/12	360
Oral tramadol	×1/5	150
Oral morphine	×1	30
SC/IV morphine	×2	15
Oral oxycodone	×2	15
SC/IV diamorphine	×3	10
Oral hydromorphone	×8	4
Fentanyl patch	×150	0.2

Table 10.5: Opiod conversion table: (equivalent doses to oral morphine)

Pain

- **P** Neuropathic, nociceptive.
- **S** Restlessness, agitation.
- **Sx** Pain.
- **I** Always look for a reversible cause (eg blocked catheter).
- **T** As per WHO analgesic ladder, if neuropathic consider amitriptyline / gabapentin.
- **C** Opioids: constipation, nausea and vomiting, hallucinations, euphoria, dysphoria, respiratory depression.

Nausea and vomiting

- **A** Obstruction, central cause, side effect of medication.
- **S** Vomiting.
- **Sx** Nausea.
- **I** Look for mechanical cause, look at drug chart.
- **T** Anti-emetics.

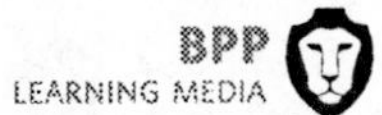

Anti-emetic (dose / route)	Mode of action	Use	Side effects / cautions
Metoclopramide 10mg TDS PO/IV/SC/IM	Peripheral pro-kinetic (5HT agonist) and central (dopamine antagonist) effects	Gastric stasis, functional bowel obstruction	Extra-pyramidal, sedation. Do not give in mechanical bowel obstruction.
Cyclizine 50mg TDS PO/IM/IV	Anti histamine (H_1), central action	Mechanical bowel obstruction, raised ICP and motion sickness	Sedation
Haloperidol 1.5–5mg PO (max 30mg/day) 2–10mg IM/IV (max18mg/day)	Dopamine antagonist	Metabolic causes of vomiting (opiod induced vomiting)	Extra-pyramidal, sedation
Levomepromazine 6.25–25mg BD PO/IM/IV/SC	Activity at multiple sites, peripheral and central	Refractory N&V, terminally ill	Sedation, postural BP drop
Ondansetron 8–16mg IV/IM	Serotonin (5HT) antagonist	Chemotherapy induced N&V. Refractory N&V	Constipation, headache, sedation. Caution in GI obstruction

Table 10.6: Anti-emetic side effects

Constipation

A Side effect of medication, decreased fluid intake / mobility, high calcium.

S Abdominal pain, agitation, restlessness.

Sx Not opening bowels.

I Serum calcium, AXR.

T Laxatives, usually co-danthramer (a faecal softener and peristaltic stimulant) or senna (stimulant) and lactulose solution (osmotic softener).

Agitation / restlessness

A Multi-factorial.

S Agitation.

I Look for reversible cause.

T Midazolam 2.5–5mg SC 4h.

Secretions

- **A** Inability to swallow normal respiratory secretions.
- **S** Gurgling.
- **T** Hyoscine butylbromide 20–120mg/24h SC.

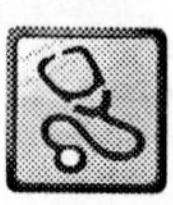

Practice Questions

Single Best Answers

1. A patient is switched from 5mg IV morphine to oral morphine. An equivalent dose for oral morphine would be

   A 5mg
   B 2.5mg
   C 10mg
   D 15mg

2. The following anti-emetic acts at the central chemoreceptor trigger zone blocking histamine.

   A Ondansetron
   B Metoclopramide
   C Haloperidol
   D Cyclizine

3. Neutropenic sepsis is defined as sepsis in a patient with neutrophils of

   A $<9 \times 10^9/l$
   B $<10 \times 10^9/l$
   C $<1 \times 10^9/l$
   D $>10 \times 10^9/l$

4. The commonest male maligancy in the UK is

   A Prostate
   B Lung
   C Colon
   D Pancreas

5. The cancer with the highest male death rates in the UK is

   A Prostate
   B Lung
   C Colon
   D Pancreas

Extended Matching Questions

A Mucositis
B Stricture formation
C Cyclophosphamide
D Vincristine
E Gabapentin
F Oral morphine
G Midazolam
H Hyoscine butylbromide

Match the statements below with the most suitable answer above.

1. Is an early side effect of radiotherapy

2. Is an appropriate medication to use in terminal agitation

3. Is an alkylating chemotherapeutic agent

4. Is an appropriate medication for terminal secretions

5. Is an appropriate medication for neuropathic pain

Answers

SBAs		EMQs	
1	C	1	A
2	D	2	G
3	C	3	C
4	A	4	H
5	B	5	E

Chapter 11

Dermatology

Dr Daniel Newton

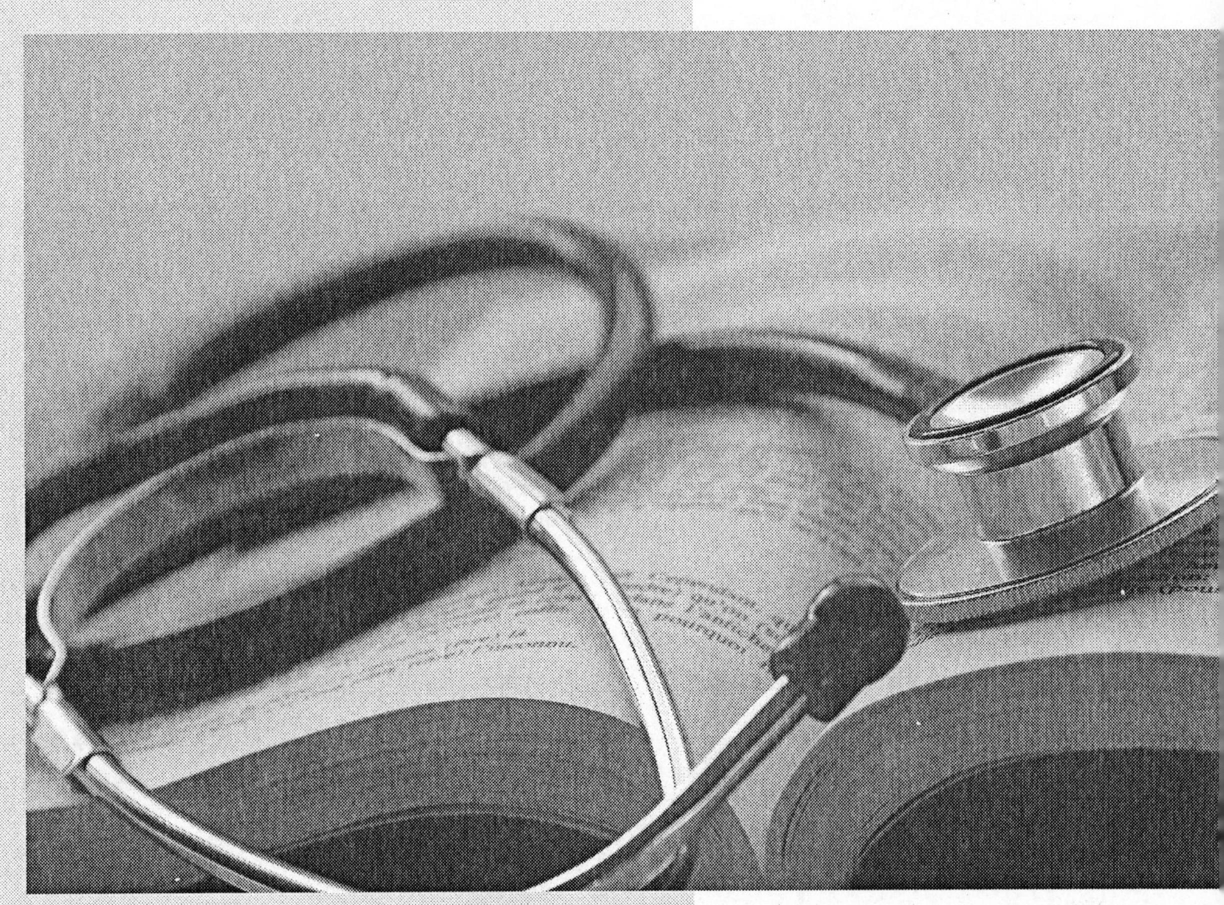

Terminology

- **Abscess**: local accumulation of pus
- **Bulla**: raised, circumscribed lesion (>0.5cm) containing serous fluid (blister) above the dermis
- **Comedone**: plug of dead epithelial material blocking pore: open (blackhead) or closed (whitehead)
- **Erythema**: blanchable redness of the skin that can be localised or generalised and is caused by dilatation of superficial blood vessels and capillaries
- **Excoriation**: scratch which has broken the surface of the skin
- **Lichenification**: skin thickening with exaggerated skin markings, as a result of repeated rubbing
- **Macule**: flat, well-defined area of altered skin pigmentation. Areas >1cm are described as patches
- **Nodule**: solid, palpable, usually subcutaneous lesion >0.5cm diameter
- **Papule**: raised, well defined lesion usually <0.5cm
- **Plaque**: raised flat-topped lesion, usually >2cm in diameter
- **Purpura**: non-blanching violaceous (purplish) discolouration of the skin due to blood that has extravasated from blood vessels. May be palpable
- **Pustule**: raised, well-defined lesion containing pus
- **PUVA**: psoralen plus Ultraviolet A
- **Vesicle**: blister less than 0.5cm diameter
- **Weal**: transient raised lesion with a pale centre and a pink margin

Common presentations

Eczema (dermatitis)

P Acute or chronic inflammation of the dermis.

A Atopy, allergic contact dermatitis (eg nickel), irritant contact dermatitis; seborrhoeic dermatitis and varicose eczema.

S Sx Erythematous and itchy, may become dry, cracked, flaky or blistering and oozing / bleeding. Excessive scratching of affected areas can lead to lichenification.

I Usually clinical diagnosis but if unclear then a biopsy can be performed. Patch testing is sometimes useful in identifying causative agent.

T *Topical:* soap substitutes, emollients, topical steroids.

Systemic: avoidance of trigger factors, oral steroids, antibiotics, anti-histamines, azathioprine (2nd line).

C Superimposed infection.

Pr Children often improve during teenage years and many resolve completely. Avoidance of known allergen / irritant should lead to complete resolution of symptoms.

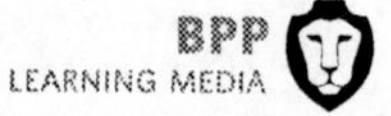

Psoriasis

P Common, chronic scaly rash. Men and women affected equally and peaks seen in teens and 50s.

A Genetic predisposition, infections can cause flares (strep sore throat precedes guttate psoriasis), drugs, smoking and alcohol are also implicated.

S Sx Well demarcated, red, scaly patches of skin. Usually symmetrical and often affects extensor surfaces. Scale is often silvery in colour. Nails affected by pitting and onycholysis. *Guttate psoriasis* presents with widespread small plaques. *Pustular psoriasis* presents with pustules on hands and feet.

I Usually clinical diagnosis.

T *Topical:* sunlight; emollients; coal tar preparations; dithranol; topical steroids.

Systemic: UVA / PUVA; methotrexate, ciclosporin.

C Psoriatic arthropathy affects 5% of those affected, associated with HLA-B27, Koebner phenomenon seen in scars.

Pr Not usually curable but often improves with compliance to treatment.

Acne vulgaris

P Inflammation of the pilosebaceous follicle.

A Almost universal amongst teenagers, affects face, neck, upper chest and back. Increased sebum production and increased growth of propionobacterium acnes.

S Comedones, papules, pustules, nodules, cysts and scarring.

I Clinical.

T Dependent on severity:

- *Mild:* topical therapies such as benzoyl peroxide, topical antibiotics.
- *Moderate:* oral antibiotics eg four to six months tetracycline/minocycline + topical benzoyl peroxide.
- *Severe:* oral retinoids (isotretinoin) 16-week course.

C Scarring, psychological impact, treatment complications (teratogenicity of isotretinoin, dry skin, hepatitis and increased serum lipids).

Pr Good if compliant with treatment. Isotretinoin leads to improvement in all cases with 60–70% experiencing no further recurrences.

Acne rosacea

P Red facial rash, commonly affects fair skinned individuals between ages 30–60. May be transient, recurrent or chronic.

A Unknown.

S Red papules and occasionally pustules on the nose, forehead, cheeks and chin. Rarely affects trunk. Often occurs on a background of dry, flaky skin. Patients commonly develop facial telangiectasia.

Sx 'Blushing' aggravated by sunlight, spicy food or alcohol.

I No specific investigations necessary.

T Avoid precipitating factors; avoid steroid creams and oil-based facial creams; oral antibiotics (tetracyclines); isotretinoin may be effective for improving resistant cases; laser treatment or surgery are also options.

C Rhinophyma and blepharophyma can develop if poorly controlled.

Pr Treatment not curative but aimed at controlling extent of disease, long-term therapy may be necessary.

Urticaria

P Group of disorders characterised by red patches and wheals on the skin. Can affect eyelids, lips and airways.

A Histamine release from mast cells causing fluid release from capillaries, usually in response to an allergen.

- Animal dander
- Drugs: anaesthetic agents, antibiotics, ACE inhibitors
- Environmental: dust, chemicals, mould, plants
- Foods: cheese, chocolate, eggs, fish, nuts, shellfish
- Idiopathic
- Infection: amoebiasis

Box 11.1: Causes of urticaria

S Sx Itchy, raised patches arising anywhere on skin (weal) surrounded by red flare. Lesions can vary in size from pinpoint to several centimetres.

I FBC: eosinophilia, skin prick testing or RAST testing.

T Avoid offending allergen; anti-histamines; oral corticosteroids. Rarely immunosuppressant therapy, UVB/PUVA. Intramuscular adrenaline if airway compromise.

Pr Can become chronic but overall good prognosis with treatment.

Lichen planus

P Chronic mucocutaneous disease that affects skin, tongue and oral mucosa.

A Unknown, thought to be due to abnormal immune reaction triggered by a viral infection or drugs.

S Sx Well defined pruritic, planar, purple, polygonal papules. Commonly affects wrists and ankles. 50% of cases have oral involvement with lacy streaks affecting the mucosa (Wickham's striae).

I Skin biopsy typically shows lichenoid tissue reaction – irregularly thickened epidermis, degenerative skin cells, basal cell degeneration, lymphocytic infiltration of subepidermal layer and melanin beneath the dermis.

T Potent topical steroids or sometimes systemic steroids are necessary for extensive disease.

C Rarely can result in squamous cell carcinoma of the mouth or genitals.

Pr 85% of cases resolve in 18 months but may recur and tends to be more persistent if the mouth or genitals are affected.

Pemphigus

P Chronic skin disease characterised by painful blistering and erosions.

A Autoimmune with autoantibodies (IgG) directed against desmoglein 1 and desmoglein 3 leading to loss of cohesion between keratinocytes in the epidermis. Peak 45–50 years.

S Sx Patient's most commonly present with oral lesions. Painful flaccid blisters and mucosal erosions. +ve Nikolsky's sign.

I Punch biopsy with direct immunofluorescence showing IgG and C3.

T Systemic corticosteroids are mainstay of treatment in suppressing disease. Immunosuppressant's and steroid sparing agents may also be used.

C Secondary infection of wounds. Side effects from high dose steroids.

Pr Aim is to control disease rather than cure and patient may require life-long steroid treatment.

Pemphigoid

P Blistering disease that more commonly affects the elderly. Blistering is immune mediated.

A Autoimmune IgG antibody mediated response against basement membrane, peak in elderly.

S Sx Tense fluid-filled blisters often arising from normal looking skin. Usually very itchy and while it can be localised it is more commonly widespread.

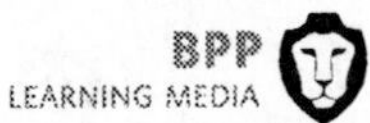

I Often clinical diagnosis but direct immunofluorescence will reveal IgG and C3 at basement membrane causing split between dermis and epidermis.

T Sterile dressings, oral steroids, other options include topical steroids, tetracycline, methotrexate and azathioprine.

C Superimposed infection; side effects of steroids / immunosuppressant drugs.

Pr Usually resolves over several months to years.

Pityriasis rosea

P Rash of unknown cause that often lasts for six weeks.

A Often follows a viral infection.

S **Sx** Begins with a single scaling patch (herald patch) before further patches or plaques appear, most commonly affects chest and back in 'christmas tree' pattern. Lesions are usually red but may appear white on darker skin due to scale.

I Usually a clinical diagnosis but biopsy sometimes needed.

T Not usually required but if rash is itchy then oral anti-histamines or topical steroids may be of benefit. Phototherapy is thought to hasten resolution.

C Usually none but skin may appear lighter for several months after resolution.

Pr Excellent: most cases resolve within six weeks and do not recur.

Infections

Cellulitis

P Bacterial infection of the sub-cutaneous tissues, more common in patients with diabetes.

A Commonest organisms β-haemolytic streptococci (strep. pyogenes) and staphylococci (staph. aureus).

S Erythema, warmth, swelling, tenderness, blistering, abscess, ulceration, pyrexia, tachycardia and other signs of sepsis.

Sx Pain and swelling of affected area, general malaise, fevers, rigors.

Ludwig's angina: cellulitis of the submandibular space (often follows dental infections).

I FBC, CRP, possible imaging to exclude DVT.

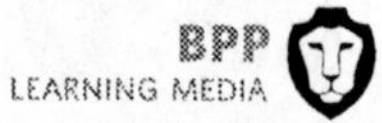

T Elevate affected limb, PO/IV antibiotics, commonly amoxicillin / benzylpenicillin + flucloxacillin, alternative options include clindamycin / ceftriaxone.

C Septicaemia, recurrent cellulitis, chronic skin discolouration.

Pr Most resolve with 10 days oral antibiotics but if systemic features or severe cellulitis present may require up to 14 days IV antibiotics.

Erysipelas

P Superficial form of cellulitis.

A Almost all cases caused by Group A β-haemolytic streptococci (strep. pyogenes).

S Well defined erythematous area with raised border. Skin is swollen and occasionally dimpled (peau d'orange appearance) and may blister.

Sx Systemic upset, rapid onset pain and redness over affected area.

I FBC (raised WCC), CRP.

T Antibiotics, usually penicillins. Oral/IV depending on degree of systemic involvement.

C Rare: distant spread via blood, post-streptococcal glomerulonephritis, cavernous sinus thrombosis.

Pr Can recur in up to one-third of cases due to persistence of risk factors and may require long-term antibiotic prophylaxis.

Scabies

P Intensely itchy rash caused by the mite sarcoptes scabiei.

A Transmitted by skin-to-skin contact with somebody else with scabies.

S Sx Itch, burrows (often seen on fingers or wrists), generalised rash, nodules and blisters on palms and soles of feet.

I None.

T Anti-scabetic (malathion, permethrin) applied topically to all areas below neck for 24-hours. Ensure all members of household are treated.

C Secondary infection.

Pr Rash usually takes up to two weeks to settle but good prognosis with compliance with treatment.

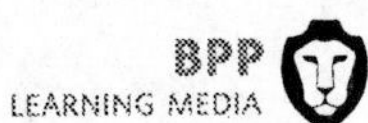

Tinea

P Fungal skin infection.

A Caused by dermatophyte (ringworm) fungus.

- *Tinea barbae:* neck and beard area
- *Tinea capitis:* scalp
- *Tinea corporis:* trunk and limbs
- *Tinea cruris:* groin
- *Tinea faciale:* face
- *Tinea manuum:* palms
- *Tinea unguium:* nails (onychomycosis)
- *Tinea pedis:* feet

Box 11.2: Tinea subtypes

S Sx Pruritic, inflamed red patches.

I Skin scrapings from active edge of lesion.

T Topical antifungals or systemic antifungals for resistant disease.

C Very contagious and can spread to other household members.

Pr Excellent.

Pityriasia versicolor

P Common skin rash where flaky, discoloured patches appear mainly on chest and back.

A Most cases caused by malassezia furfur yeast.

S Sx Occasionally itchy, well-defined patches of varying size and colour. Appear paler on darker skin and may have a fine scale to lesions.

I Usually clinical diagnosis but skin scrapings may be used.

T Topical antifungals, selenium sulphide shampoo, oral antifungals for widespread or recurrent disease.

C Occasionally discoloured skin persists after treatment.

Pr Can recur but overall excellent prognosis.

Necrotising fasciitis

P Life threatening infection of soft tissue and fascia.

A Severe cases are caused by strep. pyogenes.

S Sx Pain out of keeping with clinical features should raise suspicion. May have crepitus in affected tissues. Septic shock (pyrexia; hypotension; tachycardia). Later, area will become blistered and necrotic.

I Raised inflammatory markers, U&Es, blood cultures may give causative organism.

MRI/CT scans may reveal extent of tissue involvement.

T Broad spectrum IV antibiotics and surgical debridement.

C Extensive tissue damage may require skin grafting or even amputation. Organ damage dependent on degree of sepsis.

Pr High mortality.

Manifestations of systemic disease

Erythema nodosum

P Inflammation of fat cells beneath skin surface.

A Immune mediated and commonly associated with infections, sarcoidosis, autoimmune, pregnancy, drugs or malignancy.

- Autoimmune: inflammatory bowel disease (Crohn's, UC), Behçet's
- Drugs: OCP, sulphonamides
- Idiopathic
- Infection: strep. sore throat, TB, Hep C, leprosy
- Malignancy
- Pregnancy
- Sarcoidosis

Box 11.3: Causes of erythema nodosum

S Sx Characterised by red, tender nodules or lumps that usually occur on the shins.

I Diagnosis of underlying cause. ASO titre, autoimmune profile, TB testing may be useful.

T Should not require specific treatment as should be self-limiting therefore treatment of underlying cause is main goal. If doesn't improve potassium iodide is effective.

Pr Usually improve over three to six weeks but can become chronic.

Pyoderma gangenosum

P Neutrophilic disorder causing skin ulceration. Commonly affects lower limbs.

A Thought to be autoimmune and associated with other diseases such as inflammatory bowel disease; rheumatoid arthritis and haematological disorders (myeloma).

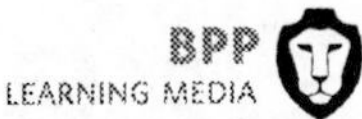

S Sx Begin as a small pustule then rapidly ulcerates. Ulcers rapidly grow in size and are typically painful with a purple border.

I None specific other than attempting to identify underlying cause.

T Topical or systemic steroids. More severe disease may require immunosuppressive treatment (tacrolimus, methotrexate, ciclosporin).

C Ulcers heal with scarring with a typical cribriform pattern.

Pr Untreated, ulcers will continue to enlarge. Treatment is usually successful but healing may take months especially if associated with vascular disease.

Dermatitis herpetiformis

P Autoimmune blistering skin condition. IgA antibodies found in dermis.

A Skin manifestation of gluten intolerance (coeliac disease).

S Sx Intensely itchy papulovesicular rash, commonly affects extensor surfaces. May arise from normal or erythematous skin.

I Skin biopsy (subepidemal blister, neutrophils and IgA seen on direct immunofluorescence); antiendomysial antibodies; tissue transglutamidase antibody (TTG).

T Gluten-free diet, dapsone usually improves itch and blistering, steroids may be necessary.

C Rarely direct complications from dermatitis herpetiformis but complications from coeliac disease and other autoimmune disease (increased incidence).

Pr Good if strict gluten-free diet adhered to.

Erythema multiforme

P Hypersensitivity reaction usually triggered by an infection.

A Herpes simplex virus and mycoplasma pneumoniae are commonest causes but other viruses and medications are also implicated.

- *Drugs:* antibiotics, sulfonamides
- *Infection:* EBV, Hep B, histoplasmosis, HSV, mycoplasma
- Lupus
- Malignancy
- Pregnancy
- Sarcoid

Box 11.4: Causes of erythema multiforme

S Sx Target lesions: well demarcated round, pink, flat lesions which become raised to form a plaque with pale ring around red centre. Mucosal membranes may also be affected.

I Clinical diagnosis.

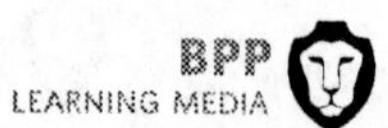

T Usually self-limiting but supportive / symptomatic measures may be necessary.

C Stevens-Johnson syndrome: systemic, severe mucosal involvement, fever, can be life-threatening.

Pr Good prognosis and heals without scarring.

Acanthosis nigricans

P Skin disorder characterised by hyperpigmented areas.

A Common causes include insulin resistance, obesity, PCOS and also seen as a paraneoplastic phenomenon (GI malignancy).

S Sx Asymptomatic, brown hyperpigmentation of the skin. Commonly affects skin folds (groins, axillae).

I Need to ascertain underlying cause – hyperisulinaemia versus malignancy.

T Treat underlying disease.

C None.

Pr Dependant on cause.

Thrombophlebitis migrans

P Recurrent, superficial thrombophlebitis.

A Often a paraneoplastic phenomenon associated with pancreatic and lung malignancy.

S Sx Tender, palpable blood vessels with overlying redness and swelling.

I Can be confirmed by doppler studies. Investigate thoroughly for underlying malignancy.

T Rest, elevation, compression stockings, NSAIDs.

C Rare but can become infected.

Pr Usually related to underlying pathological process.

Xanthelasma

P Skin lesions caused by accumulation of fat within macrophages beneath the surface of the skin. Commonly affects area around the eyes. Several different types including palpebrum, tuberous, tendinous and eruptive.

A Tend to be familial or related to high cholesterol / lipid levels in the blood.

S Sx Usually asymptomatic, soft, velvety, yellowish papules or plaques. Usually slowly enlarging.

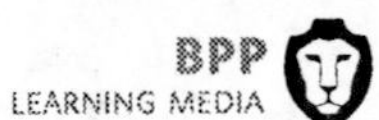

- **I** Measurement of serum lipid levels and if familial forms suspected genetic testing may be necessary.
- **T** Decrease fat intake; statins; ezetemibe; fibrates; topical trichloroacetic acid or surgical incision are options.
- **C** Increased incidence of coronary artery disease.
- **Pr** Good prognosis with treatment.

Lupus vulgaris

- **P** Persistent and progressive cutaneous manifestation of tuberculosis.
- **A** Mycobacterium tuberculosis.
- **S** Small, sharply defined reddish-brown lesions with a gelatinous consistency.
- **I** Usually confirmed by skin biopsy.
- **T** Anti-tubercular drug regime as per pulmonary TB.
- **C** Lesions occasionally cause severe disfigurement and can lead to malignancy.
- **Pr** Lesions can persist for many years.

Lupus pernio

- **P** Cutaneous manifestation of sarcoidosis.
- **A** Sarcoidosis: multisystem granulomatous disease.
- **S** Large bluish-red / purple nodules and plaques on face, hands or feet.
- **I** Skin biopsy shows granulomatous infiltration.
- **T** Often requires no treatment, corticosteroids, immunosuppressants.
- **C** Can be locally disfiguring.
- **Pr** Dependent on extent of other organ involvement. Skin lesions tend to take longer to heal.

Necrobiosis lipoidica

- **P** Rare skin disorder that affects the shins on insulin-dependent diabetics.
- **A** Unknown.
- **S** Yellowish / brown, waxy patches develop on the shins. Typically painless and slowly enlarging.

I None specific.

T Topical steroids, intralesional steroid injections, aspirin and dipyridamole, ciclosporin or PUVA treatment.

C Prone to ulceration.

Pr Dependent on extent of disease and whether lesions have ulcerated.

Granuloma annulare

P Chronic skin disease caused by granulomatous inflammation occurring within the dermis.

A Usually idiopathic but can be associated with autoimmune diseases (DM, thyroid disease, SLE) or malignancy.

S Usually a ring of small, red papules over backs of forearms, hands or feet with a tendency to joints or knuckles.

Sx Usually asymptomatic but lesions can be tender if knocked.

I Skin biopsy may be useful in confirming diagnosis.

T Often will resolve spontaneously. Other options include topical, intralesional or systemic steroids; topical imiquimod or tacrolimus. If disseminated: methotrexate, isotretinoin or dapsone may be useful.

C Chronic course, recurrence.

Pr Even if treatment clears lesions recurrence is common.

Benign skin lesions

Seborrheic keratosis

P Common, harmless wart-like growths that appear with advancing age.

A Cause unclear but are considered degenerative as the skin ages.

S Sx Painless, raised lesions with 'stuck on' appearance. May be multiple.

I Often none necessary but skin biopsy can be used to confirm diagnosis if in doubt.

T Not always necessary but can be removed by cryotherapy or curettage.

C None.

Pr Excellent.

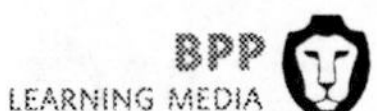

Solar keratosis

P Scaly spots that develop on sun-exposed areas.

A Due to abnormal skin proliferation due to prolonged ultraviolet exposure. More common in fair skinned individuals. They are premalignant in nature.

S Sx Usually multiple, flat or thickened scaly lesions, may be skin coloured or reddened, can be uncomfortable.

I None specific, biopsy if concerned about malignant transformation.

I Cryotherapy, curettage, 5-fluorouracil or imiquimod.

C If untreated can progress to squamous cell carcinoma.

Pr Excellent if treated and sun exposure of affected areas avoided.

Keratoacanthoma

P Dome shaped growth originating from hair follicle.

A Sun-exposed areas commonly affected, can be triggered by a minor injury.

S Sx Dome-shaped, symmetrical lesion, often surrounded by inflamed skin and capped with keratin and debris.

I Often difficult to differentiate from malignancies therefore it is important to confirm a diagnosis histologically.

T Options include cryotherapy, curettage and surgical excision.

C Rarely can recur at same site.

Pr Excellent.

Sebaceous cyst

P Lump beneath surface of skin containing thick sebum-like fluid. Can become infected.

A Usually caused by blocked sebaceous glands or hair follicles.

S Sx Usually asymptomatic lump, commonly arising on face, neck or trunk. If becomes infected then lump becomes painful, red and swollen.

I None, unless infection suspected.

T Surgical excision, can improve with applications of heat pad.

C None.

Pr Excellent.

Dermoid cyst

P Benign tumours consisting of skin cells, hair follicles and sweat glands.

A Appear in early childhood due to a defect during skin tissue development in the embryonic stage.

S Sx Firm, dough-like lumps, usually 0.5–6cm and usually occur on face, neck or scalp.

I Ultrasound scan used to plan surgical procedures.

T Surgical removal via excision biopsy.

C Dependent on size and extent of local tissue involvement.

Pr Good if surgical removal complete, can recur if not.

Lipoma

P Benign tumour composed of fat cells.

A Unknown. Possible genetic element. Trauma can trigger growth.

S Palpable soft, smooth lump beneath skin. Lump easily moved with fingers. Usually 2–10cm in size but can grow bigger.

Sx Usually asymptomatic and only noticed when they have grown large enough to become visible.

I None.

T Usually none required but can be removed surgically.

C Dercum's disease: multiple, tender lipomas.

Pr Excellent.

Malignant skin lesions

Basal cell carcinoma

P Commonest skin malignancy. Slow growing, locally invasive malignancy arising from basal cell layer of skin, very rarely metastasises.

A Excessive sun exposure. More common in fair skinned individuals. Genetic susceptibility.

S Sx Shiny, pearly nodule with 'rolled edge' and telangiectasia commonly on face, can erode into nearby structures.

I Skin biopsy.

T Surgical excision, cryotherapy, radiotherapy and chemotherapy (5-fluorouracil).

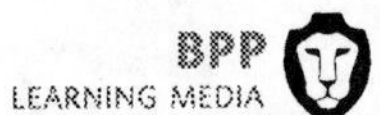

C Destruction of nearby structures if untreated, patients often have multiple BCCs.

P Excellent: invariably curable due to such low rates of metastatic spread.

Squamous cell carcinoma

P Second commonest type of skin malignancy. Originates from squamous cells in the epidermis.

A Excessive sun exposure, genetic predisposition, smoking, chronic ulceration (Marjolin's ulcer), infections (HPV).

S Sx Usually occur on sun-exposed sites and are slow-growing tender, scaly or crusted lumps, sometimes present as ulcers that don't heal.

I Biopsy of lesion.

T Surgical excision and radiotherapy.

C Can occasionally recur at the same site.

Pr Overall good prognosis but 5% of tumours will metastasise (most commonly to local lymph nodes).

Bowen's disease

P SCC-in-situ. Intraepidermal squamous cell carcinoma.

A As per squamous cell carcinoma, sun exposure and HPV.

S Sx Gradually enlarging, well demarcated erythematous plaque with an irregular border and surface crusting or scaling.

I Biopsy.

T Cryotherapy, curettage, 5-fluorouracil; imiquimod cream or photodynamic therapy.

C Recurrence is relatively common but can be treated in the same way, can progress to squamous cell carcinoma.

Pr Excellent if treated early.

Malignant melanoma

P Skin cancer caused by malignant proliferation of melanocytes.

A Genetic predisposition; sun damage; can originate from other moles. 5% of all skin cancers but highest mortality.

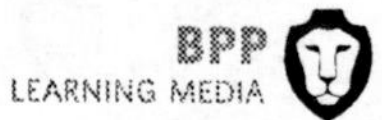

May be classified as:

- *Superficial:* superficial spreading, lentigo maligna (common on face in elderly patients), acral lentiginous.
- *Deep:* nodular melanoma, mucosal melanoma.

S **Sx** Common sites (in order of frequency) **S**kin, **E**yes, **A**nus. Worrying features of mole (below):

- **A**symmetry
- **B**order irregularity
- **C**olour variation
- **D**iameter > 6mm
- **E**volving (enlarging/changing).

I If a melanoma is suspected then the lesion should be surgically excised with a 2–3mm margin. The biopsy should then be sent for histological analysis and staging.

T Surgical excision +/- adjunctive chemotherapy or radiotherapy.

C Local and distant metastatic spread, scarring from surgery.

Pr Prognosis related to Breslow thickness (depth of tumour in millimetres) and Clark's level (more useful for melanomas <1mm Breslow depth).

Excellent prognosis for tumours <1mm depth.

Breslow thickness	Five-year survival	Clark's level
<1mm	95–100%	Melanoma confined to the epidermis (melanoma in situ)
1–2mm	80–96%	Into the papillary dermis
2.1–4mm	60–75%	Into the junction of the papillary and reticular dermis
>4mm	50%	Into the reticular dermis
		Into subcutaneous fat

Table 11.1: Malignant melanoma staging and prognosis

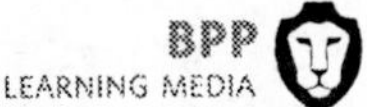

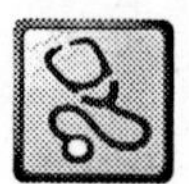

Practice Questions

Single Best Answers

1. A 60-year-old man presents to his GP with a slowly enlarging nodule on his right ear. The lesion is pearly white with fine telangectasia over its surface. There is no lymphadenopathy. What is the diagnosis?

   A Amelanotic malignant melanoma
   B Basal cell carcinoma
   C Kaposi's sarcoma
   D Seborrhoeic keratosis

2. Which of the following is the best treatment for severe nodulo-cystic acne?

   A Isotretinoin
   B PUVA therapy
   C Methotrexate
   D Oral steroids

3. Which of the following responds well to cryotherapy?

   A Malignant melanoma
   B Squamous cell carcinoma
   C Bowen's disease
   D Lupus pernio

4. A 70-year-old man presents with a lesion in the left temporal area. The lesion is small and glistening with small blood vessels crossing it.

   A Squamous cell carcinoma
   B Basal cell carcinoma
   C Keratocanthoma
   D Maliganant melanoma

5. A 20-year-old man presents with a rash on both elbows. The rash consists of well-defined erythematous plaques with adherent silvery scales.

   A Lichen planus
   B Pemphigoid
   C Eczema
   D Psoriasis

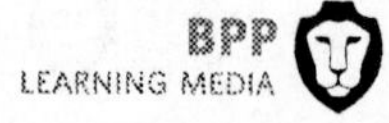

Extended Matching Questions

Cutaneous manifestations of systemic disease

A Pyoderma gangrenosum
B Erythema nodosum
C Dermatitis herpetiformis
D Erythema multiforme
E Acanthosis nigricans

For each of the following scenarios choose the **single** most likely diagnosis from the above list of options. Each option may be used more than once or not at all.

1. A 25-year-old female with Crohn's disease presents with an ulcerated lesion on her left shin that has a purple border

2. A 65-year-old with type 2 diabetes presents with hyperpigmentation of the axillae

3. A 19-year-old male university student attends GP complaining of red painful lumps on his shins. He states he recently had a sore throat.

A Skin lesions
B Malignant melanoma
C Squamous cell carcinoma
D Bowen's disease
E Basal cell carcinoma
F Seborrhoeic keratosis

For each of the following scenarios choose the **single** most likely diagnosis from the above list of options. Each option may be used more than once or not at all.

4. A 75-year-old man presents with a painless warty lesion on his back. It has a raised border giving it a 'stuck on' appearance

5. A 45-year-old lady presents with an irregular shape 'mole' which has recently increased in size and become darker in colour

6. A 70-year-old lady referred with longstanding ulcer on shin which despite satisfactory vascular studies and compression dressing does not appear to be healing.

 A Causes of skin lesions on the legs
 B Erythema nodosum
 C Erythema multiforme
 D Henoch-Schonlein purpura
 E Eczema
 F Psoriasis
 G Necrobiosis lipoidica
 H Ringworm (tinea corporis)
 I Shingles (herpes zoster)
 J Urticaria
 K Pemphigus
 L Pemphigoid

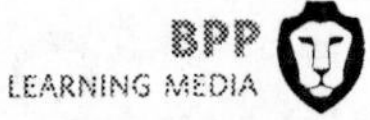

For each of the following patients choose the **single** most likely diagnosis from the above list of options. Each option may be used once, more than once or not at all.

7. A 65-year-old woman has a three-day history of a painful blistering rash on her left outer thigh. She has recently been diagnosed with breast cancer.

8. A 25-year-old woman was recently started on co-trimoxazole for a urinary infection. She is now complaining of painful, red raised lesions on both shins.

9. A 30-year-old builder has developed pink scaly patches on both knees. He has similar lesions on his elbows and scalp.

10. A 65-year-old woman has developed extensive blistering particularly involving her legs. The blisters are fragile and seem to spread under the skin surface when pressed. She feels generally unwell but has no other symptoms.

11. A 16-year-old girl presents with small purple spots on her buttocks & shins. She also has painful joints & abdomen. Urinalysis reveals proteinuria.

12. A 60-year-old man, who has had diabetes for several years, has developed a waxy yellow patch on his left shin, which is showing signs of inflammation and ulceration.

Common dermatological presentations

A Eczema
B Scabies
C Psoriasis
D Pityriasis rosea
E Malignant melanoma
F Pemphigoid
G Discoid lupus
H SLE (Systemic lupus erythematosus)
I Shingles
J Tinea
K Ringworm
L BCC (basal cell carcinoma)

For each patient below, choose the **single** most likely cause of the symptom from the above list of options. Each option may be used once, more than once or not at all.

13. A 4-year-old child with dry excoriated rash affecting the ante cubital and popliteal, fossae, the wrists and ankles.

14. A 40-year-old man with joint pains was noted to have nail pitting plus sublingual hyperkeratosis. He also had a rash on the scalp margin.

15. A 70-year-old man with itchy blisters and tense bullae over his body, especially in the flexural areas.

16. A 30-year-old lady with an erythematous rash over her cheeks and nose in the shape of a butterfly. The rash first appeared after a holiday in the Mediterranean. She also complained of hair loss and mouth ulcers.

17. A 70-year-old man under investigation for a chronic cough, weight loss and haemoptysis developed left sided chest pain followed by an area of erythema and grouped vesicles.

18. A 25-year-old man developed a rash 4cm in diameter on the right side of his chest. Several days later some smaller discrete lesions appeared on his trunk.

19. A 30-year-old lady developed a very itchy popular rash on her trunk, sides of her fingers and hands and in the webs of her fingers. Her partner also has a similar rash.

20. A 40-year-old lady noticed that a mole on her neck has increased in size, became darker in colour and started to itch. The border and edge of the mole is irregular and it has bled on a number of occasions.

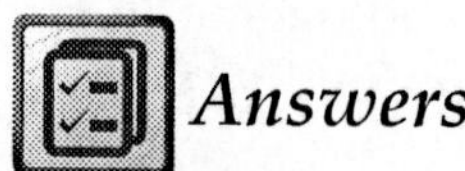

Answers

SBAs		EMQs	
1	B	1	A
2	A	2	E
3	C	3	B
4	B	4	E
5	D	5	A
		6	B
		7	H
		8	A
		9	E
		10	J
		11	C
		12	F
		13	A
		14	C
		15	F
		16	H
		17	I
		18	D
		19	B
		20	E

Chapter 12

General surgery

Mr Alexander Young and Mr John Loy

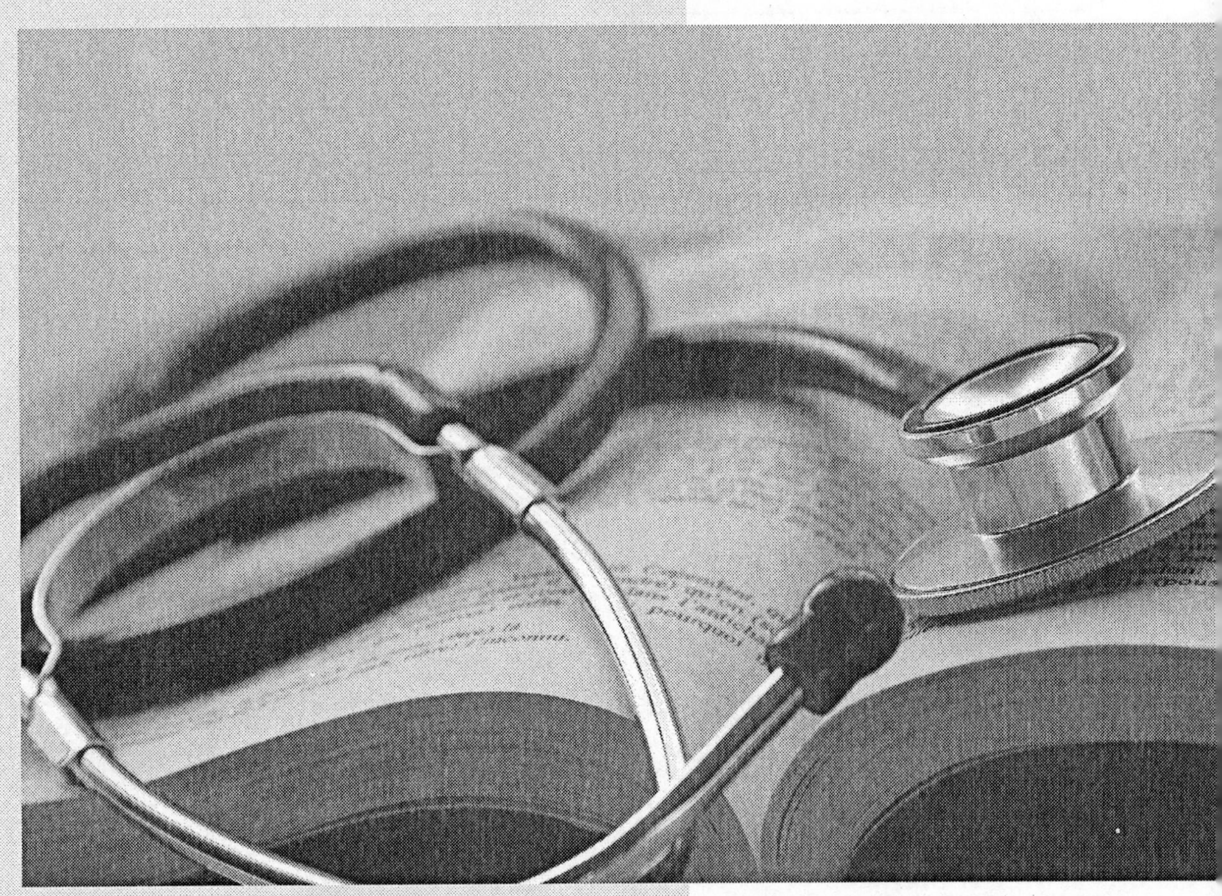

Principles of surgery

Suture material

Name	Absorption	Thread type	Use
Monocryl	Absorbable	Monofilament	Subcuticular skin closure
PDS	Absorbable	Monofilament	Abdominal wall closure
Vicryl	Absorbable	Braided multifilament	Subcutaneous fat closure, bowel anastomosis
Ethilon	Non-absorbable	Monofilament	Skin closure
Prolene	Non-absorbable	Monofilament	Arterial anastomosis
Silk	Non-absorbable	Braided multifilament	Tying drains

Table 12.1: Common sutures

Suture size

Sutures are sized using the United States pharmacopoeia (USP) scale.

Suture size (USP scale)	Suture diameter (mm)
6-0	0.07
5-0	0.10
4-0	0.15
3-0	0.20
2-0	0.30
0	0.35
1	0.40
2	0.50

Table 12.2: Suture size

Upper GI surgery

Oesophagus

Achalasia

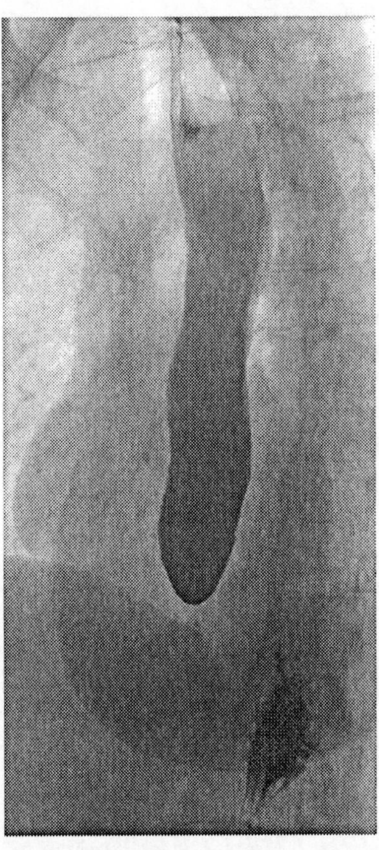

Figure 12.1: Barium swallow showing achalasia. (Reproduced with permission from SW Deanery.)

P Absence of oesophageal peristalsis and failure of relaxation of the lower oesophageal sphincter (LOS) due to degeneration of myenteric plexus.

A Peaks in young adulthood and elderly.

S Sx Slowly progressive dysphagia, liquids >solids, regurgitation as disease progresses, weight loss, aspiration, chest pain.

I Barium swallow: has classic 'birds beak' appearance with a tapered distal oesophagus and dilated mega oesophagus proximal to the constriction.

OGD: exclude benign / malignant strictures.

Oesophageal manometry: abnormally high lower oesophageal sphincter pressures.

T Endoscopic: balloon dilatation, botox injections.

Surgical: Heller's myotomy open or laparoscopic.

C Aspiration pneumonia, malignant change in distal oesophagus.

Pr Balloon dilatation successful in 80%.

Pharyngeal pouch

P Pressure causing a protrusion of mucosa between inferior constrictor and cricopharyngeus muscles, an area known as 'Killian's dehiscence'.

A Peak age elderly, associated with CVE, MND.

S Neck lump on swallowing.

Sx Regurgitation of undigested food, dysphagia, halitosis.

I Barium swallow: filling of pouch.

OGD should be avoided due to potential perforation of pouch.

T Excision of pouch and repair of muscle defect.

C Aspiration pneumonia.

Plummer-Vinson syndrome

P Web of desquamated epithelial tissue extending from oesophagus presenting as a triad of dysphagia, oesophagitis and iron deficiency anaemia.

A Peak in post-menopausal women.

S Iron deficiency anaemia: glossitis, angular stomatitis, koilonychia.

Sx Dysphagia, odynophagia.

I Bloods: iron def anaemia.

OGD: oesophageal web.

T Iron replacement, endoscopic dilatation of web.

C Increased risk of oesophageal SCC.

Pr Good with iron replacement.

Oesophageal perforation

P Perforation of the oesophagus is a surgical emergency.

A See Box 12.1.

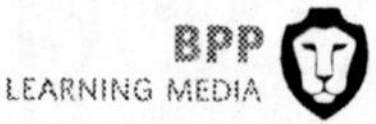

- Iatrogenic: endoscopy, intubation
- Trauma: penetrating, foreign body, ingestion caustic agent
- Malignancy
- Infection
- Boerhaave's syndrome: full thickness perforation of the oesophagus due to vomiting (Mallory-Weiss tear: partial thickness tear causing bleeding post-vomiting)

Box 12.1: Causes of oesophageal perforation

S Septic shock, surgical emphysema.

Sx Sudden onset chest pain, dysphagia, odynophagia.

I Gastrografin swallow: watersoluble contrast used over barium to show leak at point of perforation.

CXR: mediastinal surgical emphysema, air / fluid level.

T Small perforations without signs of sepsis: NBM, IV abx and fluids.

Large perforations: urgent surgical closure / resection, IV abx and fluids, nutritional support.

C Dependent on speed of treatment.

Pr If surgery for large perforations in first 24 hours mortality is 5–10%. If delayed >48 hours mortality >50%.

Oesophageal malignancy

P Squamous cell carcinoma: upper 2/3 oesophagus.

Adenocarcinoma: lower 1/3 oesophagus (Barrett's oesophagus associated).

A Increased incidence in China and Iran (possibly due to diet).

See Box 12.2.

- Achalasia
- Barrett's oesophagus: pre-malignant condition secondary to chronic GORD causing squamous to columnar metaplasia in lower oesophagus. Serial OGDs assess progression of dysplasia
- Diet high in nitrosamines
- Excess alcohol
- Smoking
- Ingestion caustic substances
- Plummer-Vinson syndrome
- Howel-evans syndrome: autosomal dominant condition causing hyperkeratosis of palms and oesophageal malignancy

Box 12.2: Causes of oesophageal malignancy

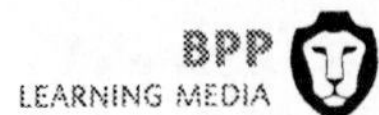

S Sx Worsening dysphagia, solids then liquids, cough, SOB, hematemesis, odynophagia.

I OGD: visualisation and biopsy for classification and grade.

CT chest, abdo, pelvis: staging by TNM.

T Surgery: curative oesophagectomy + chemotherapy.

Palliative: stent, radiotherapy, chemotherapy.

C Only one-third appropriate for surgery at presentation.

Local spread: recurrent laryngeal nerve palsy, Horner's syndrome, SVC obstruction.

Pr Five-year survival: 5%.

Hiatus hernia

P Herniation of part of stomach into the thoracic cavity through the oesophageal hiatus in the diaphragm.

Sliding (80–90%): upper stomach and gastro-oesophageal junction herniation through oesophageal hiatus.

Rolling (paraoesophageal 10%): part of fundus and / or body of stomach herniates through defect in phrenico-oesophageal membrane in diaphragm coming to lie next to the oesophagus.

A Females > males, peak >50 years. Associated with obesity, previous surgery.

S Sx Majority asymptomatic, 50% GORD in sliding HH, hiccough.

I Barium swallow, CT chest.

T Non-surgical: weight loss, treat GORD (PPI).

Surgical (indicated in rolling HH for volvulus or obstruction): open or laparoscopic reduction of hernia and repair, Nissen's fundoplication.

C Volvulus or obstruction in rolling HH.

Stomach

Pyloric stenosis

P Hypertrophy of the pylorus causing gastric outlet obstruction.

A Presents 2–7 weeks of age, commoner in boys 4:1, particularly first born, often a strong family history.

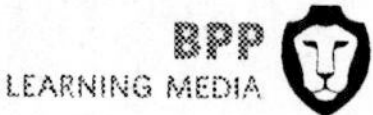

S Sx Progressive projectile vomiting (none bile stained), constant hunger after feeding, weight loss and dehydration, palpable mass (olive) in the right upper quadrant, visible peristalsis.

I Test feed.

Blood gas: hypokalaemic hypochloraemic metabolic alkalosis.

Ultrasound.

T Fluids and electrolyte correction, Ramstedt's pyloromyotomy.

Gastric carcinoma

P 90% adenocarcinoma, 5% lymphoma, 5% gastro intestinal stromal tumours (GISTs).

A 2nd commonest cancer-related death worldwide, peak age >50 years, male: female 3:1. See Box 12.3.

- H. pylori infection and chronic ulceration
- Diet high in nitrosamines (smoked fish)
- Smoking
- Alcohol
- Chronic atrophic gastritis
- Low social class
- Blood group A

Box 12.3: Risk factors for gastric carcinoma

S Troisier's sign: palpable left supraclavicular (Virchow's) lymph node suggests disseminated disease, palpable epigastric mass, succession splash, cachectic.

Sx Dyspepsia (new onset >45 years requires investigation), anorexia, weight loss, anaemia, post-prandial fullness.

Late: gastric outlet obstruction, dysphagia, upper GI bleed.

I OGD and biopsy for histology and grading, barium meal, CT/laparoscopy for staging.

T Early (T1/2 N0 M0): curative partial or total gastrectomy plus lymph node resection.

Late (T3/4 N1/2 M1/2/3): palliative chemotherapy, surgery for obstruction.

C Linitis plastica 'leather bottle' stomach in diffuse disease, transceolomic spread to ovaries 'Krukenburg tumour'.

P Five-year survival: 20%.

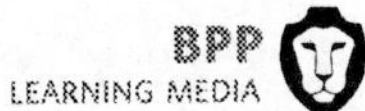

Bile ducts

Gallstones

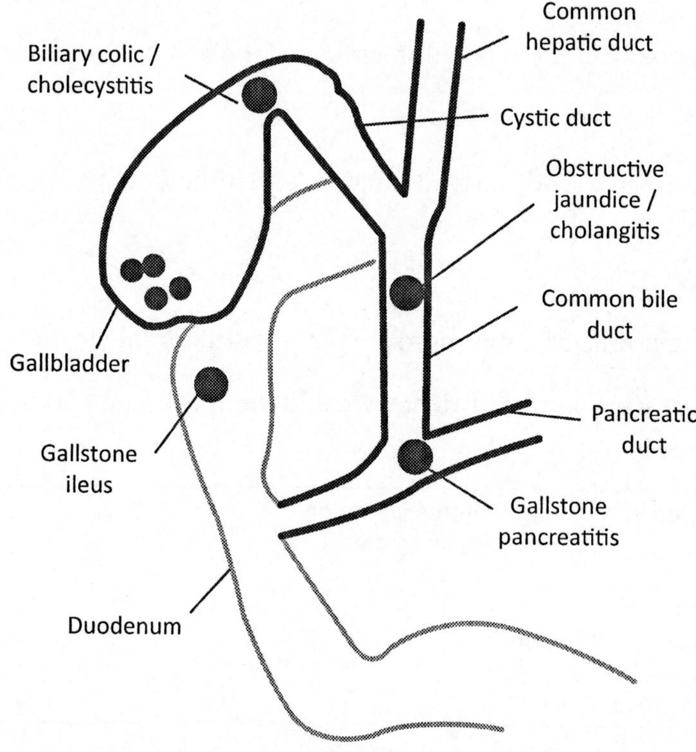

Figure 12.2: Diagram of bile ducts and stone positions

P Bile contains cholesterol, bile salts and phospholipids (lecithin). Crystallisation of these causes formation of stones, which may remain in gallbladder or become lodged at points in the biliary system causing symptoms.

A Common, classic 4Fs Fat, Fair, Fertile, Female of Forty.

Also: haemolytic disorders (pigment stones), resection of distal bowel for Crohn's disease.

- Cholesterol stones (10%): contain 80% cholesterol by weight, large (2.5cm), often solitary
- Pigment stones (10%): small, dark stones made of bilirubin and calcium salts that are found in bile. They contain less than 20% of cholesterol and are seen in haemoltytic disease
- Mixed stones (80%): typically contain 20–80% cholesterol Other common constituents are calcium carbonate, palmitate phosphate, bilirubin, and other bile pigments

Box 12.4: Types of gallstones

S Sx 90% asymptomatic.

Gall bladder stones: biliary colic, cholecystitis, gallstone ileus.

Common bile duct (CBD) stones: obstructive jaundice, ascending cholangitis.

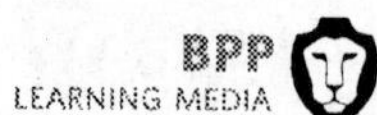

See below.

I AXR: only 10% appear on XR, USS, ERCP, MRCP.

T See below.

C See below.

Bilary colic

P Impaction of gallstone in gallbladder neck (Hartmann's pouch) or cystic duct.

A See *Gallstones*.

S RUQ and epigastric pain.

Sx Intermittent 'colicky' epigastric and RUQ pain lasting few hours, classically eased by moving, worse after eating fatty foods and at night, nausea, vomiting.

I Bloods: FBC, LFTs, amylase, U&Es.

USS abdo: location of stones, gallbladder wall thickness, oedema and duct dilatation.

T Non-surgical: NBM, IVI fluids, analgesia.

Surgical: cholecystectomy open or laparoscopic.

C Cholecystitis.

Cholecystitis

P Impaction of gallstone in gallbladder neck (Hartmann's pouch) or cystic duct causing bile to become infected with gut organisms eg E. coli.

A See *Gallstones*.

S Fever, tender, rebound, guarding RUQ.

Murphy's sign: patient catches breath on inspiration when hand placed in RUQ (only valid if –ve in LUQ).

Zachary Cope's sign: fullness in RUQ during early inflammation.

Boas' sign: hyperaesthesia below right scapula.

Sx Severe constant RUQ pain worse on moving / breathing, radiating to back and right scapula, anorexia, fever.

I Bloods: ↑ WCC, ↑ CRP, LFTs (may be elevated), U&Es, amylase.

USS: gallstones, thickened, oedematous gallbladder wall.

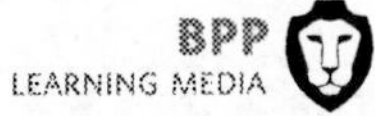

T Conservative (80% patients recover): NBM, IVI abx and fluids.

Surgery: laparoscopic (or open) cholecystectomy in first 72 hours or six to eight weeks elective cholecystectomy when inflammation reduced.

C See Box 12.5.

- Chronic cholecystitis: ongoing, non-specific symptoms following acute episode, indigestion, bloating, nausea following fatty foods
- Gallbladder mucocele: distension of gallbladder due to over secretion of watery mucoid fluid from GB wall after inflammation
- Gallbladder empyema: distension of gallbladder with frank pus. Requires IV abx and drainage to prevent perforation
- Gallstone ileus: inflammation causes cholecystoenteric fistula formation and passage of gallstone into small bowel obstructing ileum
- Perforation: perforation of the gallbladder causing biliary peritonitis

Box 12.5: Complications of cholecystitis

Obstructive jaundice

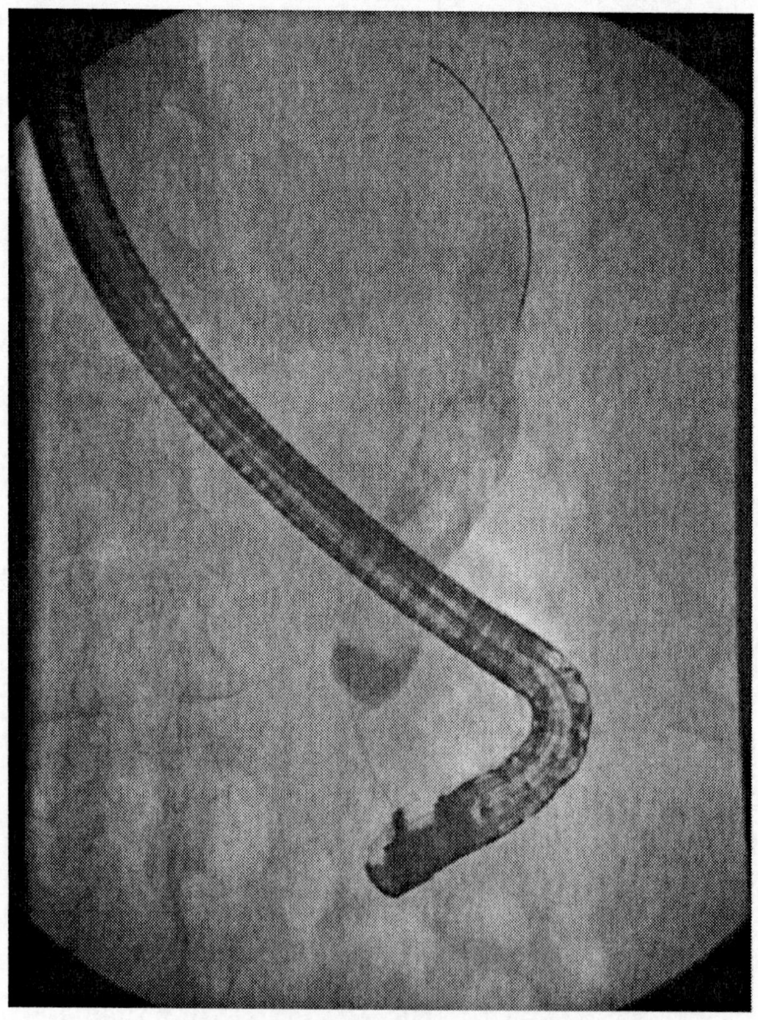

Figure 12.3: ERCP showing large CBD stone and stent

P Gallstone leaves gallbladder and becomes impacted in common bile duct causing obstruction and painful jaundice.

A See *Gallstones.*

S Dark urine, pale stools, RUQ pain.

Sx Epigastric / RUQ pain, anorexia, nausea, pruritus.

I Bloods: ↑ ALP, ↑ bilirubin (conjugated), ↑ amylase (if obstructing pancreatic duct).

Imaging: USS, MRCP, ERCP.

T **Emergency**

Endoscopy: ERCP with stone removal / sphincterotomy / stent.

Percutaneous transhepatic cholaniography (PTC): tube inserted to drain bowel if obstruction cannot be removed initially.

Surgery: open exploration of CBD with T-Tube placement to drain bile if stones cannot be removed by ERCP or PTC.

Elective

Laparoscopic (or open) cholecystectomy to prevent further episodes at six to eight weeks.

C Ascending cholangitis, acute pancreatitis.

Ascending cholangitis

P Gallstone impacted in CBD causing infection of bile ducts.

A See *Gallstones.*

S Rigors, fever, RUQ pain.

Sx Charcot's triad: jaundice, fever, RUQ pain.

Reynold's Pentad: above + hypotension and confusion.

I Bloods: ↑ WCC, ↑ CRP, ↑ ALP, ↑ ALT, ↑ bilirubin.

USS: stone in CBD, dilated CBD +/- intrahepatic system.

T Conservative: NBM, IVI abx and fluids, analgesia.

Emergency

IV abx and fluids.

Endoscopy: ERCP with stone removal / sphincterotomy / stent.

Percutaneous transhepatic cholaniography (PTC): tube inserted to drain bowel if obstruction cannot be removed initially.

Surgery: open exploration of CBD with T-Tube placement to drain bile if stones cannot be removed by ERCP or PTC.

Elective

Laparoscopic (or open) cholecystectomy to prevent further episodes at six to eight weeks.

C Acute pancreatitis.

Gallbladder carcinoma

P Majority adenocarcinomas.

A Rare. Risk factors: obesity, chronic cholecystitis.

S Sx RUQ pain, anorexia, weight loss, nausea.

I USS, CT.

T Cholecystectomy +/- chemotherapy.

Pr Poor.

Pancreas

Acute pancreatitis

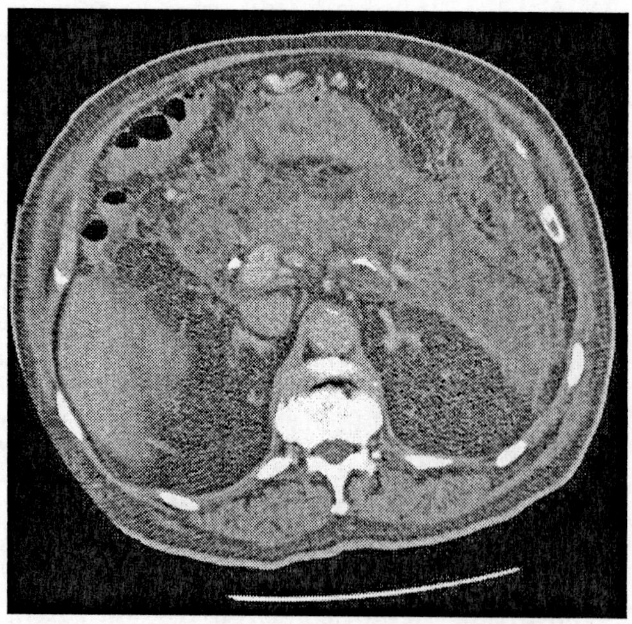

Figure 12.4: CT abdomen showing severe pancreatitis. (Reproduced with permission from SW Deanery.)

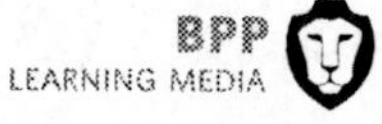

P Inflammation of pancreas with release of inflammatory cytokines and pancreatic enzymes.

A See Box 12.6.

GET SMASHED	
Gallstones (60%)	**S**teroids
Ethanol (30%)	**M**umps
Trauma	**A**utoimmune
	Scorpion Venom
	Hypthermia, **H**yperlipidaemia, **H**ypercalcaemia
	ERCP
	Drugs eg NSAIDs, thiazides, azathioprine, isoniazid

Box 12.6: Causes of acute pancreatitis

S Epigastric tenderness and guarding, septic shock.

Cullen's sign: periumbilical bruising.

Grey-Turner's sign: bilateral flank bruising indicates pancreatic necrosis with retroperitoneal bleeding.

Sx Severe epigastric pain radiating to back and relieved by sitting forward, nausea, vomiting.

I Bloods: FBC, U&E, LFTs, serum amylase >1000Iu/mL, lipase, ABG.

AXR: loss of psoas shadow indicates retroperitoneal fluid.

USS: gallstones, pancreatic fluid.

CT abdo: pancreatic inflammation, fluid.

T Immediate: resuscitate, IVI fluids, O_2 and assess severity (see prognosis), early ERCP if gallstone identified.

Transfer to HDU/ITU for monitoring of vital signs and fluid balance with nutritional support.

C Pancreatic pseudocyst, pancreatic necrosis, chronic pancreatitis (See Chapter 3 Gastroenterology), ARDS, SIRS, death.

Pr Several classification systems for severity. Glasgow Imrie, Ranson and APACHE II.

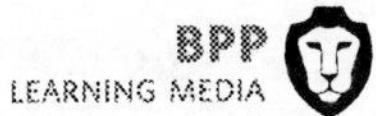

Three or more of the below in first 48 hours indicates a severe attack.	
PaO_2	<8KPa
Age	>55 years
Neutrophils	$>15 \times 10^9$/L
Calcium	<2mmol/L
Renal Function	Urea >16mmol/L
Enzymes	LDH >600iU/L / AST >2000iU/L
Albumin	<32g/L
Sugar	Glucose >10mmol/L

Box 12.7: Glasgow Imrie criteria for acute pancreatitis

Spleen

Splenic rupture

P Anatomy of the spleen: 1×3×5×7×9×11 rule. The spleen is 1″ by 3″ by 5″ in size, weighs approximately 7oz, and lies between the 9th and 11th ribs on the left side. Highly vascular.

A Commonly injured in blunt trauma, increased risk in splenomegaly.

S Sx LUQ pain, hypovolaemic shock.

I USS, CT abdo.

T Resuscitate with ATLS principles. Severe injury and haemorrhage needs urgent splenectomy.

C Increased risk of infections following splenectomy, encapsulated bacteria most dangerous.

Lower GI surgery

Small bowel

Meckel's diverticulum

P Ileal remanant of the vitellointestinal duct.

Contains ectropic gastric or pancreatic mucosa.

A Rule of 2s:

- 2% population affected
- 2 inches long
- 2 feet proximal to ileocaecal valve (on anti-mesenteric border)
- 2% are symptomatic
- 2 years of age at presentation

S Sx Most are asymptomatic. Severe rectal bleeding, may present as intussusception / volvulus or diverticulitis.

I Technetium scan: increased uptake by ectropic gastric mucosa in 70% of cases.

T Surgical resection.

Small bowel obstruction

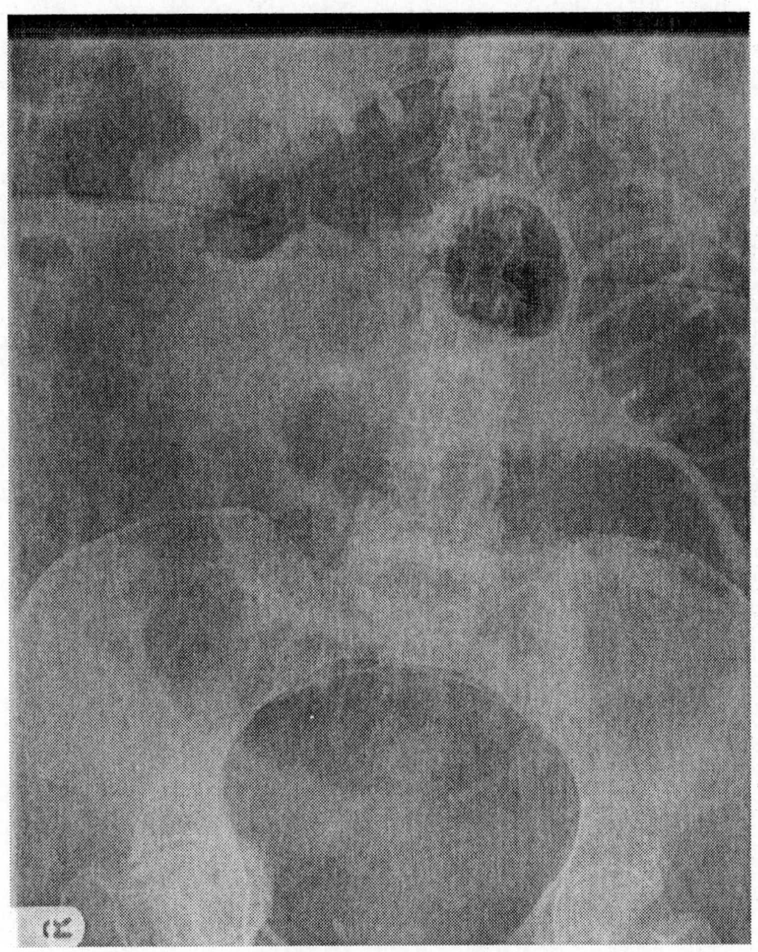

Figure 12.5: AXR showing small bowel obstruction. (Reproduced with permission from SW Deanery.)

P Blockage of small bowel.

A See Box 12.8.

- Adhesions: commonest cause due to either congenital bands or adhesions after previous abdominal surgery
- Hernias
- Tumours (especially of the caecum)
- Food bolus
- Small bowel volvulous around the mesentry

Box 12.8: Causes of small bowel obstruction (SBO)

S Distended abdomen, 'tinkling' bowel sounds, palpable masses or hernias, scars from previous surgery, empty rectum on PR.

Sx Early vomiting, central / upper abdo pain colicky in nature, abdo distension (less than in large bowel obstruction), no flatus, constipation.

I Bloods: FBC, U&Es.

Erect CXR: looking for air under diaphragm indicating perforation.

AXR: central, dilated loops of small bowel, >2.5cm (distinguished by valvulae conniventes which completely cross bowel diameter).

CT abdo: identify level and cause of obstruction.

Gastrografin follow-through: identify level and cause of obstruction.

T Immediate: NBM, nasogastric tube and IV fluids 'drip and suck', urinary catheter to monitor fluid balance.

Failure of immediate management or signs of strangulation requires surgical intervention to relieve obstruction +/- bowel resection.

C Perforation, strangulation, severe dehydration, death.

Pr Dependent on underlying cause.

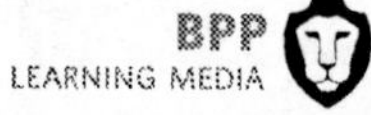

Large bowel

Large bowel obstruction

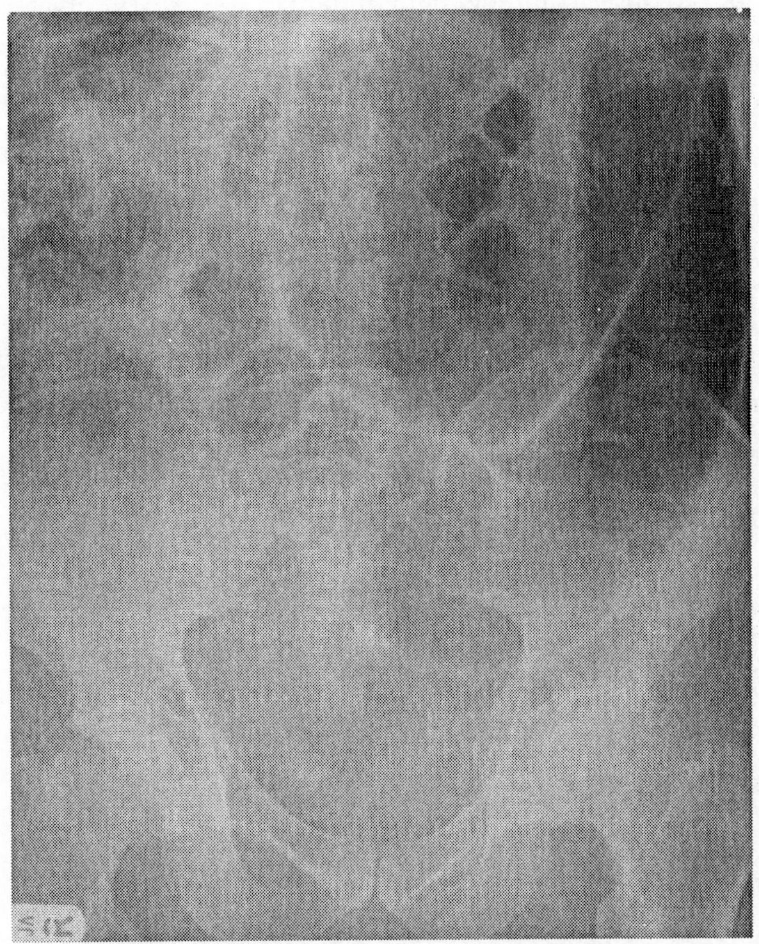

Figure 12.6: AXR showing large bowel obstruction. (Reproduced with permission from SW Deanery.)

P Obstruction of large bowel.

A Volvulus common cause. See Box 12.9.

- Intraluminal
  - Gallstone ileus
  - Food / faeces
  - Intussusception
- Bowel wall
  - Strictures
  - Tumours
  - Diverticulitis
- Extraluminal
  - Sigmoid / caecal volvulus
  - External compression

Box 12.9: Causes of large bowel obstruction

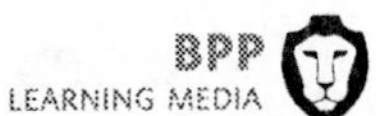

S Abdominal distension, generalised abdo tenderness, tinkling bowel sounds, palpable mass, empty rectum on PR.

Sx Constipation, no flatus in complete obstruction (flatus in partial obstruction), generalised abdo pain, late onset vomiting, dehydration.

I Bloods: FBC, U&Es.

Erect CXR: looking for air under diaphragm indicating perforation.

AXR: central, dilated loops of large bowel, >5cm (distinguished by haustral folds which partially cross bowel diameter).

CT abdo: identify level and cause of obstruction.

Gastrografin follow-through: identify level and cause of obstruction.

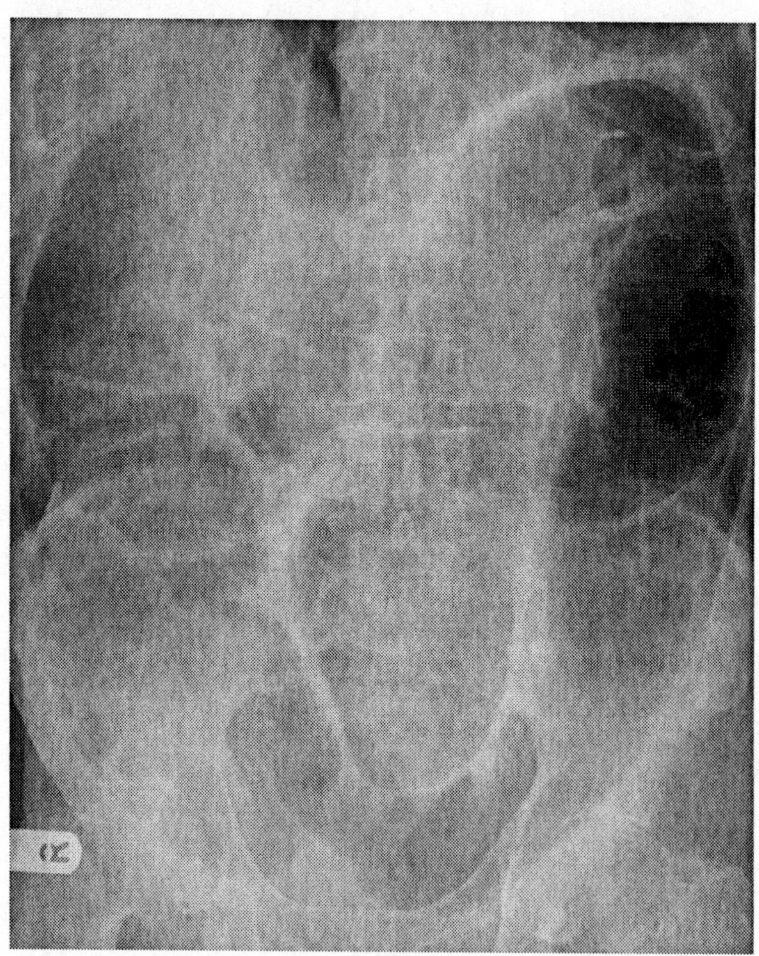

Figure 12.7: AXR showing sigmoid volvulus.
(Reproduced with permission from SW Deanery.)

T Immediate: NBM, nasogastric tube and IV fluids 'drip and suck', urinary catheter to monitor fluid balance. May not be adequate as large bowel produces 9L of fluid per day.

Treat underlying cause eg flatus tube for volvulus.

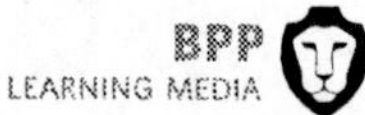

If no improvement may require surgical resection +/- resection with temporary colostomy.

C Perforation (in 20% patients ileocaecal valve remains closed increasing pressure on thin-walled caecum leading to perforation), peritonitis, severe dehydration, death.

Pr Dependent on underlying cause.

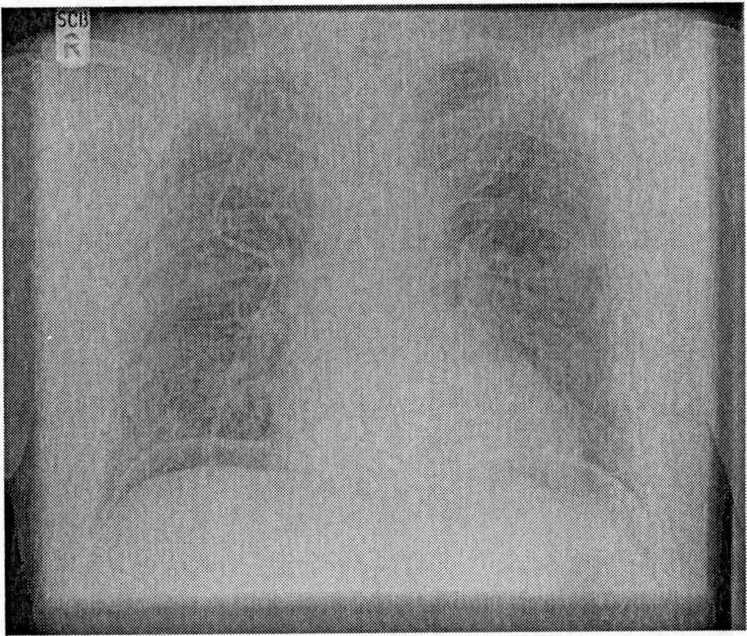

Figure 12.8: Erect CXR showing air under diaphragm caused by large bowel perforation. (Reproduced with permission from SW Deanery.)

Pseudo-obstruction / ileus

P Obstruction due to reduction / cessation of peristalsis.

Ogilvie's syndrome: acute large bowel pseudo-obstruction.

A See Box 12.10.

- Post-surgery
- Sepsis
- Hypokalaemia
- Hyponatraemia
- Uraemia
- Drugs: anti-cholinergics
- Neurological disorders

Box 12.10: Causes of ileus

S Abdo distension, generalised abdo tenderness complete absence of bowel sounds (no peristalsis).

Sx Generalised abdo pain, vomiting, constipation, no flatus.

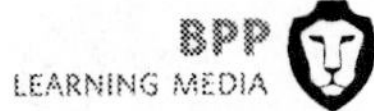

I Exclude mechanical cause as above.

Bloods: ↑ WCC, ↑ K^+, ↑ Na^{2+}, ↑ U&Es.

T Correct electrolyte disturbance, treat infection.

NBM, IVI fluids, NGT, pro-kinetics may help in some cases.

Intussusception

P Telescoping / invagination of proximal bowel into distal segment.

A Usually presents between 2 months and 2 years.

Peyer's patches are believed to be causative.

Associated with Meckel's diverticulum and HSP.

S Triad of symptoms: abdominal pain, bleeding per rectum (red currant jelly stools) and palpable mass.

Patients: may present in extremis with signs of shock and sepsis.

I AXR, USS: target lesions of telescoped bowel.

T Fluid resuscitate, triple antibiotics, NG decompression if there are signs of obstruction.

Air enema under radiological control (success rate around 85%). Contraindicated if there are signs of perforation.

Laparotomy if signs of peritonitis, perforation, or failure of air enema.

Appendicitis

P Inflammation of the appendix.

Appendiceal artery is an end-artery meaning inflammation leads to necrosis then perforation. Appendix attaches to the caecum, exact location to the caecum may differ between individuals.

A Commonest cause of emergency abdominal surgery in UK.

Uncommon at extremes of age.

Due to obstruction by faecolith (80%) or lymphoid hyperplasia.

S Fever, tachycardia, localised tenderness in RIF maximal at McBurney's point (See Box 12.11), guarding and percussion tenderness indicate peritonism, right-sided tenderness on PR.

Rovsing's sign: pain exacerbated in RIF when palpating LIF.

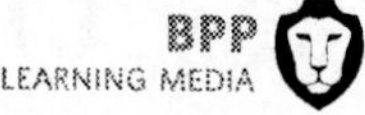

Sx Central, umbilical pain moving to RIF, worse on movement, coughing, anorexia, nausea, loose stool.

- Initially pain begins around umbilicus indicating appendiceal inflammation. Appendix and caecum localise pain poorly hence referral to umbilicus.
- Pain then localises to RIF, maximal at McBurney's point in several hours as inflammation progresses.
- McBurney's point: 1/3 distance from ASIS to umbilicus it approximates to the most common location of the appendix. Tenderness indicates irritation of overlying peritoneum as inflammation worsens.
- In a retrocaecal appendix (appendix is obscured by gas-filled caecum) RIF localisation may not occur.
- Rovsing's sign: deep palpation in LIF increases pressure in RIF around appendix exacerbating pain.

Box 12.11: Anatomy and pathology of appendicitis signs and symptoms

I Bloods: ↑ WCC, ↑ CRP, β-HCG (to exclude ectopic pregnancy). Bloods may be normal.

USS/CT abdo/pelvis (if diagnosis unclear): may show appendix mass, abscess or ovarian pathology in females.

Diagnostic laparoscopy: may be useful where there is doubt in young women who may have O&G pathology.

T IVI fluids, analgesia, IV abx if septic or perforation on appendicectomy.

Open or laparoscopic appendicectomy.

C Perforation: localised appendix abscess or generalised peritonitis. Appendix mass: omentum adheres to appendix and caecum due to inflammation.

Pr Good if diagnosed and treated quickly.

Diverticular disease

P Acquired outpouchings of colonic mucosa due to pressure at weak points in the colon where blood vessels enter colonic mucosa.

Diverticulosis: presence of asymptomatic diverticula, incidental finding.

Diverticular disease: symptomatic diverticula.

Diverticulitis: diverticula inflammation.

A Peak age 50–70 years. Associated with low dietary fibre. Commonest in sigmoid colon.

S Fever, LIF tenderness, PR: pain +/- blood.

Sx *Diverticular disease:* intermittent abdo / LIF pain, altered bowel habit.

Diverticulitis: rapid onset fever, nausea, abdo / LIF pain with altered bowel habit +/- PR bleed.

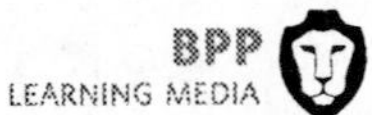

I Bloods: ↑ WCC, ↑ CRP in diverticulitis.

Gastrografin enema: assess number and location of diverticula.

CT abdo, flexi sig or colonoscopy to assess complications and exclude malignancy.

T Conservative: high fibre diet, increase fluid intake, stool softeners. IV abx for episodes of diverticulitis.

Surgical (failure of conservative treatment or perforation): resection and primary anastomosis if possible or Hartmann's procedure with anastomosis three to four months after.

C Pericolic abscess, perforation and peritonitis, fistula (colovisical, colovaginal), colonic stricture formation.

Polyps

P Group of protuberant growths into the bowel lumen. They may be benign or malignant, sessile or pedunculated.

• Adenomas: glandular tissue, have potential to undergo malignant change. Sessile > pedunculated.	
Adenoma shape and malignant potential	Adenoma size and malignant potential
• Tubular 70% all adeomas (5% become malignant) • Villous 10% all adenomas (40% become malignant) • Tubulovillous 2% all adenomas (20% become malignant)	• <1cm diameter 1% • 1–2cm diameter 10% • >40% diameter 40%
• Hamartomas: rare. May be solitary eg Juvenile polyp or multiple eg Peutz-Jegher syndrome	
• Familial adenomatous polyposis (FAP): rare autosomal dominant condition, gene on long arm chromosome 5. Hundreds of polyps cover colon and rectum. Malignant change <aged 40 years in almost all patients. Treated with prophylactic colectomy.	

Box 12.12: Polyps

Colonic malignancy

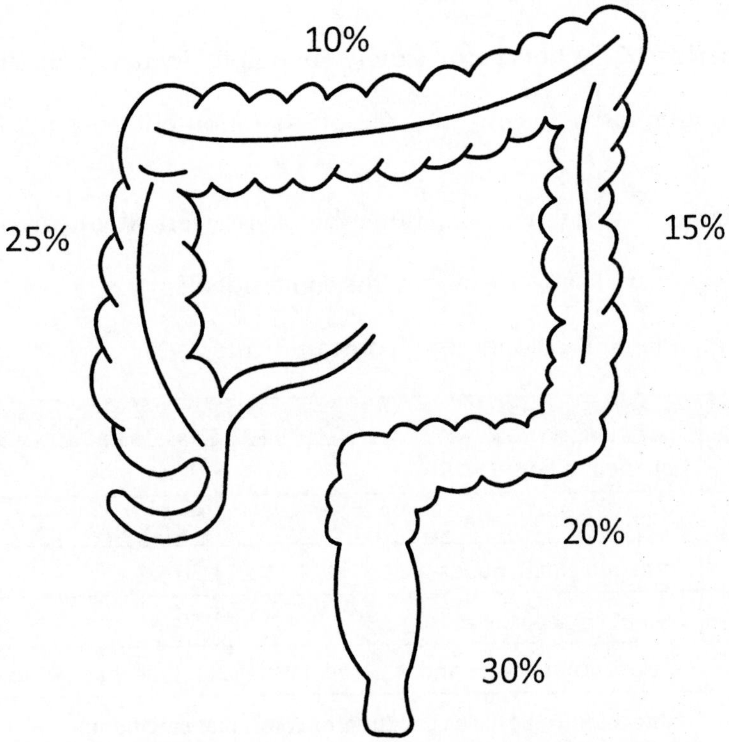

Figure 12.9: Distribution of colorectal cancer

P Most are adenocarcinomas. Adenoma to carcinoma sequence due to mutated tumour suppressor genes and activated oncogenes. See Figure 12.9.

A Second highest incidence and mortality rates in UK, male:female 3:1, peak age 45–65. See Box 12.13.

- Low fibre / high fat diet
- Chronic Colonic UC or Crohn's Disease (risk higher in UC)
- Radiation
- Colonic polyps
- Familial adenomatous polyposis (FAP): see above
- Hereditary non-polyposis colon cancer (HNPCC): autosomal dominant condition with increased incidence of right sided carcinomas but few polyps (non-polyposis)
- Family history of colorectal cancer

Box 12.13: Risk factors for colorectal cancer

S Anaemia, palpable abdominal mass, lymphadenopathy, PR: palpable mass, blood.

Sx Right-sided: Iron deficiency anaemia (may be only sign), weight loss.

Left-sided: change in bowel habit, tenesmus, PR bleeding. Emergency presentation (40%): obstruction, perforation.

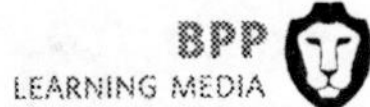

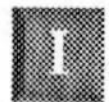 Bloods: iron deficiency anaemia.

Tumour markers: CEA not useful acutely but helpful in managing disease progression.

CT abdo: non-invasive, useful in acute presentation but does not allow biopsy, also TNM staging.

Flexible sigmoidoscopy: visualisation + biopsy for left-sided tumours.

Colonoscopy: visualisation + biopsy for right-sided.

Gastrografin enema if colonoscopy contraindicated.

Dukes' grade	Spread	Five-year survival
A	Confined to bowel wall	90%
B	Through bowel wall	70%
C	Spread to lymph nodes	30%
D	Distant metastases	5%
NB Grade D added to Dukes' classification later and is based on clinical rather than pathological evidence.		

Table 12.3: Dukes' classification of colorectal carcinoma

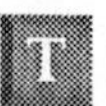 Based on staging, curative resection if no mets.

Right-sided: right hemicolectomy.

Left-sided: left hemicolectomy.

Sigmoid rectum: anterior resection.

Anorectal: abdomino-perineal resection.

+/- Adjuvant / neo-adjuvant chemo / radiotherapy.

C Obstruction, perforation.

Pr See Table 12.3.

Stomas

Colostomy	Ileostomy
• These can be end or loop colostomies, temporary or permanent. • Usually sited in the left iliac fossa and tend to be flush with the skin. • They have solid faeces and the bag needs changing usually once a day.	• Situated in the right iliac fossa and has a spout. • Discharges liquid effluent continuously and the bag may need changing several times a day. • The spout protects the surrounding skin from the corrosive nature of the effluent. • Ileostomies can be temporary, such as a defunctioning loop ileostomy after a left sided colon resection and anastomosis or permanent, after a total colectomy for inflammatory bowel disease.

Box 12.14: Colostomy versus ileostomy

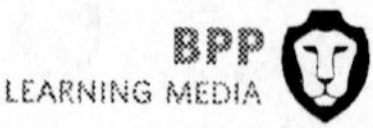

Hernias

P Abnormal protrusion of a viscus through its containing wall into an abnormal position.

A Usually due to a weakness or defect in the containing cavity, can be congenital or acquired.

C *Irreducible*: cannot be pushed back into original cavity, often due to a narrow neck or adherence of contents to the sac wall.

Obstructed: hernia contains obstructed but viable bowel.

Strangulated: hernia contents' blood supply is compromised.

Inguinal hernias

- Oblique passage from deep to superficial inguinal rings
- Contains spermatic cord and ilioinguinal nerve in males, round ligament and ilioinguinal nerve in females
- Deep inguinal ring: defect in transversalis fascia, lies 1cm above midpoint of inguinal ligament, immediately lateral to inferior epigastric artery
- Superficial inguinal ring: defect in inguinal ligament, lies above and medial to pubic tubercle
- Boundaries of inguinal canal (**MALT**)
  - Roof: internal oblique and transversus abdominis **M**uscle fibres
  - Anteriorly: external oblique **A**poneurosis and internal oblique
  - Floor: Inguinal **L**igament
  - Posteriorly: **T**ransversalis fascia

Box 12.15: Anatomy and boundaries of inguinal canal

P Protrusion of abdominal cavity contents through inguinal canal.

Direct: protrudes through a weakness in posterior wall of the canal appearing medial to inferior epigastric artery.

Indirect: passes through the deep ring, along the inguinal canal and (if large) into the scrotum lying lateral to the inferior epigastric artery.

A Commonest abdominal hernia, ♂:♀ 8:1.

Risk factors: raised intra-abdominal pressure eg obesity, chronic cough, straining or weakness of wall eg age, congenital.

S Hernia palpable above and medial to pubic tubercle, cough impulse, may be red and tender if strangulated.

Clinical distinction between direct and indirect inguinal hernias. See Box 12.16.

Sx Noticeable lump and groin pain both increasing on coughing / straining.

- Reduce hernia and apply finger pressure over deep inguinal ring (mid-point of inguinal ligament – half-way between ASIS and pubic tubercle)
- Ask the patient to cough
- Pressure over deep ring should maintain reduction of indirect hernia (passes through deep ring) on coughing
- Direct inguinal hernia will bulge out despite pressure over deep ring medial to point of pressure (passes through weakness in posterior wall of canal)

Box 12.16: Direct versus indirect inguinal hernias on examination

I Usually clinical diagnosis, CT or herniography if doubt.

T Conservative: weight loss, groin truss.

Surgical: laparoscopic or open hernia repair with mesh.

C Obstruction, strangulation (less frequent than femoral).

Pr Bilateral hernias frequent.

Femoral hernia

- Medial compartment of femoral sheath (covers femoral artery, vein and canal but not nerve)
- Canal contains: fat, lymphatics and Cloquet's lymph node
- Opens superiorly into abdomen via femoral ring
- Boundaries of femoral ring and canal:
  - Anteriorly: inguinal ligament
  - Posteriorly: pectineal ligament
  - Laterally: femoral vein
  - Medially: lacunar ligament

Box 12.17: Anatomy of femoral canal

P Protrusion of abdominal contents through femoral canal.

Femoral ring is narrow and lacunar ligament forms a sharp medial border increasing the risk of strangulation and irreducibility, see Box 12.17.

A ♀>♂ due to wider pelvis.

S Hernia palpable below and lateral to pubic tubercle, difficult to reduce, no cough impulse, may be red and tender if strangulated.

Sx Small lump, 30% present as emergencies due to risk of strangulation and obstruction.

I Clinical diagnosis.

T Always require surgical repair due to risk of strangulation.

C High risk of strangulation and obstruction.

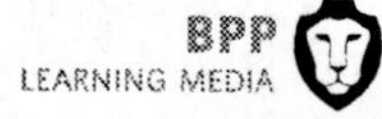

Incisional hernia

P Protrusion of viscus through the scar / incision of previous operation or injury with skin intact.

Most have a large neck so minimal risk of strangulation.

A Risk factors include: surgical closure technique, wound infection, steroids, malnutrition, elderly, increased abdominal pressure (obesity, cough).

S Lump at site of scar.

Sx Noticeable lump.

I Clinical diagnosis.

T Conservative: weight loss, groin truss.

Surgical: reduction and mesh or suture repair.

C Risk of recurrence despite repair.

Rectum and anus

Haemorrhoids

P Dilation and displacement of endoanal vascular cushions. Greek term meaning 'running-blood'.

Typically occur at sites of main anal blood vessels (3, 7 and 11 o'clock in supine / lithotomy position).

See Box 12.18.

- External: arise below dentate line
- Internal: arise above dentate line and sub-classified as:
  - Grade I: bleeding only
  - Grade II: prolapse, reduce spontaneously
  - Grade III: prolapse, require manual reduction
  - Grade IV: permanently prolapsed

Box 12.18: Classification of haemorrhoids

A Associated with: constipation, obesity, straining, childbirth, aging.

S Anaemia, lump at anal margin, usually not palpable on PR.

Sx Internal: painless rectal bleeding (no sensory fibres above dentate line), post-defecation bleeding (blood on toilet paper), feeling of a lump.

External: perianal pain, pruritus ani.

I Proctoscopy / sigmoidoscopy: visualise haemorrhoids.

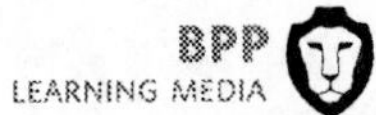

T Conservative: stool softeners, reduce intra-abdominal pressure.

Surgical: phenol oil injection, rubber band ligation, cauterisation / cryotherapy as an outpatient, haemorrhoidectomy if continued symptoms after above.

C External: thrombosis, internal: strangulation.

Pr 70–90% respond to band ligation or sclerotherapy.

Anal fissure

P Mucosal ischaemia secondary to internal sphincter muscle spasm results in painful fissure.

90% posterior midline, 10% anterior midline.

A Possibly associated with passage of hard stools, 5% associated with intersphincteric abscess.

S Visible fissure, sentinel pile (external hypertrophic skin tag).

Sx Pain on defecation, bright red PR bleeding, pruritus ani.

I Clinical diagnosis.

T Conservative: stool softeners, local anaesthetic cream, GTN cream relaxes anal sphincter, 50% heal spontaneously.

Surgery: anal dilatation or sphincterotomy.

C Need to exclude other causes of fissures eg Crohn's, TB, syphilis.

Anorectal abscess

P Infection in one of the anal crypts resulting in abscess formation.

E. coli if from pelvic infection, staph aureus if from hair follicle infection.

Classified by location: perianal (60%), ischiorectal (20%), intersphincteric (5%), supralevator (4%).

A Risk factors include: immunosuppression, diabetes, Crohn's.

S Fever, fluctuant abscess mass visible.

Sx Severe pain limiting ability to sit, exacerbated by defecation.

I Examination under anaesthetic (EUA): to assess abscess due to pain.

CT/MRI for intersphincteric and supralevator abscesses.

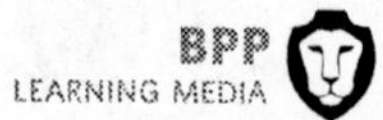

T IV abx, incision and drainage under GA.

C Fistula-in-ano formation.

Fistula in-ano

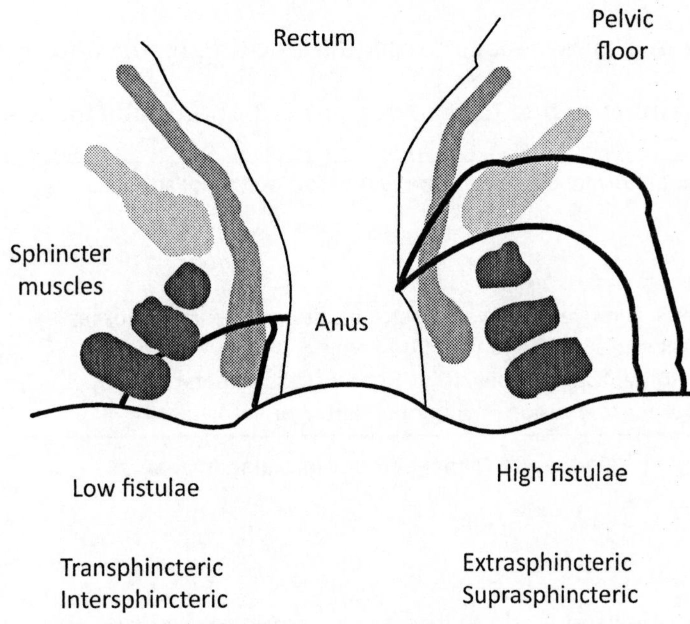

Figure 12.10: Fistulae-in-ano

P Abnormal connection between anorectal lining and perineal or vaginal skin.

Goodsall's rule: an external opening situated posterior to the transverse anal line will open into the anal canal in the midline posteriorly, an anterior opening will follow a curved path to open in the midline.

- Low fistulae
  - Intersphincteric (70%)
  - Transphincteric (25%)
- High fistulae
  - Suprasphincteric (5%)
  - Extrasphincteric (<1%)

Box 12.19: Parks' classification of anal fistulae

A Majority arise from previous anorectal abscess.

Risk factors: radiotherapy, Crohn's TB, malignancy.

S Pustular discharge from tract opening, visible opening on skin with surrounding erythema, recurrent fevers / sepsis.

Sx Perianal pain, perianal discharge.

I EUA: to visualise fistula.

MRI pelvis: assess passage of fistula.

T IV abx.

Low fistula in ano: open with fistulotomy.

High fistula in ano: two-stage procedure opening fistula and inserting seton suture.

C Post-op incontinence due to involvement of puborectalis muscle.

Fistula: abnormal connection between two epithelial surfaces

SNAP

- **S**epsis: remove source, protect skin, drain concurrent abscesses
- **N**utrition: optimise to promote healing
- **A**natomy: fistulography, CT/MRI to visualise tracts
- **P**roceed: to excision, laying open and / or seton suture

Box 12.20: Management of fistulae in general

Pilonidal abscess

P Hair follicle infection leads to abscess or sinus formation with hair trapped in sinus, 'Pilonidal' = 'nest of hair'.

Usually occurring in midline of buttock clefts.

A ♂:♀ 4:1, risk factors: hirsuitism, long-seated periods.

S Purulent discharging sinus, fever.

Sx Recurrent pain and discharge.

I Clinical diagnosis, MRI to assess sinus path.

T Conservative: abx, hygiene advice.

Surgical: incision and drainage of abscess / sinus under GA

Rectal prolapse

P Prolapse of rectum through anus.

Partial thickness: only mucosa prolapsed.

Full thickness: all wall layers prolapsed.

A Risk factors: post-menopausal, multiparous women, constipation, chronic straining, cystic fibrosis.

S Sx Partial thickness: small visible mass, mucous discharge, pruritus ani, small PR bleeding.

Full thickness: visible external prolapsing mass following defecation, reduced sphincter tone, PR bleeding.

I Sigmoidoscopy.

T Conservative: stool softeners, avoid straining.

Partial: phenol injection, banding.

Full thickness: Delorme's procedure or transabdominal rectopexy.

Anal carcinoma

P 80% squamous cell carcinoma, rest are melanoma, lymphoma and adenocarcinoma.

A Uncommon, 300 cases per year in UK.

Associated with HPV infection causing anal warts, increased incidence in homosexuals.

S Sx Perianal pain and bleeding (50%), palpable mass (only in 25%), faecal incontinence, palpable superficial inguinal nodes.

I EUA with biopsy, CT/MRI to assess spread.

T 50% respond to radiotherapy, surgical resection if this fails.

C Rectovaginal fistula.

Pr Five-year survival: 50%.

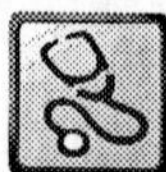 Practice Questions

Single Best Answers

1. The following occurs in small bowel obstruction:

   A Early vomiting
   B PR bleeding
   C Palpable groin mass
   D Dysphagia

2. What percentage of anal carcinomas are SCC?

   A 10%
   B 40%
   C 50%
   D 80%

3. What percentage of gallstones are visible on AXR?

   A 45%
   B 80%
   C 10%
   D 25%

4. The commonest cause of pancreatitis is:

   A Gallstones
   B Alcohol
   C ERCP
   D Steroids

5. Meckel's diverticulum is located

   A Two feet from the ileocaecal valve
   B Two feet from the splenic flexure
   C Two inches from the appendix
   D Two inches from the hepatic flexure

6. The following has the highest malignant potential:

   A Tubular adenoma
   B Villous adenoma
   C Tubulovillous adenoma
   D Hamartoma

7. The following is the correct Dukes' classification grade.

   A Grade A and 60% five-year survival
   B Grade D and 30% five-year survival
   C Grade B and 70% five-year survival
   D Grade C and distant metastases

8. 90% of gastric carcinomas are:

   A Adenocarcinomas
   B Squamous cell carcinomas
   C Lymphomas
   D Stromal cell tumours

9. McBurney's point is:

   A 1/3 distance from ASIS to pubic tubercle
   B 2/3 distance from umbilicus to ASIS
   C 2/3 distance from pubic tubercle to umbilicus
   D 1/3 distance from umbilicus to ASIS

10. The following appears medial to the inferior epigastric artery on operation:

   A Direct inguinal hernia
   B Indirect inguinal hernia
   C Femoral hernia
   D Incisional hernia

Extended Matching Questions

Colostomies and ileostomies

A Ileal conduit
B Defunctioning loop ileostomy
C End ileostomy
D Parastomal hernia
E Prolapsed colostomy
F Hartman's procedure: end colostomy
G Loop colostomy
H Subtotal colectomy and end ileostomy

For each of the following scenarios, choose the **single** most likely diagnosis from the above list of options. Each option may be used once, more than once or not at all.

1. A 69-year-old patient has a midline scar and stoma in the right iliac fossa, where there is urine in the bag.

2. An 85-year-old man presented with perforated diverticular disease in the sigmoid colon. After resuscitation he had an emergency procedure.

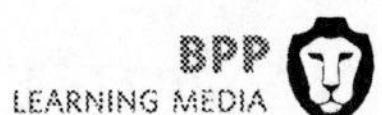

3. A 65-year-old man undergoes elective excision of a rectal carcinoma and primary anastomosis. He is left with a stoma.

4. A 25-year-old man with a history of ulcerative colitis, deteriorates and requires an emergency operation to treat the disease. He is left with a stoma.

5. A 72-year-old woman has disseminated malignancy of the colon. She presents with abdominal distension and increasing constipation. She has a procedure before going on to palliative care.

Dysphagia

A Achalasia
B Carcinoma of oesophagus
C TIA
D Thyroid goitre
E Myasthenia gravis
F Inflammatory oesophageal stricture
G Plummer-vinson syndrome
H Carcinoma of bronchus
I Hiatus hernia
J Pharyngeal pouch

For each of the following scenarios, choose the **single** most likely diagnosis from the above list of options. Each option may be used once, more than once or not at all.

6. A 35-year-old woman has a ten-year history of low retrosternal dysphagia and painless regurgitation of food in the mouth.

7. A 65-year-old woman has progressive low retrosternal dysphagia, initially to solids, but now also to liquids over the last four months. There has also been loss of appetite and 3kg weight loss.

8. A 45-year-old lady presents with high retrosternal dysphagia. She has spoon-shaped nails and is noted to be pale.

9. A 40-year-old man presents with dysphagia that worsens as he eats. He has droopy eyelids and sometimes has difficulty in speaking.

10. A 50-year-old man has a 20-year history of acid sometimes regurgitating into his mouth from his stomach; more recently he has low retrosternal dysphagia at times.

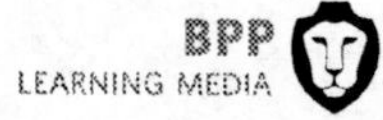

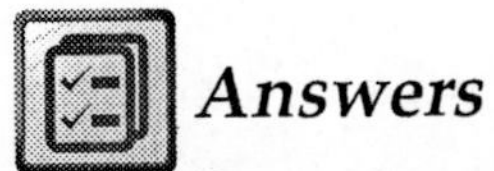

Answers

SBAs		EMQs	
1	A	1	A
2	D	2	F
3	C	3	B
4	A	4	H
5	A	5	G
6	B	6	I
7	C	7	B
8	A	8	G
9	B	9	E
10	A	10	F

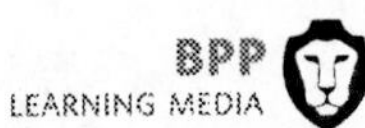

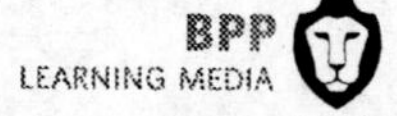

Chapter 13

Vascular surgery

Mr Alexander Young and Mr John Loy

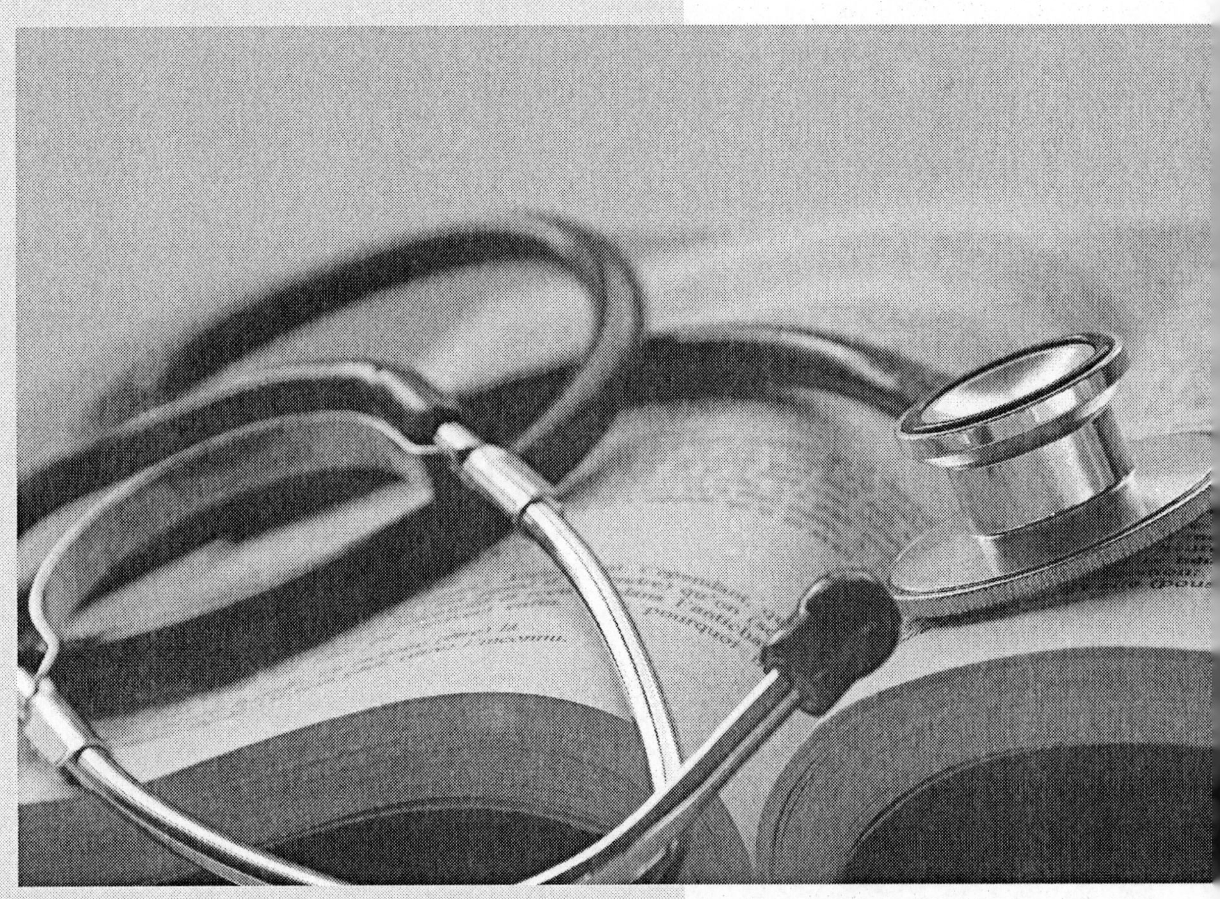

Key investigations

- **ABPI**: ankle brachial pressure index. Usually BP is higher in legs than arms. In diabetes calcification of vessels can give falsely elevated results
  >1 = normal
  0.9-0.6 = claudication
  0.6-0.3 = rest pain
  <0.3 = critical ischemia
- **Angiography**: injection of radiolucent dye into arteries to highlight areas of occlusion
- **Duplex USS**: ultrasound test that uses duplex technique to analyse flow in arteries and veins and to identify occlusion
- **Hand-held doppler**: useful tool for quickly listening to arterial or venous flow through vessels. Arteries normally have a biphasic flow sound with monophasic indicating occlusion or poor flow.

Peripheral vascular disease

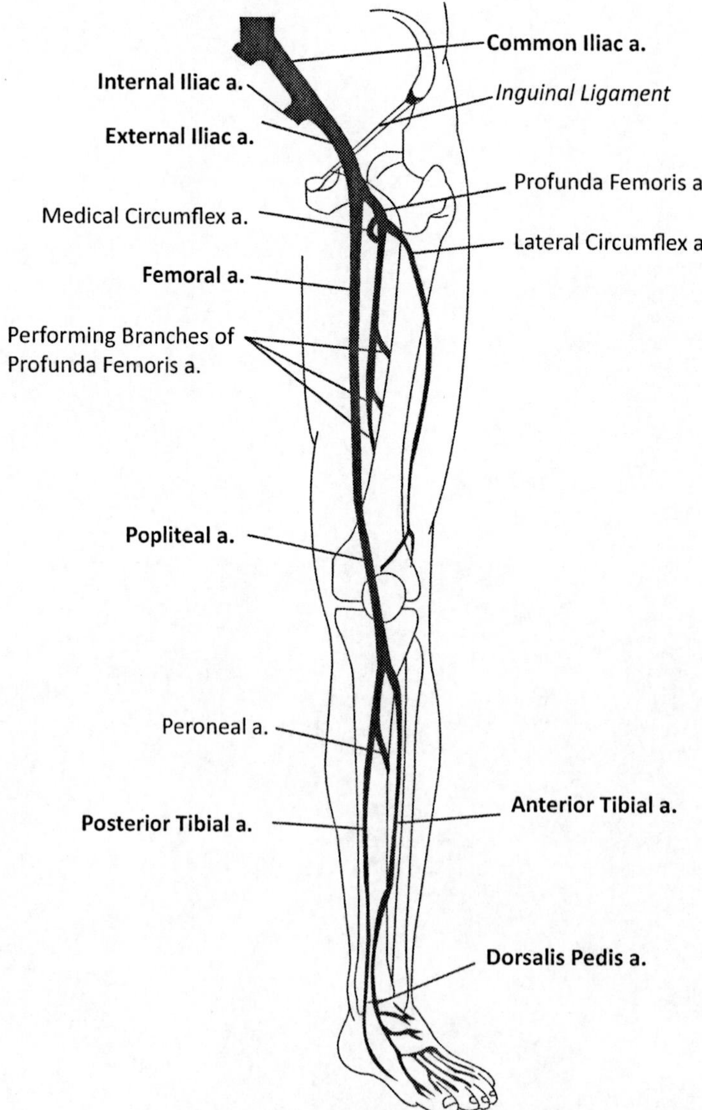

Figure 13.1: Arteries of the lower limb

Acute limb ischaemia

P Sudden onset arterial occlusion with no time for collateral vessel formation (unless pre-existing occlusive disease) resulting in inadequate perfusion to distal tissues.

A See Box 13.1.

- Acute thrombosis in-situ (60%)
  - Acute occlusion in a vessel with pre-existing atherosclerosis
  - Risk factors: dehydration, malignancy, hypotension, prothrombotic disorders
- Emboli (30–40%)
  - Cardiac cause (80%): AF, MI, prosthetic / damaged heart valves
  - Also from aneurysm, tumour, foreign body
- Other causes
  - Trauma, peripheral aneurysm (popliteal), dissecting aneurysm

Box 13.1: Causes of acute limb ischemia

S Sx See Box 13.2 'The Six Ps'.

Thrombosis in-situ: history of intermittent claudication, slower onset, no embolic source, contralateral limb affected.

Embolic: no claudication history, rapid onset with complete occlusion, cardiac source eg AF, murmur, MI.

Onset of fixed mottling of skin implies irreversibility.

The Six **P**s

- Pain
- Pallor
- Pulselessness
- Perishing cold
- Paraesthesia
- Paralysis

Box 13.2: Signs and symptoms of acute limb ischemia

I FBC, clotting, glucose, G&S, ECG: dysrhythmias, CXR.

T *Immediate*: oxygen and IVI fluids, analgesia and heparinise, treat underlying cardiac conditions.

Thrombosis in-situ: thrombolysis, angioplasty, bypass surgery.

Embolic: embolectomy, thrombolysis.

Amputation if irreversible.

C Loss of limb (40%): irreversible tissue damage at 6 hours, death (20%), complications from thrombolysis: CVE, retroperitoneal bleed.

Pr Dependent on underlying cause, generally poor.

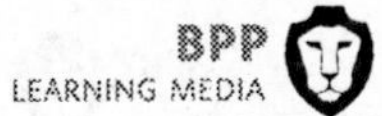

Chronic lower limb disease

P Gradual atherosclerotic arterial occlusion of aorto-iliac, femoral, popliteal or calf vessels with collateral vessel formation. Presents as intermittent claudication (perfusion inadequate for exercise) or critical limb ischemia (perfusion inadequate for basal metabolic requirements).

A 7% of men >50 years develop intermittent claudication.

1/3 improve, 1/3 remain stable and 1/3 deteriorate.

Risk factors: see Table 13.1.

Fixed	Modifiable
• Male • Elderly • Family history of atherosclerosis • Type 1 diabetes	• Obesity • Smoking • Hypertension • Hyperlipidaemia • Type 2 diabetes

Table 13.1: Fixed and modifiable risk factors for chronic lower limb disease

S Sx *Intermittent claudication:* pain on exercising affected limb and relieved by rest, claudication distance = pain on walking a fixed distance, site of pain depends on locations of stenosis:

- Aortic bifurcation → buttock pain
- External / internal iliac → thigh pain
- Femoral / popliteal → calf pain
- Leriche's syndrome → buttock pain and impotence due to aorto-iliac occlusion

Critical limb ischemia: rest pain worse at night and on elevation, relieved by hanging leg over side of bed.

European Working Group on Critical Limb Ischemia (1991) defined CLI as:

- Rest pain for >2 weeks not relieved by simple analgesia or
- Presence of gangrene / ulceration or
- Doppler ankle pressure <50mmHg (<30mmHg toe in diabetics)

- I: Asymptomatic
- II: Intermittent claudication (ABPI 0.9–0.6)
- III: Rest pain (ABPI 0.6–0.3)
- IV: Ulceration / Gangrene (ABPI<0.3)
- III & IV = Critical Limb Ischemia (CLI)

Box 13.3: La Fontaine Classification of Lower Limb Ischemia

I Clinical diagnosis, FBC, glucose, clotting, ↑ BP, ABPI <1, monophasic hand-held doppler signal, duplex doppler USS, angiography, MRA.

T *Risk factor modification*: exercise, smoking cessation, statins, anti-hypertensives, anti-glycaemics.

Endovascular: angioplasty +/- stent.

Surgery: bypass grafts, amputation.

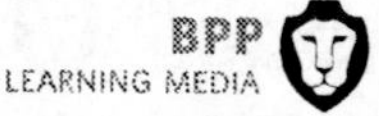

C Loss of limb.

Pr 10% IC and 50% CLI require amputation at five years.

20% IC and 50% CLI mortality at five years from IHD.

Chronic upper limb disease

P Occlusion of flow in arteries of the upper limb.

A See Box 13.4.

Buerger's disease: inflammation and occlusion of medium-sized arteries. Common in young, male, heavy smokers. May present with severe Raynaud's.

Subclavian steal syndrome: retrograde flow in the vertebral artery due to proximal stenosis. The arm is supplied at the expense of verterobasilar circulation reducing hindbrain perfusion. May present with dizziness, syncope or arm claudication.

Takayasu's arteritis: see *Rheumatology* chapter.

Thoracic outlet obstruction: compression of the neurovascular bundle at the superior thoracic outlet. May present with arm claudication, paraesthesia, pain or weakness exacerbated by elevating arm.

Trauma or axillary irradiation causing stenosis.

Box 13.4: Causes of chronic upper limb ischemia

S Sx Arm claudication, weakness, digital ischaemia or gangrene.

I XR C-spine, monophasic hand-held doppler USS, arterial duplex USS.

T *Buerger's disease:* smoking cessation, cervical sympathectomy.

Thoracic outlet obstruction: excision of 1st rib (improves symptoms in 90%).

Raynaud's disease

P Peripheral digital ischaemia due to vasospasm, worse in cold.

A Raynaud's disease is idiopathic occurring in females.

Raynaud's phenomenon associated with autoimmune and connective tissue disorders.

S Sx Digits classically change colour in stages, often triggered by cold: white (ischaemic), blue (cyanosis), red (hyperaemic).

I Clinical diagnosis, look for underlying cause.

T Smoking cessation, gloves in cold, sympathectomy.

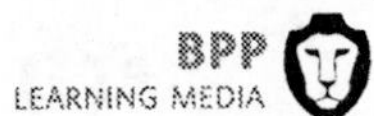

C Necrosis of digits if severe.

Carotid artery disease

P Atherosclerosis at bifurcation of common carotid artery.

Produce TIA/CVE due to embolus from plaque (80% strokes ischaemic).

A CVE incidence is 2/1,000 in the UK with 15% due to atherosclerosis of carotid arteries.

S Carotid bruit (detectable in 10% patients).

Sx Amaurosis fugax, TIA, crescendo TIAs, CVE.

I Glucose, lipid profile, carotid artery duplex USS, MRA.

T *Medical:* aspirin, reduce hypertension, cholesterol, blood sugar, smoking cessation.

Surgery: carotid endarterectomy (CEA) under GA or LA: see Box 13.5.

> Evidence supports CEA for symptomatic patients with severe (70–99%) stenosis and is moderately useful for symptomatic patients with moderate (50–69%) stenosis.
>
> - *ECST (Europe) and NASCET (USA) Trials:* for patients with 70–99% symptomatic stenosis the risk of stroke reduced by 15% at five years post-CEA compared to medical therapy only. Smaller risk reduction of 7% at five years for symptomatic patients with 50–69%.
> - *ACST (UK) and ACAS (USA) Trials:* some benefit for asymptomatic patients with >70% stenosis but number needed to treat to prevent one stroke is 22.
> - *GALA Trial:* compared general anaesthetic (GA) to local anaesthetic (LA) for CEA and found no significant difference.

Box 13.5: Indications and evidence for carotid endarterectomy

C Stroke, death.

Pr Good if prompt investigations and referral.

Mesenteric disease

P Atherosclerosis or embolus obstructing arteries supplying bowel.

Usually SMA thrombus (35%) or embolus.

A AF with abdo pain suggests mesenteric ischemia.

S Tender abdomen, weight loss.

Sx Abdominal pain after eating, fear of eating, PR bleeding, shock.

I FBC, U&Es, ABG, lactate, mesenteric angiography, CT abdo.

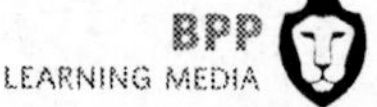

T Lapartomy and bowel resection for infarcted bowel.

C Total ischaemic bowel usually fatal.

Aneurysms

P Abnormal, localised dilatation of an artery.

True aneurysm: wall of aneurysm contains all three-layers of the vessel wall (intima, media and adventitia).

False / pseudo aneurysm: 'pulsating haematoma', wall formed by overlying connective tissue or adventitia only.

A Male:female 10:1, oestrogen protective, associated with atherosclerosis, smoking, hypertension, family history.

- True
  - Fusiform: dilatation affects whole circumference of the artery
  - Saccular: dilatation affects only part of the circumference
- False: pulsating haematoma, usually due to trauma. Transmits pulse but does not expand / contact itself
- Congenital
  - Berry aneurysms
- Acquired
  - Atheromatous peripheral aneurysm: eg popliteal, femoral, AAA (see below)
  - Mycotic aneurysm: associated with any bacteraemia weakening vessel wall (eg salmonella, subacute endocarditis)
  - Syphylitic aneurysm: seen in progressive syphilis infection, tends to affect thoracic aorta and arch

Box 13.6: Types of aneurysms

Abdominal aortic aneurysm (AAA)

P Atherosclerotic or inflammatory. 95% are infrarenal.

A More common in males, 3% >50 years.

S 40 % detected incidentally and are asymptomatic, pulsatile mass.

Sx Back / loin pain (may mimic pyelonephritis), rupture causes shock, severe pain and collapse.

I USS, CT abdomen.

T See Box 13.7.

Non-surgical: lower hypertension, glucose, cholesterol, smoking cessation.

Surgical: open repair with synthetic graft, endovascular repair with graft (EVAR).

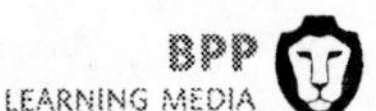

Small aneurysms trial: aneurysms <5.5cm do not require surgical repair
• Aneurysms <5.5cm: six-monthly USS surveillance • Aneurysms >5.5cm or expanding by >1cm/year: surgical repair

Box 13.7: Management of AAA

C Risk of rupture increases with aneurysm diameter.

- <5.5cm = <1%/year
- >5.5cm = 25%/year

Death, renal failure, ischaemic bowel, limb loss.

Pr Rupture mortality 50–80% even with surgery.

Popliteal aneurysm

P Atherosclerosis in popliteal artery.

A Commonest peripheral aneurysm, occurs in 10% patients with AAA, >50% bilateral.

S Sx Often asymptomatic, pulsatile mass, distal ischaemia with thrombosis or embolus.

I Duplex USS.

T Reduce risk factors, bypass surgery.

C Thrombosis / embolus is biggest complication leading to distal ischaemia and potential limb loss, rupture.

Pr Good if treated early.

Aortic dissection

P Tear in the intima layer of the aorta allowing blood to flow between the layers forcing them apart. Tear can extend antegrade or retrograde. Retrograde spread can produce aortic incompetence and MI. See Box 13.8.

A Male:female 2:1, peak in 6th–7th decade.

Associated with hypertension, Marfan's, Ehlers-Danlos, Turner's, syphilis infection.

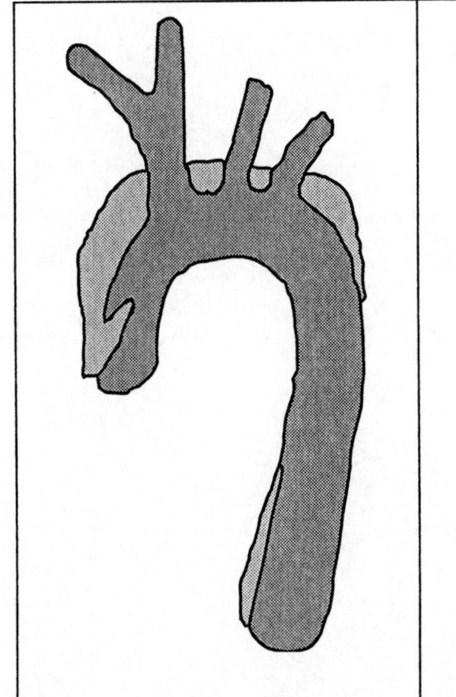	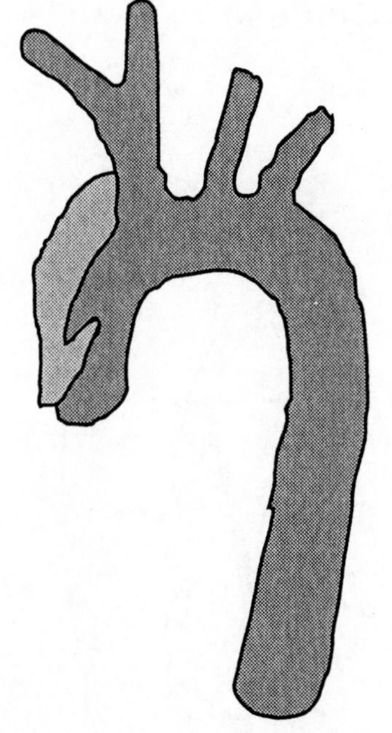	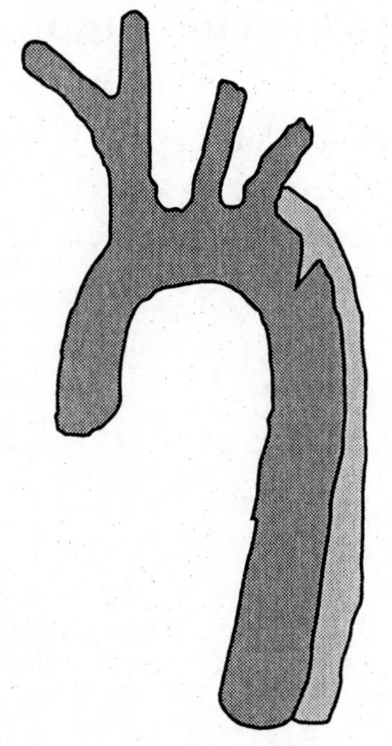
Stanford Type A (ascending aorta) DeBakey I (60%) (ascending aorta + descending aorta)	Stanford Type A (ascending aorta) DeBakey II (10%) (confined to ascending aorta)	Stanford Type B (descending aorta) DeBakey III (30%) (confined to descending aorta, beyond subclavian artery)

Box 13.8: Stanford and DeBakey classifications of aortic dissection

S Unequal pulses / BP, shock, aortic regurgitation in retrograde tear.

Sx Sudden onset tearing chest pain radiating to between scapula (96%), limb weakness.

I FBC, G&S, CXR: widened mediastinum, ECHO, CT/MRI, ECG.

T Stanford Type A: emergency requiring surgery to replace affected part with graft.

Stanford Type B: medical control of hypertension.

C Death, CVE, MI, limb ischemia.

Pr 80% mortality in Stanford Type A, 50% of patients die before getting to hospital.

Venous and lymphatic disease

Varicose veins

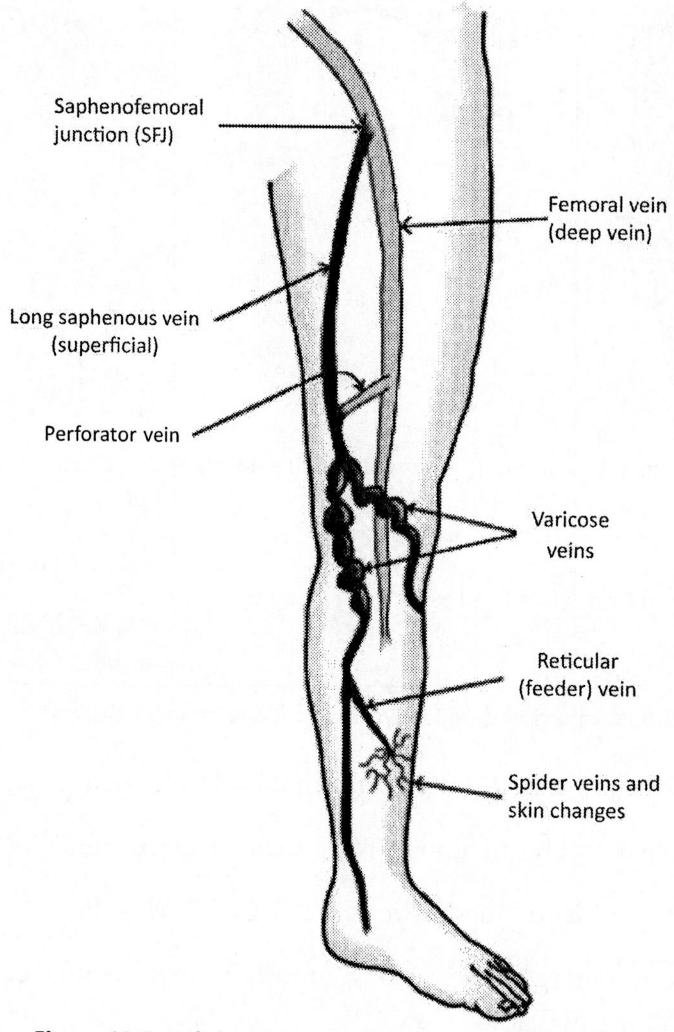

Figure 13.2: Left leg varicose veins in long saphenous system (short saphenous vein on lateral calf running to saphenopopliteal junction)

P Tortuous, dilated veins due to failure of one-way valves in perforator vessels which connect superficial to deep venous systems.

Superficial veins will join either the long saphenous or short saphenous veins.

Perforators are located in calf and at saphenofemoral, saphenopopliteal and mid-thigh points.

A Affects 20% population, female:male 10:1.

Primary idiopathic or secondary due to pelvic mass (eg pregnancy, pelvic tumour) or venous damage (eg post DVT).

S Tortuous dilated veins, large 'blow-out' veins at sites of incompetence, cough impulse, tap impulse on percussion, superficial 'spider' veins, venous skin changes (varicose eczema, brown pigmentation due to haemosiderin deposition, lipodermatosclerosis).

Sx Often asymptomatic, tender, cramp-like pain worse at end of day.

I Hand-held doppler: listens for reflux over SFJ and SPJ while squeezing calf, a biphasic signal on releasing calf squeeze indicates reflux and incompetence.

Tourniquet test: tourniquet applied to thigh, patient stands, if veins below tourniquet fill up incompetent perforators are below that level.

Trendelenburg test: direct digital pressure is applied rather than a tourniquet.

Venous duplex USS: gold standard.

T *Medical:* compression stockings.

Surgery: venous stripping, local avulsions, foam sclerotherapy, laser ablation.

C Eczema, thrombophlebitis, lipodermatosclerosis, ulcers.

Lymphoedema

P Failure of lymphatic drainage causing oedema.

A Primary at birth or in teens (Milroy's syndrome) or secondary due to infection, malignancy, trauma or radiotherapy.

S Oedematous limb, lymphadenopathy in infection / malignancy.

Sx Swollen, heavy limb.

I Clinical diagnosis.

T Medical: compression garments / bandages, manual drainage.

Surgical: bypass, excision of tissue.

C Cellulitis, lymphangitis, ulcers.

Ulcers

Arterial

P Break down in epithelial surface due to underlying chronic ischemia.

A Atherosclerosis.

S Punched-out edge, deep, sloughy base, signs of limb ischemia (six Ps).

Sx Painful at rest, ulceration over pressure areas: toes, lateral malleolus, heels.

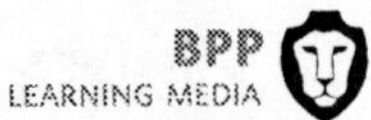

I Biopsy, investigate for chronic limb ischemia.

T Treat underlying cause of ischemia, debridement, skin graft, amputation if severe.

C Necrosis, loss of limb.

Diabetic

P Due to neurovascular complications of diabetes.

Pure neuropathic ulcers (45%), ischaemic ulcers (10%), mixed neuroischaemic ulcers (45%).

A Diabetes with neuropathy (peripheral / Charcot's Joints), previous ulceration, visual impairment, living alone, peripheral vascular disease.

S Sx Sensory loss with unrecognised local trauma, pulses may be intact or absent, painless ulceration over pressure areas and areas of trauma: toes, balls of feet, malleoli.

I Glucose, biopsy, ABPI may be falsely elevated due to calcification of vessels, XR for osteomyelitis.

T Treat infection if present, treat underlying ischaemia and diabetes, amputation.

C Infection, gangrene, amputation.

Venous

P Break down in epithelial surface due to chronic venous insufficiency.

A Chronic venous disease, post-thrombotic limb.

S Sloped edge, shallow, granulation tissue at base, surrounding venous eczema, lipodermatosclerosis.

Sx Painless at rest, painful on palpation.

I Venous duplex USS, biopsy.

T Compression stockings, treat underlying venous disease, debridement and skin graft if severe.

C Marjolin's ulcer: SCC in chronic venous ulcer, infection.

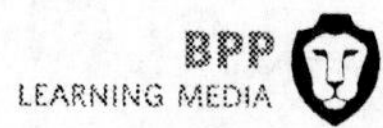

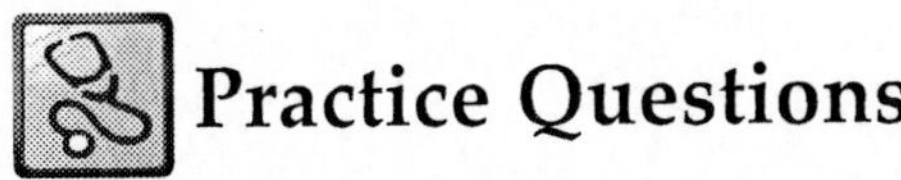

Practice Questions

Single Best Answers

1. What percentage of AAAs occur below the renal vessels?

   A 10%
   B 45%
   C 75%
   D 95%

2. In aortic dissection which of the following requires urgent surgical treatment?

   A Stanford Type B
   B Stanford Type A
   C DeBakey III
   D La Fontaine I

3. Arterial ulcers are usually:

   A Painless at rest
   B Associated with a glove and stocking peripheral neuropathy
   C Deep
   D With rolled edges

4. Regarding popliteal aneurysms:

   A They are less common than femoral artery aneurysms
   B The main complication is rupture
   C 25% are bilateral
   D They occur in 10% of AAAs

5. Regarding abdominal aortic aneurysms:

   A They present with pain and a pulsatile mass in 90% cases
   B They may mimic pyelonephritis
   C The Small Aneurysms Trial advised surgery in aneurysms <4.5cm
   D They are more common in females

6. The following ABPI reading is consistent with intermittent claudication.

   A <0.1
   B 0.3–0.6
   C >1
   D 0.6–0.9

7. The major cause of acute limb ischaemia is

   A Acute thrombus in-situ
   B Embolus
   C Trauma
   D Infection

8. Features of critical limb ischaemia include

   A Pain on exercise relieved by simple analgesia
   B Doppler ankle pressure >50mmHg
   C Presence of gangrene
   D Asymptomatic

9. The following is true regarding carotid artery disease.

   A CEA should be offered to symptomatic patients with stenosis >70%
   B The GALA trial showed local anaesthetic to be superior to GA when performing CEA
   C A carotid bruit is detectable in 80% patients
   D 80% of stokes due to carotid artery disease are haemorrhagic

10. The classic digital colour changes in Raynaud's are:

   A Blue, White, Red
   B Red, White, Blue
   C White, Red, Blue
   D White, Blue, Red

Extended Matching Questions

Vascular presentations

A Dissecting aortic aneurysm
B AAA
C Intermittent claudication
D Critical limb ischaemia
E Buerger's disease
F Mesenteric ischaemia
G Carotid artery disease

For each of the following scenarios choose the **single** most likely diagnosis from the above list of options. Each option may be used once, more than once, or not at all.

1. A 22-year-old male smoker presents with severe Raynaud's phenomenon.

2. A 74-year-old smoker has thigh pain after walking 100 yards which is relieved by rest.

3. A 65-year-old man with AF reports abdominal pain after eating and stomach cramps.

4. A 64-year-old man states that he suffered a visual disturbance 'like a curtain coming down' over his left eye, which resolved.

5. A 58-year-old diabetic man has been referred in by his GP with suspected left pyelonephritis. He complains of left groin pain radiating to his back.

6. A 59-year-old lady attends A&E complaining of a sudden tearing pain in her chest and back. On examination she has unequal pulses.

7. A 68-year-old male smoker presents with left calf pain that is present at rest but relieved by hanging his leg out of his bed at night.

Ulceration

A Arterial
B Venous
C Marjolin's ulcer
D Diabetic
E BCC

For each of the following scenarios choose the **single** most likely diagnosis from the above list of options. Each option may be used once, more than once, or not at all.

8. A 70-year-old lady presents with a large ulcer over her medial malleolus. The ulcer is shallow with sloping edges.

9. An 84-year-old lady with a long history of venous ulceration of her left leg is referred in by her GP as one ulcer has recently extended and changed shape with eversion of its edges.

10. A 60-year-old male smoker with poorly controlled diabetes presents with a deep, painful ulcer over his lateral malleolus. ABPI on that leg is 0.9.

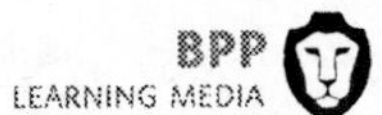

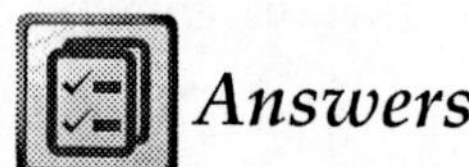

Answers

SBAs		EMQs	
1	D	1	E
2	B	2	C
3	C	3	F
4	D	4	G
5	B	5	B
6	D	6	A
7	A	7	D
8	C	8	B
9	A	9	C
10	D	10	A

Chapter 14

Breast surgery

Miss Jane Carter and
Miss Sarah Vestey

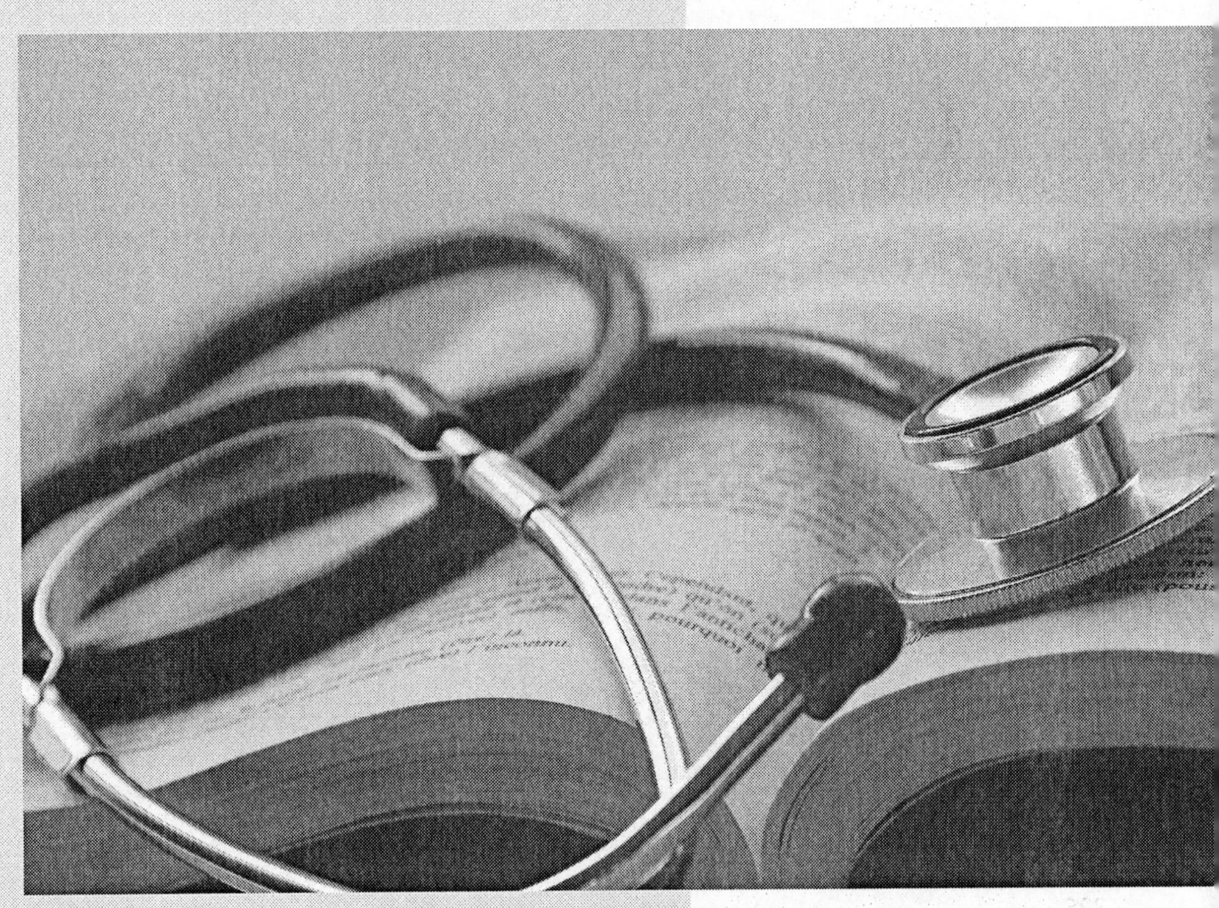

Key investigations

Ultrasound

- Effective diagnostic tool using high frequency sound waves
- Detects focal breast lesions
- Women <40 years as primary investigation
- Used in conjunction with mammography in women >40 years
- Not good at detecting pre-invasive cancer, so not recommended for screening
- Used routinely to guide biopsies
- Used in the pre-operative assessment of axillary lymph nodes in women with breast cancer

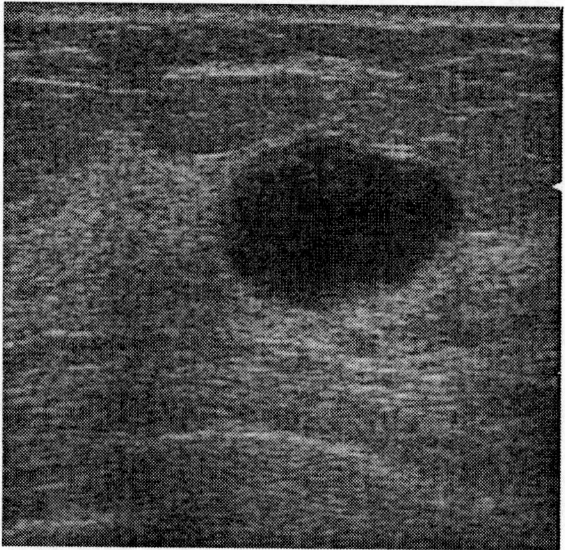

Figure 14.1: Cyst seen on ultrasound (well defined mass). (Reproduced with permission from SW Deanery.)

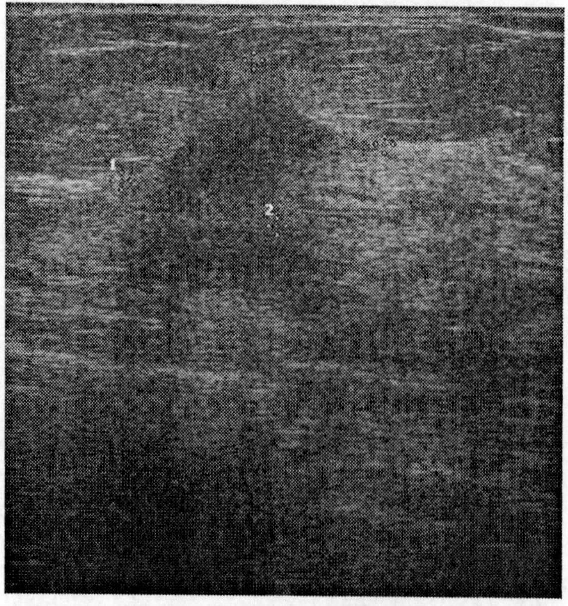

Figure 14.2: Cancer seen on ultrasound (ill defined mass). (Reproduced with permission from SW Deanery.)

Magnetic resonance imaging (MRI)

- Very sensitive but less specific imaging modality
- Used routinely in the assessment of extent / focality of tumours that are not well shown on mammogram (such as lobular cancers)
- Used in the imaging of women with breast implants and in screening of women under 40 at very high risk of developing breast cancer (eg gene defects)

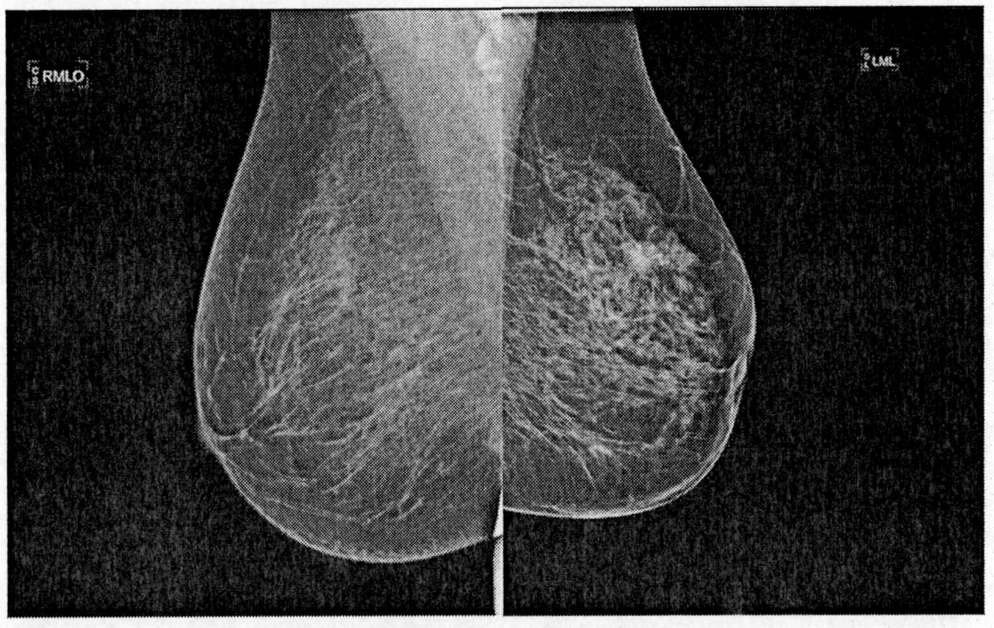

Figure 14.3: Mediolateral oblique (MLO) view
Right breast: normal tissue, left breast: abnormal density in upper breast (cancer).
(Reproduced with permission from SW Deanery.)

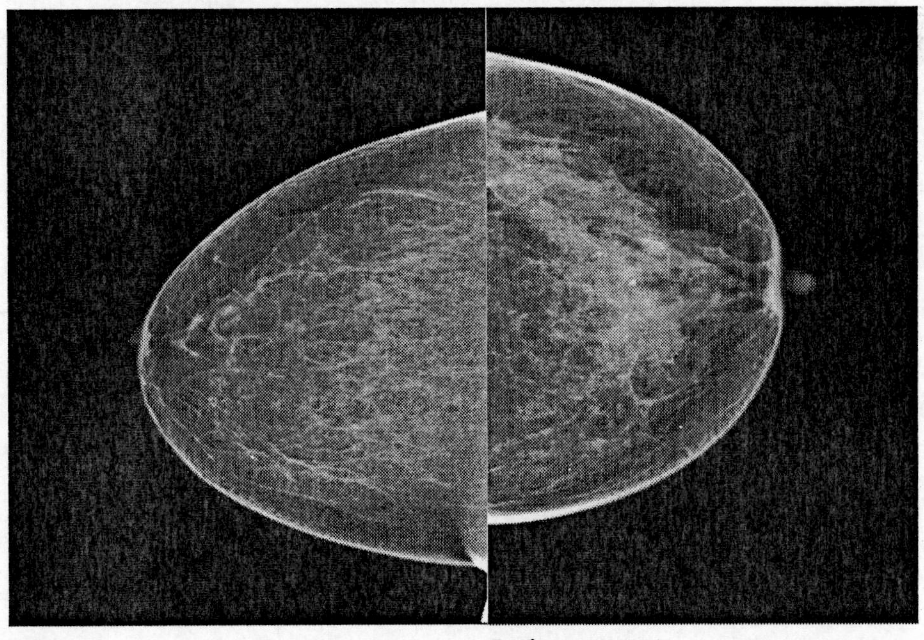

Figure 14.4: Craniocaudal (CC) view
Right breast: normal tissue, left breast: extensive microcalcification (DCIS)
(Reproduced with permission from SW Deanery.)

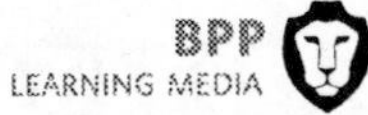

Computed tomography (CT)

- Used in staging systemic spread of breast cancer and measuring response of metastatic disease following treatment

Core biopsy

- Provides histological information
- A small core of tissue from a mass is removed with a cutting needle
- The needle is combined with a mechanical device
- Several cores are removed from a mass or an area of microcalcification, usually under USS guidance

Fine needle aspiration (FNA)

- Provides cytological information
- No longer the mainstay but particularly useful for pre-operative staging of lymph nodes
- Needle aspiration can differentiate between solid and cystic lesions
- A needle is introduced into a lesion and suction is applied by withdrawing the plunger of a syringe
- Multiple passes are made through the lesion
- The material is then spread onto microscopy slides and sent for cytology

	1	2	3	4	5
Palpation (P)	No lesion	Benign lesion	Atypia	Suspicious	Malignant
Mammography (M)	No lesion	Benign lesion	Atypia	Suspicious	Malignant
USS (U)	No lesion	Benign lesion	Atypia	Suspicious	Malignant
Cytology (C)	Blood and fat	Benign epithelial cells	Atypia	Suspicious	Malignant
Histology (B)	Normal breast tissue	Benign lesion	Atypia	Suspicious	Malignant B5a – Pre-invasive B5b – Invasive

Table 14.1: Classification of breast lesions

For example documentation would be:

A lipoma P_2, M_1, U_1, C_1, B_1.

A fibroadenoma P_2, M_2, U_2, C_2, B_2.

A cancer P_5, M_5, U_5, C_5, B_5.

Breast lesions

Fibroadenoma

P Over proliferation of stromal and glandular breast tissue.

A Arising in the terminal duct lobular unit in adolescent women. Occur due to changes in oestrogen levels.

Commonly presents in 20s.

S Discrete, mobile, smooth and rubbery mass.

Sx Usually palpable, painless lump or incidental finding on breast imaging.

I History, clinical examination, imaging, core biopsy.

T Usually conservative.

Excision is recommended (in >25 year-olds) if there is significant increase in size, distortion of the breast occurs, tumour size >4cm, any histological concern of phyllodes tumour.

Pr Majority in women >40 years will not change in size (50%), some will get smaller or resolve (40%) and a small number will increase in size (10%).

Phyllodes tumour

P (Cystosarcoma Phyllodes). Fibroepithelial tumour that is typically a large, fast growing mass formed from periductal stromal cells.

Many clinical and pathological features of a fibroadenoma.

A May be considered benign (common), borderline or malignant (both rare) depending on histologic features.

Benign tumours can convert to malignant over time.

S Can be very fast growing.

Sx Firm, palpable, smooth mass.

I History, clinical examination, imaging, core biopsy.

T Wide local excision of lesion with clear margins.

C Risk of developing sarcoma.

Pr Favourable, with local recurrence occurring in approximately 15% of patients overall and distant recurrence in approximately 5% to 10% overall.

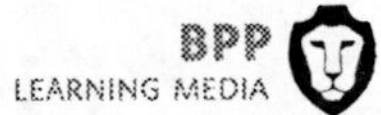

Cyst

P Distended and involuted lobules seen most frequently in older pre-menopausal women.

A Hormonally related.

Commonly presents in early 40s or those on HRT.

S Smooth, round and discrete breast lump.

Sx Tenderness, incidental finding on screening.

I History and clinical examination, confirmed by USS.

Mammogram if >40 years (1–3% chance of incidental carcinoma).

T If symptomatic: aspirate to dryness (to check lump has resolved), if bloody contents send for cytology then review three to six weeks post procedure to check not refilled.

C Often recurrent.

Pr Cyst formation usually ceases after menopause.

Duct papilloma

P Very common, considered as aberrations rather than true benign neoplasms.

A Three forms.

Commonly solitary-duct discrete.

Rarely multiple or juvenile papillomas.

Commonly presents in >40s.

S Single duct discharge.

Sx Serous nipple discharge (occasionally bloody), painless.

I History, clinical examination, mammogram.

T Microdochectomy (surgery to excise the involved duct) to exclude a papillary tumour.

Pr Minimal, if any, malignant potential.

Duct ectasia

P Benign condition affecting the major breast ducts in the subareolar region. Ducts dilate and shorten with age. Dilated ducts contain coloured (green, brown, creamy) secretions.

A Smoking, older women.

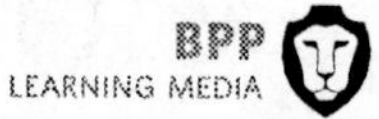

S Slit like end of nipple.

Sx Multi-duct, multi-coloured nipple discharge, nipple inversion (sometimes evertable).

I History, clinical examination, imaging.

T Reassurance, rarely major duct excision (Hadfield's procedure).

Pr No increased risk of breast cancer.

Fat necrosis

P Injured adipocytes incite a foreign body giant cell reaction with subsequent fibrosis and calcification forming a mass.

A May occur from a bruise or injury to the breast, previous breast surgery or radiotherapy. Many women may not remember any specific injury.

S Difficult to distinguish from carcinoma, dimpling, mass, oil cyst.

Sx Painless lump.

I History, clinical examination, imaging, core biopsy.

T Reassurance, may need follow up imaging as slow to resolve.

Pr No increase in risk of developing breast cancer.

Lipoma

P Encapsulated nodules of mature adipose tissue.

A No definitive link between trauma and lipoma formation. Often multiple on trunk and inherited tendency (Dercum's disease).

S Soft, lobulated, localised mass in the subcutaneous tissue or within the breast itself.

Sx Lump, sometimes tender.

I History and clinical examination, mammography +/- FNA.

T Reassure, excision if rapid increase in size to exclude liposarcoma.

Pr Rare to undergo sarcomatous change.

Gynaecomastia

P The growth of glandular tissue in males, generally located around the nipple, benign, usually reversible.

Compared with pseudogynaecomastia, which is fatty breast enlargement and is cosmetic only.

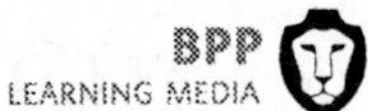

A Two age peaks: puberty and old age.

Imbalance of oestrogens and androgens.

S Firm disc of retro-areolar tender tissue.

Sx Progressive breast enlargement, without pain or tenderness.

Unilateral eccentric, tender, hard or ulcerating lesions suggest underlying pathology may be breast cancer.

I (To exclude breast cancer or hormone secreting causal tumour). History, clinical examination, imaging, core biopsy.

Bloods: LFTs, renal and thyroid function, hormone levels.

T A short course of Tamoxifen / aromatase inhibitor.

Surgical removal if resistant to treatment.

C Can reoccur, may undergo scarring / fibrosis if present long term, psychological consequences.

Pr No increased risk of breast cancer, but may be a sign of an underlying cancer elsewhere.

Puberty	Older age	Misc
Cannabis	Idiopathic	Hormone secreting tumours – Testicular / Pituitary
Alcohol	Medications	
Anabolic steroids	Liver / Renal disease	
	Testicular failure	

Table 14.2: Common causes of gynaecomastia

Breast pain

Cyclical

P Most common type of breast pain caused by the normal monthly changes in hormones.

A Unknown, younger age group.

Theories include excess prolactin production, excess oestrogen, insufficient progesterone and abnormal fatty acid profiles.

Approximately 2/3 of all patients presenting with mastalgia.

S Often none.

Sx Discomfort, heightened awareness, fullness and heaviness of the breast three to seven days prior to menstrual period.

I History and clinical examination to exclude musculoskeletal causes or mass lesion.

Mammograms not needed in uncomplicated cases.

T Reassurance if imaging is negative. Check for correctly fitting bra. Short course of tamoxifen in severe cases (10mg od).

Evening Primrose Oil may help, but trials demonstrate a similar effect to placebo.

Pr Not a symptom of breast cancer.

Non-cyclical

P Breast pain with a time pattern that is not associated with cyclical ovarian function.

A Older, post menopausal women. Is mostly musculoskeletal.

Age 40s is hormone related.

Affects 1/3 of all patients presenting with mastalgia.

S As for cyclical breast pain.

Sx As for cyclical breast pain.

I History and clinical examination to exclude cysts.

Imaging: mammogram / USS (if focal symptoms).

T Sports bra, simple analgesia eg NSAIDs.

Pr Very rarely a symptom of breast cancer.

Infection

Lactating mastitis

P (Puerperal mastitis). Inflammation in the breast in connection with pregnancy, breast feeding or weaning. Thought to be caused by blocked milk ducts or milk excess.

A Staphlococcus aureus (most common), s. epidermidis and streptococci.

S Erythema, oedema, warmth, cracked nipple or skin abrasions may be seen.

Sx Pain, swelling, tenderness, systemic illness.

I History, clinical examination, USS.

T Appropriate antibiotics.

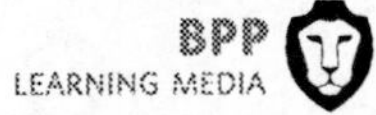

Abscess: multiple aspirations (under LA), incision and drainage. Encouraged to continue breast feeding.

C Recurrence, milk stasis, abscess formation.

Pr Breast cancer may coincide with mastitis or develop shortly afterwards. All suspicious symptoms that do not completely disappear must be investigated.

Lifetime risk for breast cancer is significantly reduced for women who were pregnant and breastfeeding.

Non-lactating mastitis

P (Non-puerperal mastitis). Inflammatory lesions of the breast occurring unrelated to pregnancy and breastfeeding.

A *Periareolar (central)* infection: active inflammation around non-dilated subareolar breast ducts (periductal mastitis).

Common in smokers aged 30s, anaerobic organisms.

Peripheral non-lactating breast abscesses are less common. Associated with diabetes, rheumatoid arthritis, steroid treatment, granulomatous lobular mastitis, and trauma.

S Erythema, oedema, warmth.

Sx Pain, swelling, tenderness, mass, nipple retraction or discharge, systemic illness.

I History, clinical examination, USS.

T Stop smoking, appropriate antibiotics.

Abscess: aspiration, incision and drainage.

If recurrent: excision of diseased duct.

C Recurrence, abscess formation, mammary duct fistula.

Pr Mastitis episodes do not appear to influence lifetime risk of breast cancer.

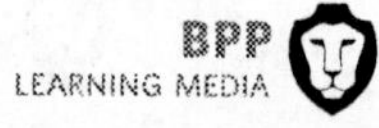

Malignant breast disease

Breast screening

- The condition screened for should be an *important* one.
- There should be an *acceptable treatment* for patients with the disease.
- The facilities for *diagnosis and treatment* should be available.
- There should be a recognised *latent or early symptomatic stage.*
- There should be a *suitable test or examination*, which has few false. positives (specificity) – and few false negatives (sensitivity).
- The test or examination should be *acceptable to the population.*
- The cost, including diagnosis and subsequent treatment, should be *economically balanced* in relation to expenditure on medical care as a whole.

Box 14.1: Principles of a screening programme (WHO)

Purpose: To detect evidence of pre-invasive or invasive cancer in asymptomatic women.

Age: Current UK guidelines, age 50–70 years. In the process of age extension to 47–73 years.

Process: Women are invited to attend by GP practice cohort every three years, women over 73 years of age can request imaging.

Raised risk patients commence yearly mammograms age 40 until screening age. Very high-risk patients have a yearly MRI between 30–40 years, then annual mammograms until screening age.

Imaging: Two view mammograms.

Results: Routine recall for normal imaging.

Abnormal imaging: core biopsy, discussion at MDT with results and further management as appropriate.

Ductal carcinoma in-situ (DCIS)

P 80% of non-invasive cancer. Malignant cells that have not yet breached the duct basement membrane.

The next step is micro-invasion.

Classified as low grade, immediate or high grade (high grade having the highest risk of conversion to invasive disease).

A See *Invasive carcinoma*.

S Commonly no signs therefore it is mostly found through breast screening. DCIS seen as micro-calcification on mammogram.

Sx Usually asymptomatic, occasionally presents with a mass, nipple discharge or Paget's disease.

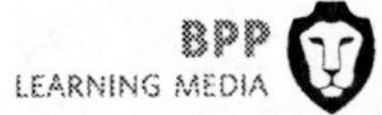

I Screening mammogram, stereotactic (image guided) core biopsy.

If symptomatic: history, clinical examination, mammogram, core biopsy.

T *Surgery:* wide local excision / mastectomy, depending on extent / proportion of breast involved, if >5cm consider mastectomy.

Adjuvant radiotherapy considered in high grade DCIS to reduce local recurrence.

C Risk of subsequent carcinoma, majority of these will be in the same breast.

Approximately 1/3 of screen detected DCIS will already have an invasive focus.

Pr If untreated, the natural course varies according to the grade of the DCIS.

Low grade: approximately 60% risk of progression to invasive disease within 40 years.

High grade: approximately 50% risk of progression to invasive disease within 7 years.

Lobular carcinoma in-situ (LCIS)

P Benign proliferative condition, but higher risk pleomorphic variant should be considered as DCIS, disease tends to be multifocal, multicentric, and bilateral.

A Some association with use of HRT.

S LCIS is non-palpable and has no consistent features on breast imaging.

Sx Often none.

I Often an incidental finding during a breast biopsy for a separate mammographic abnormality or palpable mass.

T Additional screening mammograms.

C Risk of subsequent carcinoma, 50–60% of these will be in the same breast.

Pr 15–20% of women will develop invasive breast cancer in the same breast. 10–15% will develop invasive cancer in the contralateral breast.

Paget's disease of nipple

P Pre-invasive disease (DCIS) spreading from the major ducts onto nipple skin, causing eczematous change.

A As for DCIS.

S Skin changes: red, itchy, inflamed, starts centrally, nipple may be destroyed.

Sx As above, there may or may not be an associated lump.

I History and clinical examination, mammogram, punch biopsy.

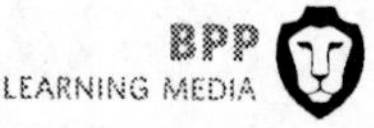

T As for DCIS.

C As for DCIS.

Pr As for DCIS.

Invasive carcinoma

P Arises in the terminal duct lobular unit (TDLU) of the breast.

Non special type

- *Ductal (80%):* often small and picked up by screening

Special types

- *Lobular (≈20%):* often multifocal and extensive, usually not high grade, poorly visualised on mammography
- *Mucinous*: thick mucin at centre of lump
- *Tubular*: low grade

Box 14.2: Classification

A Increasing age, early menarche, late menopause, nulliparity, late age at first birth (>35 years), BRCA1/2 gene, radiation exposure, OCP and HRT use, obesity, family history.

Breast feeding contributes to reducing overall risk.

Tumour grade:

- Grade I: well differentiated.
- Grade II: moderately differentiated.
- Grade III: poorly differentiated.

Grade I tumours have a better prognosis than Grade III tumours, the latter being associated with a five-year survival of approximately 45%.

S Lump, asymmetry, nipple inversion, nipple discharge, skin changes.

Sx Palpable lump, rarely painful.

I History and clinical examination, imaging, core biopsy.

T See Table 14.2.

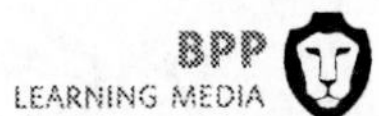

Local	Systemic
• Surgery – **Breast:** wide local excision, mastectomy – **Axilla:** sentinel node biopsy, axillary clearance • Radiotherapy – Usually 50 grays given in fractions	• **Hormonal** – **Selective oestrogen receptor modulator (SERM):** Tamoxifen (all ages) – **Aromatase inhibitor (AI):** Anastrozole / letrozole (post menopausal only) • Chemotherapy – **Anthracycline based:** FEC (most common) – **Taxanes:** TAC (node +ve disease) • Herceptin

Table 14.3: Treatment of breast cancer

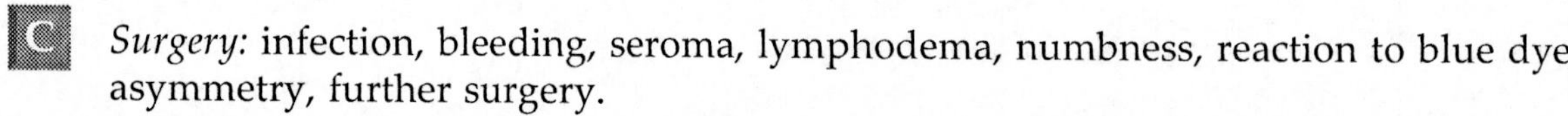

C *Surgery:* infection, bleeding, seroma, lymphodema, numbness, reaction to blue dye, asymmetry, further surgery.

Radiotherapy: local skin reaction, fatigue.

Hormones: Tamoxifen – hot flushes, endocrine malignancy, DVT, stroke. AI – osteoporosis.

Chemotherapy: neutropenic sepsis, fatigue, nausea and vomiting, hair loss, decreased appetite, bruising, oral mucositis.

Herceptin: decline in heart function, infusion reactions.

Pr *Multifactoral:* axillary node status, tumour grade, tumour size, lymphovascular invasion (LVI), hormone receptors (ER/PR), and human epidermal growth factor receptor-2 (HER2). Generally computerised databases give statistics with / without adjuvant treatment. See Box 14.3.

Poor prognostic factors

- High grade / large size
- Young age
- During pregnancy / breast feeding
- ER –ve
- Her2 +ve
- Triple –ve (ER –ve, PR –ve, Her2 –ve)
- Lymph node +ve

Box 14.3: Adjuvant online / Nottingham prognostic index (NPI)

Breast reconstruction

What: Creation of new breast shape using surgery.

When: Following mastectomy / wide local excision / uneven breast development / risk reducing surgery.

Why: To restore breast shape, psychological factors.

Types: **Simple implant:**

Tissue expander under pectoral muscle +/- dermal sling.

- *Pros:* Simple surgery, no scar elsewhere.
- *Cons:* Not after radiotherapy, often needs symmetry surgery to contralateral side, further surgery in the future to replace implant.

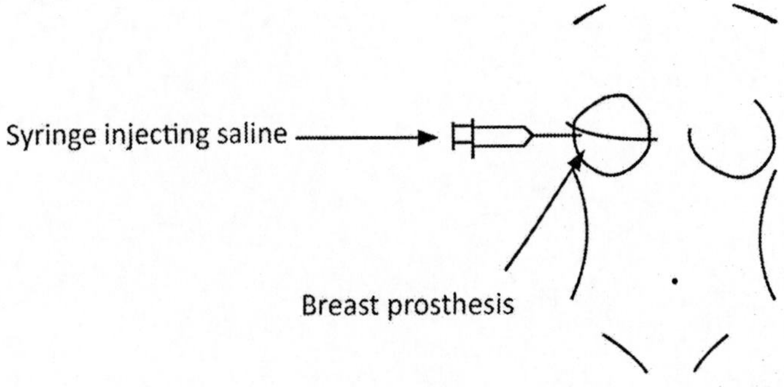

Figure 14.5: Simple implant reconstruction

Latissimus dorsi (LD flap):

Uses latissimus dorsi muscle, skin and fat from back. Thoracodorsal vessels remain attached in the axilla.

Without implant (autologous / extended)

- *Pros:* More natural look and feel to the breast, can reconstruct smaller breasts without an implant.
- *Cons:* Scar on back, some upper body weakness.

With implant

- *Pros:* Reconstructs larger breasts with good ptosis.
- *Cons:* Scar on back, weakness, implant will need replacing in the future.

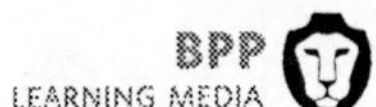

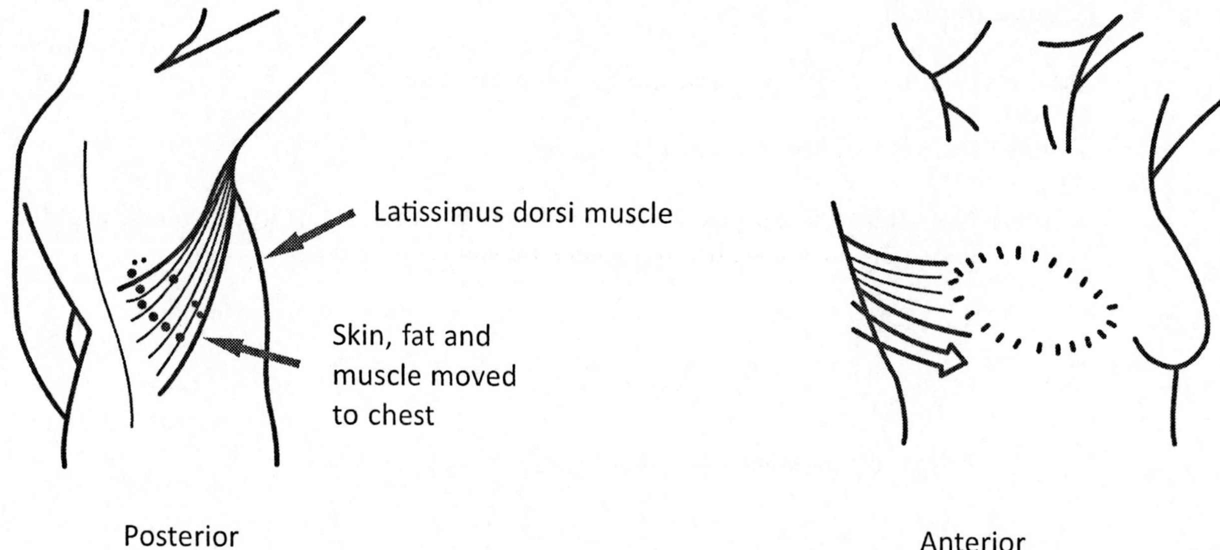

Figure 14.6: LD flap

Abdominal flaps*:*

Transverse Rectus Abdominis Muscle flap (TRAM)

Uses rectus abdominis muscle, either on a pedicle or as a free flap, taken under the skin on the abdomen and chest to form a new breast.

- *Pros:* Autologous tissue, no need for implant, abdominoplasty.
- *Cons:* Can only reconstruct one side, weakness, hernia, flap loss, large scar, long recovery.

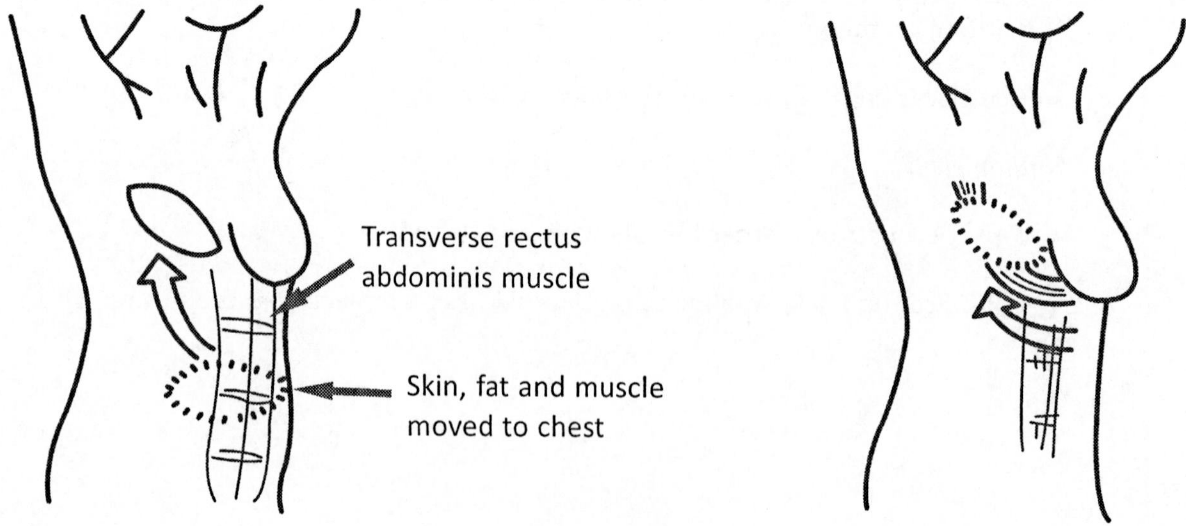

Figure 14.7: TRAM flap

Deep Inferior Epigastric Perforator flap (DIEP)

Uses skin and fat only from the lower abdomen along with the deep inferior epigastric artery and veins to form the new breast shape. Vessels attached in the axilla / chest wall using microvascular surgery.

Pros: No muscle used so the strength of the abdomen is not affected. Autologous tissue, no need for implant, abdominoplasty, can reconstruct bilaterally.

Cons: Flap loss, large scar, long recovery.

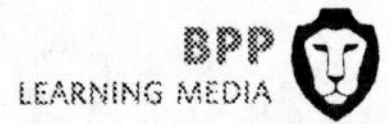

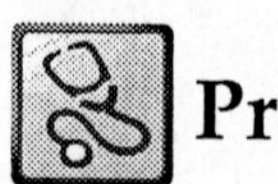

Practice Questions

Single Best Answers

1. What is the breast imaging investigation of choice in women <40 years?

   A CT
   B USS
   C MRI
   D Mammogram

2. What is the most common painless, palpable breast lump presenting in a woman aged in her 20s?

   A Phyllodes tumour
   B Cyst
   C Fibroadenoma
   D Lipoma

3. Profuse serous nipple discharge from a single duct suggests

   A Duct papilloma
   B Paget's disease
   C Duct ectasia
   D Lactating mastitis

4. An oil cyst is a feature of which one of the following?

   A Duct ectasia
   B Lipoma
   C Fat necrosis
   D Duct papilloma

5. Which of the following has malignant potential?

   A Fibroadenoma
   B Cyst
   C Duct ectasia
   D Phyllodes tumour

6. Which of the following is not a cause of gynaecomastia?

   A Smoking
   B Liver disease
   C Testicular tumour
   D Spironolactone

7. The common organism causing lactational mastitis is:

   A S. epidermidis
   B S. aureus
   C Streptococci
   D E. coli

8. The current age range of breast screening in the UK is:

   A 30–50
   B 45–65
   C 50–70
   D 53–73

9. The proportion of pre-invasive breast cancer that is ductal in origin is:

   A 80%
   B 70%
   C 20%
   D 30%

10. What is the most common type of invasive cancer?

    A Lobular
    B Ductal
    C Mucinous
    D Tubular

11. What is the feature of DCIS seen on mammography?

    A Irregular mass
    B Benign calcification
    C Smooth mass
    D Microcalcification

12. Which of the following is an additional treatment / investigation for DCIS?

    A Radiotherapy
    B Sentinel node biopsy
    C Chemotherapy
    D Hormones

13. Which one of the following increases a woman's risk of developing breast cancer?

    A Late menarche
    B Early menopause
    C Nulliparity
    D Breast feeding

14. Which of the following indicate a worse prognosis in breast cancer?

    A ER +ve
    B Grade III disease
    C Older age
    D Her2 –ve

15. Osteoporosis is a common side effect of which mode of treatment for breast cancer?

    A Aromatase inhibitor
    B Tamoxifen
    C Radiotherapy
    D Herceptin

Extended Matching Questions

Benign disease

A Fibroadenoma
B Cyst
C Phyllodes tumour
D Fat necrosis
E Lipoma

For each of the following scenarios choose the **single** most likely diagnosis from the above list of options. Each option may be used once, more than once, or not at all.

1. A 40-year-old woman presenting with a painful breast lump.

2. A 55-year-old woman presenting with several small lobulated lumps, one of which is in the breast.

3. A woman presenting with a lump and bruising to her breast.

Breast pain and infective disease

A Cyclical pain
B Non-cyclical pain
C Lactating mastitis
D Non-lactating mastitis

For each of the following scenarios choose the **single** most likely diagnosis from the above list of options. Each option may be used once, more than once, or not at all.

4. A woman presenting with breast pain and arthritis of the neck.

5. A woman smoker presenting with periareolar inflammation.

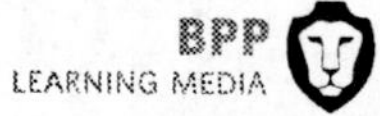

Malignant disease

A DCIS
B Invasive ductal carcinoma
C Paget's disease
D Invasive lobular carcinoma

For each of the following scenarios choose the **single** most likely diagnosis from the above list of options. Each option may be used once, more than once, or not at all.

6. A woman presenting with an eczematous nipple and thickening of affected skin on mammogram.

7. A woman with a strong family history and a BRCA1 gene mutation presents with alteration in breast shape and skin tethering.

8. A woman found to have easily palpable multifocal breast lumps not seen on mammography.

9. A woman presenting with a breast lump, having had previous excision of high grade DCIS ten years before.

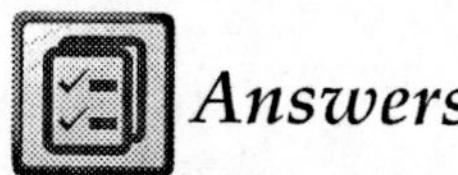

Answers

SBAs		EMQs	
1	B	1	B
2	C	2	E
3	A	3	D
4	C	4	B
5	D	5	D
6	A	6	C
7	B	7	B
8	C	8	D
9	A	9	B
10	B		
11	D		
12	A		
13	C		
14	B		
15	A		

Chapter 15

Endocrine surgery

Mr Dermot Mallon

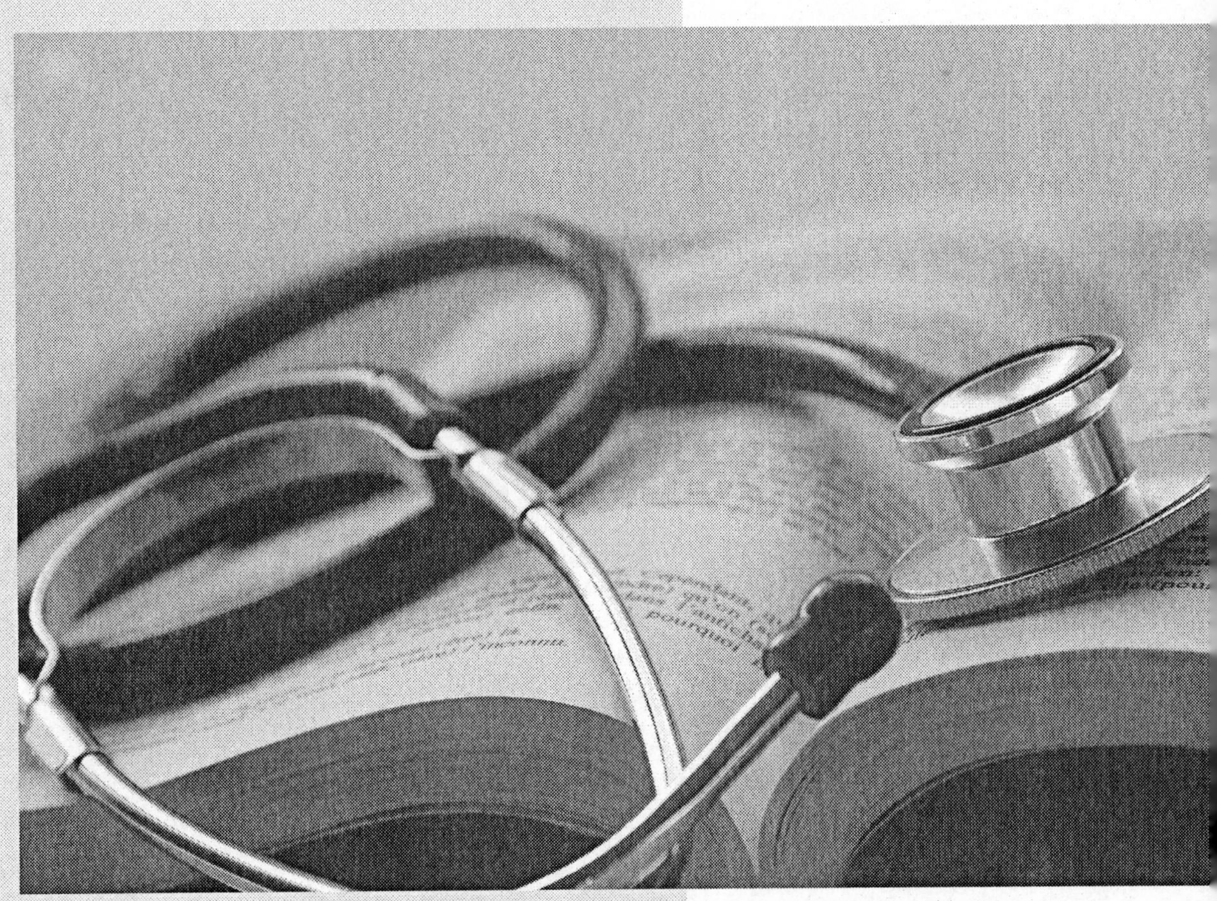

Neck lumps

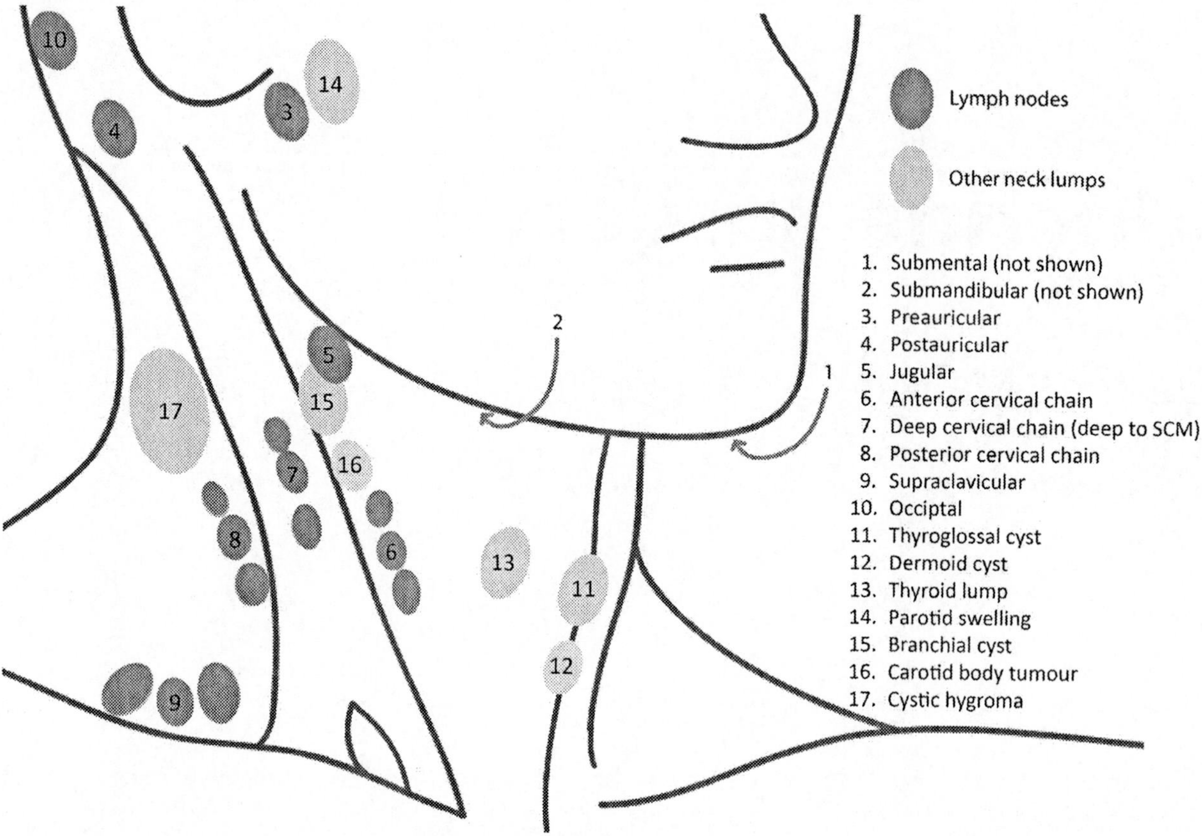

Figure 15.1: Neck lumps

Midline

Dermoid cyst

A Benign congenital hamartoma forms cyst at site of embryonic cleft closures that contains tissue normally present in skin such as sebaceous glands, sweat glands and hair follicles.

S Painless midline lump found in lateral third of eyebrow, face, scalp and trunk and is tethered to skin, vast majority apparent by age of five years.

Sx Mostly asymptomatic.

I Clinical diagnosis is usually made however FNA and USS may be used to differentiate from other causes of neck lumps.

T Excision is treatment of choice.

C Cyst may get infected.

Pr With complete resection no further follow-up is required.

Thyroglossal cyst

A From remnant of tract formed by the migration of the thyroid from foramen caecum at the base of the tongue to cricoid.

S Midline lump most commonly in third decade, moves with tongue protrusion.

Sx Usually asymptomatic, painful and swollen if infected.

I Thyroid function tests, FNA, USS / MRI to ensure presence of normal thyroid gland.

T Sistrunk procedure which involves removal of median third of hyoid bone to prevent recurrence.

C Infection, may be associated with ectopic thyroid tissue and therefore risk of malignancy.

Pr Recurrence rate approximately 8%.

Anterior triangle

Branchial cyst

A Congenital malformation most commonly due to aberrant development of second Branchial cleft.

S Smooth, painless, slowly enlarging lump anterior to sternocleidomastoid most commonly on the left hand side, may develop as a sinus with opening onto the skin.

Sx Of asymptomatic, cosmetic, may become infected.

I Largely a clinical diagnosis. FNA to exclude SCC.

T May use sclerotherapy however treatment of choice is surgical excision when not infected after 3 months of age.

C Recurrent infection with fibrotic changes resulting in compromise of local structures eg hypoglossal and accessory nerve.

Pr Recurrence is <5% although this increases if history of infection.

Carotid body tumour (Chemodectoma)

P Paraganglioma of the carotid body, which helps, regulate pH, blood O_2 and CO_2 levels and is located at the bifurcation of the carotid artery.

A Three subtypes are recognised: sporadic (85%), familial (10%) and hyperplasic (5%).

Hyperplastic is seen in those with chronic hypoxia seen in COPD and high altitude.

S Slow growing anterior triangle neck lump which is fixed in the vertical plain.

Sx Usually asymptomatic; pressure on adjacent cranial nerves may cause dysphagia, dysphonia or Horner's syndrome.

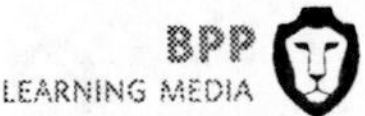

I Duplex USS and / or angiography to determine relationship with carotid arteries and for contralateral pathology.

CT / MRI / Endoscopy can be used to assess for local invasion.

T Surgical resection is preferred in young patients, radiotherapy may be used in older patients.

Pre-operative embolisation may be employed in larger (>4cm) tumours.

C May cause CN palsies through local invasion most commonly CN X and XII.

Surgery is inherently risky due to proximity of vascular structures. The rate of malignancy is below 5%.

Pr Recurrence is seen in between 5–10%.

Pharyngeal pouch

P Oesophageal outpouching through a weakness at Killian's dehiscence above cricopharyngeal and below inferior pharyngeal constrictor muscles.

Also known as Zenker's diverticulum.

A The diverticulum is caused by intra-oesophageal pressure at the place of weakness. Cranial nerve dysfunction, smoking, excess alcohol, GORD and increasing age are risk factors.

S Crepitus of a neck lump, reducible lump.

Sx Mass effect causing dysphagia, regurgitation from pouch and halitosis. May change in size with swallowing.

I Barium swallow.

T Surgical or endoscopic myotomy of cricopharyngeus to unite lumen of diverticulum with oesophagus.

C May rupture if endoscopy inadvertently inserted.

Pr Despite elderly cohort the morbidity of endoscopic repair is safe with a recurrence of <3%.

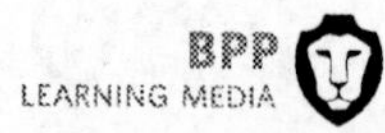

Posterior triangle

Cervical rib

P Normal variant with extra rib from cervical vertebrae.

S May cause thoracic outlet syndrome with occlusion of subclavian artery and vein and impingement of brachial plexus nerves. Rib may be palpable.

Sx Mostly asymptomatic, may cause thoracic outlet syndrome with motor and sensory changes, ischaemic pain or venous congestion.

I Apparent on chest radiograph.

T Conservative approach with physiotherapy or behavioural changes. If refractory or neurosurgical symptoms then surgical removal of rib.

C Permanent loss of function.

Pr Excellent in uncomplicated patients.

Cystic hygroma

P A lymphangioma, which is a lymph-filled cyst caused by a congenital malformation of lymphatic drainage.

A Congenital aberration of vestigial lymph channels.

S Posterior triangle, painless, soft and compressible lump that transilluminates. Overlying skin may have a bluish tinge.

Sx Usually asymptomatic unless infected where it may expand in size and become painful.

I Clinical examination can be augmented with CT / MRI / USS to determine the anatomy of the lesion and demonstrate a cystic lesion and its association with nearby structures.

T Surgical excision if persistent although they may rarely resolve spontaneously.

C Potential for expansion with compromise of neighbouring structures, the trachea in particular.

Pr Recurrence does not happen if no macroscopic disease remains.

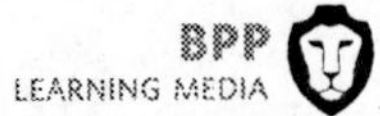

Goitre

- Iodine deficiency
- Defect in thyroxine synthesis
- Grave's disease
- Hashimoto's thyroiditis
- Lymphoma
- Thyroid amyloidosis

Box 15.1: Causes of goitre

- Grave's disease (in those where radioiodine treatment has failed or is not appropriate)
- Treatment of multiple benign or malignant thyroid tumours
- Treatment of compressive symptoms
- Cosmetic

Box 15.2: Indications for thyroidectomy

Complications of thyroidectomy

- Damage to external branch of the superior laryngeal nerve
  - Most common complication, often asymptomatic it may cause a change in voice
- Damage to recurrent laryngeal nerve
  - Motor supply to all intrinsic muscles of larynx (except cricothyroid) and therefore disruption on one side causes altered voice while bilateral disruption causes the vocal cords to rest in mid-adduction which may cause airway obstruction
- Thyrotoxic storm
  - In those with hyperthyroidism, simple manipulation of the gland or stress of surgery causes raised thyroid hormone and consequent increased sympathetic tone and metabolism.
- Treatment is with beta-blockers and iodine-based fluid to reduce thyroid hormone release.
- Post-operative bleeding and haematoma formation
  - Devastating complication as rapidly expanding haematoma can compromise airway.
- Hypoparathyroidism due to inadvertent parathyroidectomy
- Post-operative hypothyroidism

Thyroid tumours

Benign

Colloid nodule

P Also know as a macrofollicular adenoma. Most common benign growth consisting of normal thyroid tissue. They are colloid-filled and are lined by a fibrous capsule. They do not spread beyond the thyroid.

A Thyroid adenomas have been associated with Hashimoto's disease, radiation exposure and iodine deficiency.

S Firm, painless lump within thyroid gland.

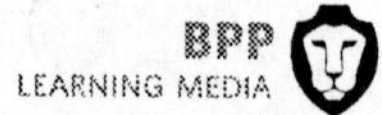

Sx Usually asymptomatic.

I Ultrasound, fine needle aspiration, thyroid function tests.

T Treatment for confirmed colloid nodule is not required unless causing compression or cosmetic problems.

C Compression on neighbouring vessels.

Pr Excellent, they have no malignant potential and do not recur if removed.

Follicular adenoma

P Benign neoplasm of thyroid tissue held within a capsule.

A Thyroid adenomas have been associated with Hashimoto's disease, radiation exposure and iodine deficiency.

S Firm, painless lump within thyroid gland.

Sx Usually asymptomatic.

I Ultrasound, fine needle aspiration, thyroid function tests, Isotope scanning with radioactive iodine. Hot nodules are unlikely to be cancerous while cold nodules are associated with a 15% risk of malignancy.

T FNA is unable to differentiate between follicular adenoma and carcinoma and therefore excision is often necessitated.

C Thyroidectomy is associated with damage to recurrent laryngeal nerve, which affects phonation, hypocalcaemia due to parathyroid gland loss and hypothyroidism.

Pr Adenomas have a low potential for recurrence.

Malignant

Papillary carcinoma

P Tumour of thyroid epithelial cells. Accounts for 70% of thyroid malignancy most commonly seen in children and women less than 40 years old.

A Associated with radiation exposure and (as with most thyroid neoplasia) females > males.

S Painless neck lump that may grow quickly. Cervical lymphadenopathy is present in one-third of patients at presentation.

Slow growing, late spread to lymph nodes.

Sx Often asymptomatic or may have thyroid lump(s).

I — Thyroid function tests, USS, FNA, isotope scanning with I^{131}, CT / MRI to evaluate potential spread.

T — Total thyroidectomy indicated if tumours >1cm, bilateral involvement or a suggestion of metastatic spread.

Lobectomy may be performed if there is no suggestion of metastasis and the tumour is <1cm.

Tumours tend to be multicentric and therefore total thyroidectomy is preferred.

Post-operative I^{131} after which thyroid replacement therapy is required. Cervical lymph nodes are also removed.

C — Metastatic spread is most commonly via lymphatics and therefore assessment with US / FNA of cervical lymph nodes is necessary.

Pr — Potentially curable with resection. Tend to spread relatively early. Ten-year survival is greater than 90%.

Follicular carcinoma

P — Tumour of thyroid epithelial cells with vascular and capsular invasion c.f. follicular adenoma.

A — Accounts for 10–20% of thyroid cancer. Radiation exposure is best-documented risk factor. May occur in nodular goitre.

S — Painless neck lump that may grow quickly and is rarely seen in young patients (<30 years old). Early haematogenous spread to liver, lung and therefore respective signs should be sought eg hepatomegaly.

Sx — Painless lump in neck. Potential for symptoms due to spread to liver, lung and bone.

I — Thyroid function tests, isotope scan, CT / MRI scan of neck. Notably FNA cannot differentiate between follicular adenoma and follicular carcinoma.

T — Total thyroidectomy under same criteria as for papillary cancer. Lobectomy is utilised more often because follicular carcinoma is less likely to be multi-focal than papillary carcinoma. T4 is given to suppress TSH secretion to reduce risk of recurrence.

C — Haematogenous spread seen in 20% of patients at presentation.

Pr — Ten-year survival is approximately 80%.

Medullary carcinoma

P — Tumour of calcitonin producing parafollicular C cells.

A — Accounts for 5% of thyroid cancer. Sporadic in 80% of cases, the remainder is associated with MEN IIa/IIb.

S — Hard enlargement within thyroid. Cervical lymphadenopathy noted in over 50% of patients at presentation.

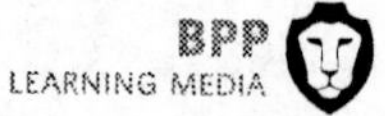

Sx If not related to familial syndrome is often asymptomatic. May have symptoms of altered calcium level. Apart from lump often asymptomatic.

I Serum calcitonin is raised, FNA, genetic screening for MEN syndromes, parathyroid hormone level 24-hour urine catecholamine to exclude parathyroid adenoma and pheochromocytoma.

USS examination of neck lymph nodes.

T Total thyroidectomy is indicated with removal of affected lymph nodes.

C Raised calcitonin levels may cause calcium abnormalities. May be associated with MEN IIa/b syndrome. May also secrete ACTH and is therefore a rare cause of acromegaly.

Pr Much poorer if associated with MEN syndromes where survival above 45 years of age is rare.

Prognosis at 10 years generally less than 50%.

Anaplastic carcinoma

P Highly malignant undifferentiated tumour that is locally invasive and highly metastatic potential especially to lung.

A Rare and sporadic, seen most commonly in elderly patients. 25% have history of differentiated thyroid Ca.

S Rapidly growing goitre that may be painful. Local invasion may cause recurrent laryngeal nerve palsy resulting in a hoarse voice. Horner's syndrome may result from local invasion of sympathetic chain.

Sx Goitre, neck pain, cough, tracheal compression resulting in stridor and oesophageal compression causing dysphagia.

I FNA or open biopsy, CT to assess local invasion, compression of local structures and for presence of metastatic disease.

T Ensure safe airway, may require intubation or tracheostomy. Resection is rarely possible due to extent of invasion however it may be used to relieve pressure symptoms.

C Frequent due to local invasion and also pulmonary metastasis.

Pr Extremely poor with survival of 20% at one year and <5% at five years.

Thyroid lymphoma

P Tumour of lymphoreticular tissue of the thyroid, Non-Hodgkin's lymphoma is the most frequent.

A 5% of thyroid cancer. Most commonly associated with autoimmune thyroiditis although may also a *de novo* lymphoma.

S Goitre with 'doughy' texture

Sx Often asymptomatic, may have compression symptoms (dysphagia, dyspnoea, stridor) from goitre, 'B' symptoms typical of lymphoma.

I Full blood count, FNA / core biopsy to determine lymphoma subtype, CT scan for staging.

T Treatment is as per most other lymphomas with chemoradiotherapy.

C Bone marrow involvement is a rare complication.

Pr Chemoradiotherapy is often curative.

With localised lymphomas survival is nearly 90% at five years.

Papillary	70% thyroid malignancies Young age of onset (<40 years) Females > males Spread to lymph nodes occurs late 90% ten-year survival
Follicular	10–20% thyroid malignancies Middle aged onset (40–60 years) Females > males Early haematogenous spread to bone, lungs, liver 80% ten-year survival
Medullary	5% thyroid malignancies Sporadic or part of MEN IIa/b Equal sex incidence and occurs at any age Occurs in parafollicular C cells secreting calcitonin 50% ten-year survival
Anaplastic	Rare Elderly patients Females > males (3:1) Rapid growth and early local invasion with spread via lymph Very poor prognosis, 20% survival at one year
Lymphoma	5% thyroid malignancies Females > males (3:1) May present with stridor or dysphagia due to goitre 90% five-year survival for local disease

Table 15.1: Summary of thyroid carcinoma

Other endocrine tumours

Carcinoid tumour

P Rare neuroendocrine tumour of enterochromaffin-like cells of the gut wall.

Classified by foregut (which includes mediastinum, lungs and trachea), midgut or hindgut origin, affect multiple sites such as lung, mediastinum and liver. In children the appendix is most commonly affected.

Often secrete vasoactive peptides that give rise to carcinoid syndrome.

A Stomach carcinoid may be caused by pernicious anaemia and chronic atrophic gastritis secondary to gastrin hypersecretion. Associated with MEN Type 1 and Peutz-Jeghers syndrome.

S Highly dependent on size and site of tumour.

Sx Often asymptomatic, may cause symptoms of peptic ulcer disease.

If metastases outside the portal system, then the vasoactive peptides may cause flushing and tachycardia.

I The serotonin metabolite, Urinary 5-HIAA, is often raised.

CT / MRI and ideally PET scanning of the GI tract, somatostatin-receptor scintigraphy is increasingly being used. Upper and lower GI endoscopy may also be employed for biopsy.

T Octreotide reduces symptoms, chemotherapy, chemoembolisation of liver metastasis, surgical resection of tumours.

C Generally carcinoid tumours have high propensity for metastasis. Tricuspid insufficiency due to endocardial fibrosis that may result in heart failure.

Pr If tumour is completely resected then excellent prognosis can be expected.

Multiple endocrine neoplasia (MEN) Type I

P Parathyroid gland adenomas occur in all patients coupled with pancreatic neuroendocrine tumours (50%) and pituitary tumours (35%).

Also associated with carcinoid tumours and adrenal cortex tumours.

A Abnormality in MENIN gene.

S Hypercalcaemia (hypotonia, hyporeflexia, volume depletion). Pituitary lesions: diplopia, bitemporal hemianopia, galactorrhoea, and amenorrhoea.

Skin lesions (angiofibromas, lipomas).

Pancreatic hormone hypersecretion: gastrinomas (peptic ulcer disease), insulinomas (hypoglycaemia).

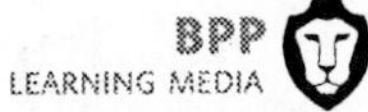

Sx Variable and often vague. Hypercalcaemia symptoms (lethargy, weakness, polyuria, constipation, nausea), neck lump, dyspepsia.

I Serum calcium and hormone (insulin, gastrin, PTH etc) profile, blood glucose, FNA of neck pathology, CT / MRI for pituitary and pancreatic neoplasia.

Genetic studies of patient and family may be considered.

T Correct hypocalcaemia and fluid balance.

Parathyroid adenoma: Parathyroidectomy (leaving no more than 15% of parathyroid tissue in forearm of patient).

Pituitary adenoma: dopamine agonists for prolactin hypersection, transphenoidal hypophysectomy if medical therapy fails.

Cutaneous lesions: surgical removal, cryotherapy.

C Pancreatic cell tumours have high rate of malignancy Acromegaly and Cushing's disease may be caused by GH and ACTH release by medullary carcinomas.

Pr Life expectancy of individual with MEN Type I is around 50 years of age.

Multiple endocrine neoplasia (MEN) Type II

P *MEN 2a*: syndrome characterised by medullary thyroid carcinoma (100%), phaeochromocytoma (50%), parathyroid hyperplasia (25%).

MEN 2b: as 2a with marfanoid appearance and without parathyroid hyperplasia.

A Mutation in RET proto-oncogene which is inherited in an AD manner.

S *Medullary thyroid carcinoma:* neck lump, evidence of hypocalcaemia, signs of compression of local structures such as trachea and veins.

Phaeochromocytoma: hypertension, orthostatic hypotension, and papilloedema.

Parathyroid hyperplasia: signs of hypercalcaemia.

Sx Medullary thyroid carcinoma and parathyroid hyperplasia may cause symptoms of calcium dysregulation and neck lump. Phaeochromocytoma causes triad of pounding headache, palpitations and episodic sweating and anxiety.

I FNA of neck lump, serum calcium and PTH, urinary catecholamines, CT neck / abdomen.

Genetic testing required if suspected and if confirmed family must also be genetically screened.

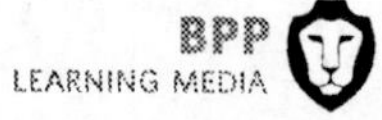

T If RET mutation present then prophylactic thyroidectomy is indicated.

Hypertension of phaeochromocytoma is treated with alpha-blockade followed by surgical resection.

Parathyroid hyperplasia necessitates removal of 3 ½ parathyroid glands and autotransplantation of remainder into the forearm (in case of further surgery).

C Potential for malignant spread of phaeochromocytoma and medullary carcinoma.

Pr Life expectancy approaches normal after thyroidectomy for inevitable medullary carcinoma.

MEN 1 (PPP)
- Parathyroid tumour: ↑ Ca^{2+}
- Pancreatic islet cell tumour: gastrinoma, insulinoma, VIPoma
- Pituitary tumour: ↑ GH/Prolactin

MEN 2a (TPP)
- Thyroid medullary carcinoma (100%)
- Parathyroid tumour (50%): ↑ Ca^{2+}
- Phaechromocytoma (25%)

MEN 2b (TPM)
- Thyroid medullary carcinoma (85%)
- Phaechromocytoma (50%)
- Mucosal neuroma (100%)
- \+ Marfanoid appearance

Box 15.3: MEN summary

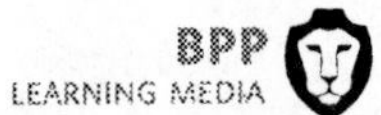

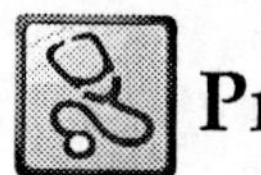

Practice Questions

Single Best Answers

1. FNA is **not** useful in diagnosing which of the following?

   A Follicular carcinoma
   B Medullary carcinoma
   C Colloid nodules
   D Anaplastic carcinoma

2. Which of the following does not occur in papillary carcinoma?

   A Tumour may be multifocal
   B Spread to nodes is rare
   C Cell of origin is thyroid follicular cell
   D Age influences prognosis

3. Which statement is incorrect regarding thyroid neoplasms?

   A A solitary thyroid nodule is more likely to be neoplastic than multiple
   B Follicular carcinoma has a tendency for vascular invasion
   C Commonest cause of 'cold' nodule on radio iodine scan is carcinoma
   D Medullary carcinomas are associated with APUD cells

4. What is the commonest complication of thyroidectomy for medullary carcinoma?

   A Recuurent laryngeal nerve palsy
   B Hypocalcaemia
   C Wound infection
   D Haemorrhage

5. Which of the following is a remnant of the descent of the thyroid from foramen caecum?

   A Thyroglossal cyst
   B Dermoid cyst
   C Branchial cyst
   D Pharyngeal pouch

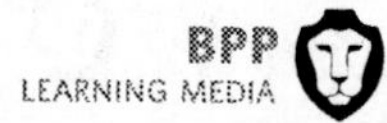

Extended Matching Questions

Diagnosis of neck lumps

A Hodgkin's lymphoma
B Lymphadenopathy 2° to infection
C Lymphadenopathy 2° to malignancy
D Carotid body tumour
E Thyroid cancer
F Thyroiditis
G TB lymphadenitis
H Thyroid goitre
I Salivary gland tumour
J Parotitis
K Mumps
L Thyroglossal cyst
M Pharyngeal pouch
N Glandular fever

For each of the following scenarios choose the **single** most likely diagnosis from the above list of options. Each option may be used once, more than once, or not at all.

1. An 80-year-old man presents with symptoms of dysphagia. He has been a lifelong smoker. On examination there is a reducible mass that seems to squelch over the lateral aspect of the anterior triangle.

2. An anxious 19-year-old female presents with a lump in the neck. She has lost 3kg in three months. On examination there is lymphadenopathy on both sides of the neck and larger nodes on the right. Her pulse is 96 regular; thyroid function tests are normal.

3. A 17-year-old male presents with a one-week history of fever, malaise, pain on swallowing and has noticed lumps in his neck. On examination a tender scrotal swelling is also noted.

4. A 58-year-old male presents to his GP with a lump in the neck. He reports that he suffered from a mild upper respiratory infection in the previous week and has lost three stone in the last two months. On examination there is a hard mobile lump in the supraclavicular fossa.

5. An 18-year-old girl presents with a midline swelling in the neck which has recently become tender. It moves on swallowing and on protusion of the tongue.

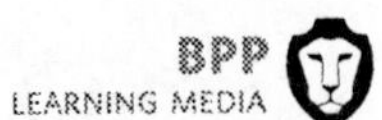

Thyroid cancer

A Medullary carcinoma
B Follicular carcinoma
C Papillary carcinoma
D Anaplastic carcinoma
E Lymphoma
F Follicular adenoma

For each of the following scenarios choose the **single** most likely diagnosis from the above list of options. Each option may be used once, more than once, or not at all.

6. Rare, affecting elderly population with extremely poor prognosis

7. Can only be differentiated from follicular carcinoma on histology

8. Secretes calcitonin

9. Commonest thyroid malignancy

10. Spread is via blood

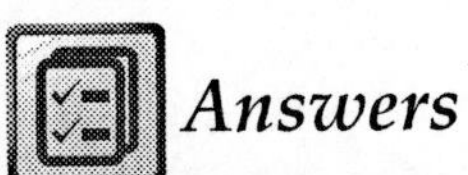

Answers

SBAs		EMQs	
1	A	1	M
2	B	2	A
3	C	3	K
4	B	4	C
5	A	5	L
		6	D
		7	F
		8	A
		9	C
		10	B

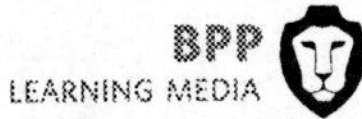

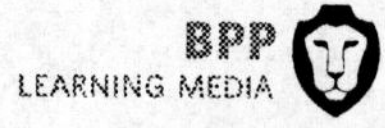

Chapter 16

Urology

Mr John M Henderson

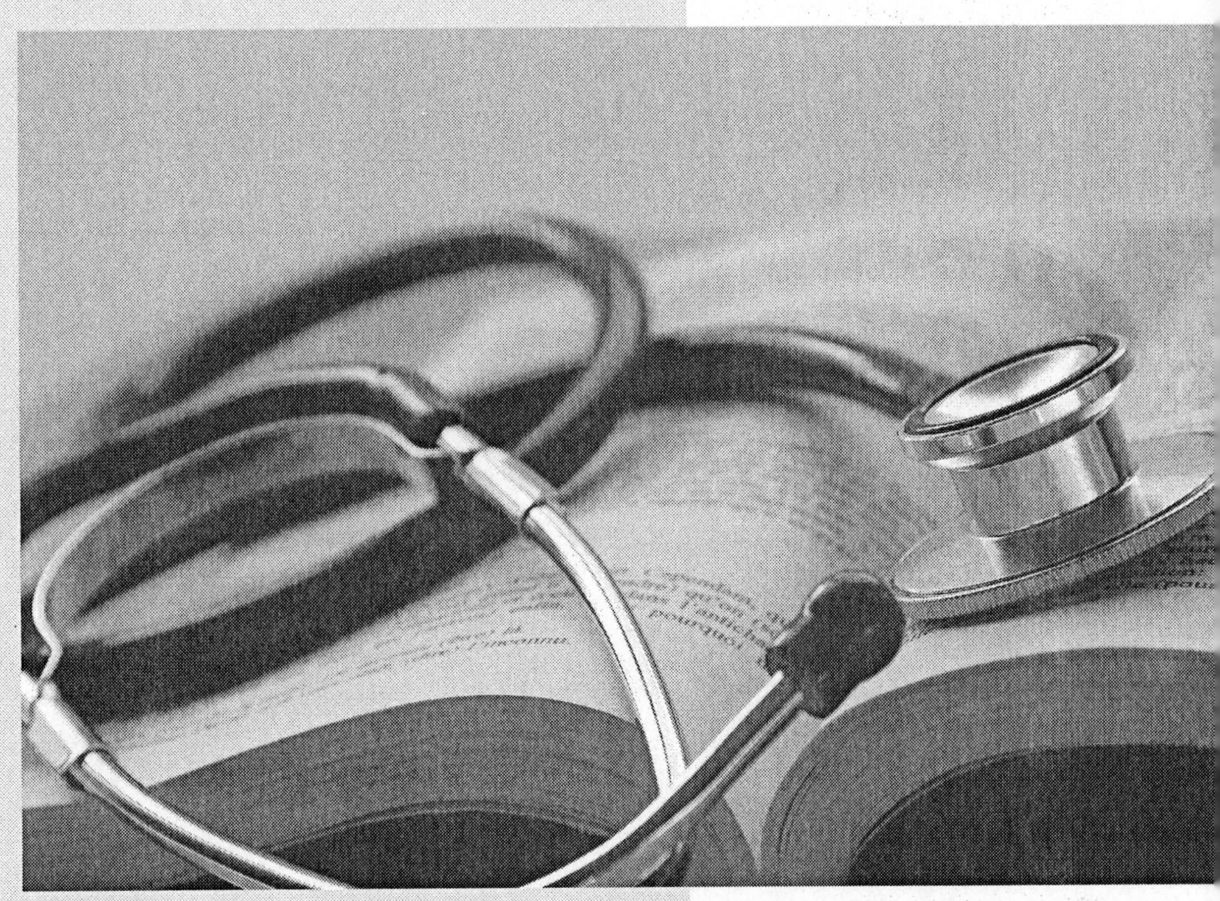

Key investigations

- **CT**: used without contrast to image for calculi (CTKUB) or with contrast for cancer staging or investigation of haematuria
- **Cystoscopy**: endoscopic visualisation of the bladder via the urethra. Can be done with flexible or rigid cystoscope
- **Dimercaptosuccinic acid (DMSA) scan**: measures split renal function and demonstrates renal scarring
- **Intravenous urography**: contrast given intravenously and interval plain X-rays taken of the kidneys, ureters and bladder (KUB)
- **Mercaptoacetyltriglycine (MAG3) renogram**: determines the presence of renal obstruction and measures split renal function
- **Midstream urine (MSU)**: cultured for bacterial growth and sensitivity to various antibiotics
- **Prostate Specific Antigen (PSA)**: an enzyme produced by normal and malignant prostatic tissue which can be measured in the blood
- **Transrectal ultrasound (TRUS) and biopsy**: obtains histological tissue from the prostate for suspected prostate cancer
- **Ultrasound**: used to image all parts of the urinary tract
- **Urinalysis:** dipstick testing for blood, protein, leucocytes, nitrites and pH
- **Urine cytology**: urothelial cells are shed in the urine and can be examined under the microscope. Abnormal cells can indicate cancer
- **Uroflowmetry**: measurement of flow rate (FR) and post void residual (PVR)
- **Urodynamics**: bladder and abdominal pressure are measured to derive detrusor (bladder muscle) pressure during bladder filling and voiding

Haematuria

Haematuria

P Presence of blood in urine.

A Cancer (bladder, kidney, renal pelvis, ureter, prostate).

Calculi (kidney, ureter, bladder).

Infection, inflammation, BPH, nephrological, trauma, foreign body, A/V malformation.

Sx Visible / macroscopic haematuria – seen by the patient.

Non-visible / microscopic – blood on dipstick / microscopy.

S Examine for abdominal mass. DRE to examine prostate.

I MSU (all), cystoscopy (all), ultrasound (all), IVU or CT urogram (for visible haematuria).

T Specific to cause.

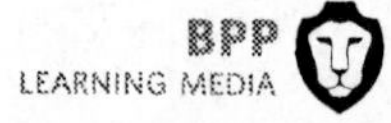

C Large volume haematuria may cause haemodynamic compromise.

Pr Likelihood of urological cancer – visible haematuria (30%), non-visible (5%).

Renal tract

Renal tract stones

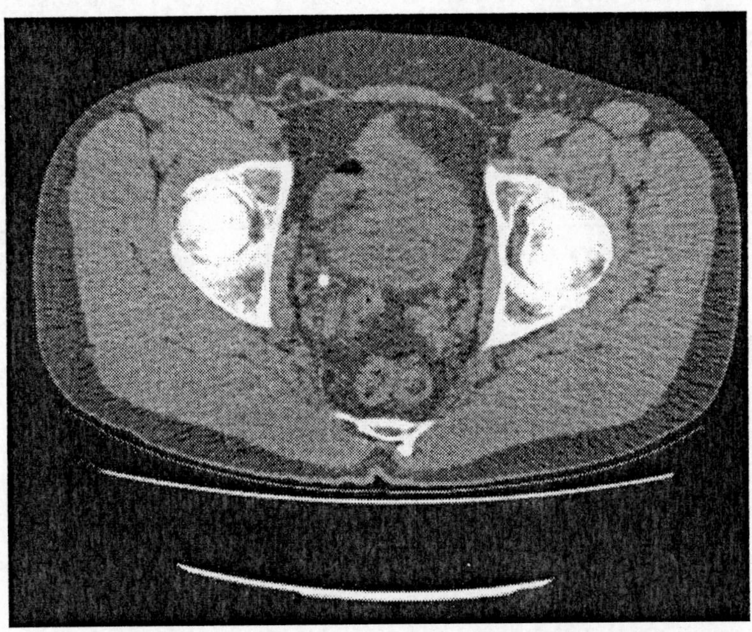

Figure 16.1: CTKUB showing 5mm calculus at right VUJ. (Reproduced with permission from SW Deanery.)

P Formation of calculus in renal tract.

A Various (see Table 16.1).

Sx Loin pain in acute phase, may be incidental finding on imaging Recurrent UTIs.

S Always exclude abdominal aortic aneurysm (AAA): may present with loin pain and haematuria.

I Non-contrast CT (NCCT/CTKUB) if available.

Urinalysis, U&Es, Ca^{2+}, uric acid, 24-hour urine collection in high risk patients.

T Analgesia, conservative with alpha-blocker (relaxes ureteric smooth muscle) awaiting spontaneous passage if calculus small. Extracorporeal shock wave lithotripsy (ESWL).

Ureteroscopy (URS) and fragmentation of stone.

Percutaneous nephrolithotomy (PCNL).

Oral chemolitholysis for uric acid stones (urinary alkalisation).

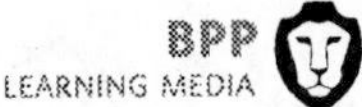

C Requirement for urgent renal decompression (ureteric stent or percutaneous nephrostomy): infected, obstructed kidney (look for signs of sepsis), obstructed single kidney.

Pr Once patient has formed a stone, higher risk of subsequent stone formation.

Type	Radiological characteristic	Prevalence	Predisposing factors
Calcium oxalate	Radio-opaque	85%	Hypercalcaemia, hyperoxaluria
Calcium phosphate and oxalate	Radio-opaque	10%	Renal tubular acidosis
Uric acid	Radiolucent	5–10%	Gout, myeloproliferative disorders
Struvite	Relatively radiolucent	2–20%	Infection
Cystine	Relatively radiolucent	1–2%	Cystinuria

Table 16.1: Types of renal tract stones

Ureteric obstruction

P Obstruction to free flow of urine down the ureter.

A Benign (calculus) or malignant (prostate / bladder / ureteric tumour). Obstruction may be extrinsic (eg lymphadenopathy), intramural (eg TCC) or intrinsic (eg calculus).

Sx Renal failure, anuria if bilateral or solitary kidney.

S Examine for cause – DRE for prostatic malignancy.

I U&Es. Renal tract ultrasound / CT.

T ABCDE resuscitation, medical treatment of hyperkaelamia (insulin /dextrose).

Relief of obstruction: percnephrostomy or stents.

C Renal failure and death.

Pr Life threatening if untreated.

Urinary tract infection

(See also Chapter 4 *Renal.*)

P Bacterial infection of urine.

A E. coli, klebsiella, proteus.

Sx Dysuria, frequence, incontinence.

S Suprapubic tenderness.

I Midstream urine (MSU) for culture and antibiotic sensitivities.

T Course of appropriate antibiotics. Trimethoprim, Nitrofurantoin, Cephalexin.

C Pyelonephritis, renal scarring.

Pr Recurrent UTI (>2 infections in 6 months).

Kidney disease

Pyelonephritis

P Renal infection, often ascending from the lower urinary tract.

A E. coli, klebsiella, proteus, enterobacter.

Sx Flank pain, fever, vomiting.

S Temperature, loin tenderness.

I FBC, U&Es, CTKUB/US to exclude obstructed renal tract.

T Oral antibiotics if well, IV antibiotics if unwell.

C Pyonephrosis (renal abscess), perinephric abscess (abscess around the kidney). Both usually require drainage.

Pr Renal scarring.

Renal tumours

P Renal cell carcinoma (RCC) (see paeds for Wilms' tumour).

A 3% cancers, Von Hippel-Lindau (VHL): 50% develop RCC.

Sx Haematuria (50%), loin pain, malaise.

S Palpable mass, hypertension, weight loss, left varicocele (RCC obstructing drainage to left renal vein, right renal v. drains directly to IVC).

I FBC: polycythaemia, anaemia, U&Es, ↑ Ca^{2+}, LFTs, triple phase contrast CT.

T Surveillance, radical nephrectomy (partial or whole): usually laparoscopic, immunotherapy.

C Recurrence, local disease to renal vein, IVC, adrenals, mets to bone, lung ('canon ball lesions') and lymph.

Pr Calculate from scoring methods eg Leibovich score.

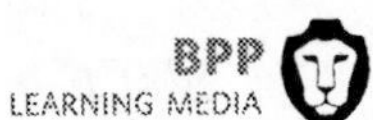

Kidney transplant

P An option for end-stage renal failure (ESRF).

A Diabetes, renovascular disease, glomerulonephritis.

Sx Uraemia, oliguria.

S Donors may be living or deceased.

I Assessment of the donor (HIV, hepatitis B&C, CMV, CJD).

Assessment of the kidney (MI, DM, malignancy, DMSA, Cr clearance).

Assessment of the recipient (ABO blood group, HLA).

T Transplantation with immunosuppression.

C Rejection (hyperacute, acute, chronic).

Pr Close follow up by transplant team.

Bladder

Bladder malignancy

P TCC, SCC, adenocarcinoma.

A Smoking, occupational exposure (aniline dyes).

Sx Haematuria (visible or non-visible), lower urinary tract symptoms (LUTS), incidental finding on imaging.

S Abdominal / PV or PR mass.

I Flexible cystoscopy, upper tract imaging (CT Urogram or ultrasound and IVU).

T Initially transurethral resection of bladder tumour (TURBT): excision of tumour and obtains histology of tumour.

C Bleeding.

Bladder perforation:

- Extraperitoneal: usually heal with catheter
- Intraperitoneal: requires laparotomy to repair and exclude injury to abdominal viscera

Pr Low grade non-muscle invasive tumours: surveillance +/- MMC.

High grade non-muscle invasive tumours: BCG.

Muscle invasive tumours (T2): cystectomy or radical radiotherapy.

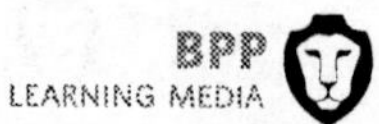

Prostate

Benign prostatic hyperplasia

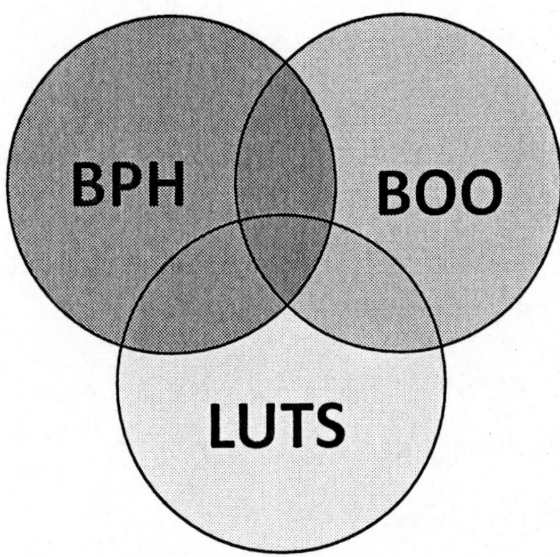

Figure 16.2: Overlap between benign prostatic hyperplasia (BPH), bladder outflow obstruction (BOO) and lower urinary tract symptoms (LUTS)

P Lower urinary tract symptoms caused by prostatic obstruction.

A Hyperplasia of prostatic transition zone cells with resultant bladder outflow obstruction.

Sx LUTS: hesitancy, intermittency, poor flow, incomplete emptying.

S Palpable bladder, DRE: prostate may be normal or enlarged.

I Assessment score (eg IPSS).

PSA after counselling (surrogate marker for prostate volume), urinalysis, uroflowmetry, U&Es.

T Conservative: 'watchful waiting'.

Medical therapy: alpha blocker, 5-alpha reductase inhibitor (5ARI).

Combination therapy (both of the above).

Surgical: transurethral resection of prostate (TURP), laser prostatectomy (HOLEP / PVP), open (Millin's) prostatectomy.

C Progression of symptoms, chronic retention (high / low pressure).

Alpha blocker – retrograde ejaculation, postural hypotension.

5 ARI loss of libido.

TURP: retrograde ejaculation, erectile dysfunction, incontinence, failure to void.

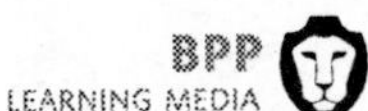

Pr One-third improve, one-third stable, one-third deteriorate.

Prostatitis

P Infection or inflammation of the prostate.

A See Table for classification.

Sx Perineal pain, may radiate down legs. LUTS: dysuria, frequency, poor flow.

S Exquisitely tender prostate in acute phase.

I MSU, TRUS to exclude prostatic abscess.

T Antibiotics for ABP eg ciprofloxacin.

Alpha blockers, NSAIDs, 5ARI.

C Chronic pelvic pain syndrome.

Pr Depends on type and response to treatment.

Type	Description
I	Acute bacterial prostatitis (ABP)
II	Chronic bacterial prostatitis (CBP)
III	Chronic pelvic pain syndrome (CPPS) A: inflammatory B: non-inflammatory
IV	Asymptomatic inflammatory prostatitis

Table 16.2 Prostatitis grading

Prostate malignancy

P Malignant cells in the prostate gland.

A Growth of malignant tissue under influence of testosterone and dihydrotestosterone.

Sx Asymptomatic, PSA screening, LUTS, haematuria, bone pain.

S Abnormal DRE, lymphatic obstruction.

I Renal function, TRUS and biopsy for Gleason grading score, MRI, bone scan.

T Active surveillance (low risk cancer).

Radical prostatectomy (open / laparoscopic / robotic).

Radiotherapy: external beam (EBRT) or brachytherapy (radioactive seeds implanted in prostate).

Androgen Deprivation Therapy (ADT): LHRH analogues, antiandrogens, oestrogens, steroids.

Chemotherapy.

C Urinary symptoms, bone pain.

Pr Depends on grade / stage.

Testes

Testicular torsion

P Twisting of the spermatic cord compromising blood supply to the testis.

A Extravaginal (neonatal): twisted spermatic cord.

Intravaginal (any age): 'bell clapper testis' where tunica vaginalis inserts high on spermatic cord allowing testis to rotate freely.

Sx Sudden onset of pain, sometimes preceded by mild trauma, vomiting.

S Testis may be lying higher and horizontal due to the cord twisting .

I None, surgical exploration if diagnosis is suspected.

T Three point fixation (orchidopexy) of both testes to prevent re-torsion.

Can also fix in Dartos pouch.

C Unrecognised torsion results in testicular ischaemia within approximately six hours.

Pr Good with early diagnosis.

Torsion of Hydatid of Morgagni

P Twisting of testicular appendage leads to pain.

A Embryological remnant of Müllerian duct.

Sx Very similar to those of testicular torsion.

S May have 'blue dot' sign.

I None.

T Often need to explore, excision of torted hydatid.

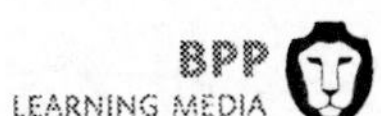

C None.

Pr Difficult to differentiate clinically from testicular torsion.

Epididymal cyst

P Fluid filled cyst on the epididymis.

A Arise from the collecting tubules of the epididymis.

Sx Scrotal swelling.

S Cystic swelling arising from the epididymis.

I Ultrasound.

T Conservative.

Surgical excision (avoid in young men who wish to preserve fertility).

C Recurrence, scrotal pain.

Pr Good.

Epididymo-orchitis

P Inflammation of epididymis and / or testis.

A Young men: usually chlamydia or gonorrhoea.

Older men: usually secondary to UTI.

Pure orchitis can be caused by mumps and is associated with parotitis.

Sx Swollen, tender erythematous epididymis and / or testis, may be associated with LUTS.

S Vanishingly rare diagnosis in non-sexually active teenagers or younger, consider torsion.

I MSU, ultrasound to exclude collection, urethral swab.

T Antibiotics (doxycycline where chlamydia likely), analgesia.

C Testicular infarction, abscess formation, infertility.

Pr Can progress to chronic form of disease with persistent pain.

Hydrocele

P Collection of fluid in the tunica vaginalis.

A Primary or secondary (epididymo-orchitis, torsion, varicocele operation).

Sx Scrotal swelling.

S Transilluminable swelling around testis.

I Ultrasound if any doubt and to confirm normal underlying testis.

T Observation.

Aspiration – not recommended as recurrence likely.

Surgical treatment (Lord or Jaboulay technique).

C Recurrence, scrotal pain.

Pr Good.

Varicocele

P Dilatation of pamniform plexus of veins.

A Rarely, left sided varicocele can be due to pressure on insertion of left testicular vein into left renal vein by renal tumour.

Sx Often asymptomatic. Pain, infertility, atrophy.

S 'Bag of worms' on examination, often disappears on lying down.

I Ultrasound can confirm.

T Ligation or occlusion of internal spermatic veins, embolisation.

C Infertility (20%): treating varicocele may help.

Recurrence.

Pr Good.

Testicular cancer

P Malignant cells in testis.

A Germ cell tumors: 90% (eg seminoma, teratoma).

Sex cord stromal tumours: <10% (eg Sertoli cell, Leydig cell tumours).

Sx Hard mass in body of testis.

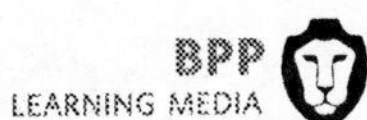

S History of cryoptorchidism, Klinefelter's syndrome (increase risk).

Abdominal mass.

I Ultrasound testes, tumour markers: alpha-fetoprotein (AFP), beta-human chorionic gonadotrophin (hCG), lactate dehydrogenase (LDH).

CT chest / abdomen / pelvis for metastases.

T Radical inguinal orchidectomy initially.

Surveillance.

Chemotherapy with cisplatin, eposide, bleomycin.

Retroperitoneal Lymph Node Dissection (RPLND).

Radiotherapy.

C Progression of disease.

Pr Stratify prognosis based on histology, presence of metastases, tumour markers.

Penis

Penile malignancy

P Malignancy of penis.

A Human papilloma virus (HPV) is risk factor for SCC.

Premalignant conditions – balanitis xerotica obliterans (BXO), erythroplasia of Queyrat, Bowen's disease.

Sx Firm mass palpable on penis.

S Examination of mass and inguinal lymph nodes.

I Biopsy of mass (if diagnosis in doubt).

MRI of penis, CT scan for lymphadenpathy.

T Surveillance.

CO_2 or Nd:YAG laser.

Wide local excision.

Glansectomy with inguinal lymphadenectomy.

Partial / total penectomy.

Chemo / radiotherapy.

C 92% of recurrence within five years, close follow up essential.

Pr Cure rate 80%.

Phimosis

P Inability to retract the foreskin.

A Normal foreskin may not retract until late childhood.

Balanitis Xerotica Obliterans (BXO).

Sx Painful, scarred foreskin which may tear on retraction.

S As above.

I None.

T Medical: strong topical steroid.

Surgical: frenuloplasty, prepucioplasty, dorsal slit, circumcision.

C Change in cosmesis and sensation.

Pr Good.

Paraphimosis

P Inability to return to foreskin from a retracted position back over the glans.

A May be iatrogenic eg foreskin not returned after catheterisation.

Sx Painful retracted oedematous foreskin.

S 'Ballooned' foreskin.

I None.

T Gentle manual reduction (often successful).

Dundee technique: multiple needle punctures of oedematous foreskin to reduce swelling.

Ice or granulated sugar (works by osmosis) can also be effective.

Dorsal slit if other techniques fail. Circumcision can be difficult acutely and is usually performed at a later stage.

C May require surgical treatment.

Pr May recur – elective circumcision usually warranted.

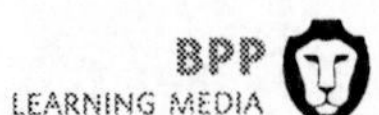

Erectile dysfunction

P Persistent inability to maintain an erection sufficient for sexual performance.

A Iatrogenic: radical prostatectomy (cavernosal nerve injury).

Cardiovascular: diabetes.

Sx Nocturnal tumescence may help differentiate physiological and psychological causes.

S Physical examination and DRE, penile curvature (eg Peyronies), hypogonadism, cardiovascular and neurological examination.

I Often none required. Blood tests: glucose tolerance test, lipid profile, testosterone, PSA, endocrinological investigation.

Vascular studies.

T Specific to cause.

Psychosexual therapy, testosterone replacement therapy.

Phosphodiesterase 5 (PDE5) inhibitors: sildenafil, tadalafil, vardenafil (contraindicated with nitrate use – hypotension).

Vacuum constriction device (VCD) with constriction band at base of penis.

Intracavernosal injections: alprostadil.

Penile prosthesis.

C PDE5 inhibitors: headache, flushing, visual abnormalities.

Intracavernosal injections: priapism (prolonged erection), penile pain.

Penile prosthesis: mechanical failure, infection.

Pr Variable.

Priapism

P Prolonged penile erection not accompanied by sexual desire.

A Primary / idiopathic.

Secondary: trauma, sickle cell, thromboembolic, drugs (alpha blockers, antidepressants, antigoagulants), neurological.

Sx High flow (non-ischaemic): mild pain, turgid.

Low flow (ischaemic): severe paid, rigid.

S Cavernosal blood gas is arterial in high flow, venous in low flow.

I FBC, sickle test, cavernosal blood gas.

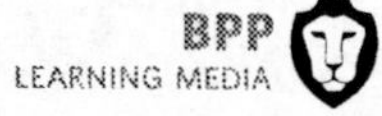

T Conservative: ice, ejaculation, exercise.

Corporeal aspiration ×2.

Intracorporeal injection of phenylephrine.

Arterial embolisation or ligation (high flow).

Surgical shunt: cavernoglandular, cavernospongiosal, cavernosaphenous.

C Can be recurrent (stuttering priapism).

If untreated: cavernosal necrosis.

P Good if treated early, poor if not.

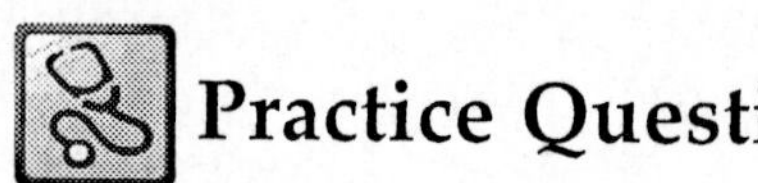

Practice Questions

Single Best Answers

1. Which of the following is a contraindication for PDE5 inhibitor usage?

   A Previous radical prostatectomy
   B Addison's disease
   C Concomitant nitrate use
   D Alpha-1 antitrypsin deficiency

2. Which of the following medications can cause retrograde ejaculation?

   A Alpha-blocker
   B 5ARI
   C PDE5 inhibitor
   D SSRI

3. Which of the following is the strongest risk factor for testicular cancer?

   A Smoking
   B Cryptoorchidism
   C Testicular trauma
   D Vasectomy

4. A 14-year-old boy presents with a four-hour history of right testicular pain waking him from sleep. What is the next step?

   A Ultrasound
   B Scrotal exploration
   C Oral antibiotics and observe
   D CT scan

5. What is the most common cause of epididymoorchitis in a heterosexual 25-year-old man?

   A E. coli
   B Gonorrhoea
   C Amiodarone
   D Chlamydia

6. Which is the most common type of renal calculus?

   A Calcium oxalate
   B Uric acid
   C Struvite
   D Indinavir

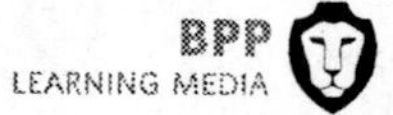

7. Which of the following is associated with the 'blue dot' sign?

   A Testicular torsion
   B Hydrocele due to trauma
   C Varicocele
   D Torted Hydatid of Morgagni

8. Which of the following can be used to treat priapism?

   A Solifenacin
   B Phenylephrine
   C Zuidex
   D Carbemazepine

9. The treatment of which of the following has been shown to improve fertility?

   A Varicocele
   B Hydrocele
   C Inguinoscrotal hernia
   D Scrotal sebaceous cysts

10. Which genetic condition increases the chance of renal cell carcinoma?

   A Cystic fibrosis
   B Thalassaemia
   C Von Hippel-Lindau
   D Kleinfelter's

11. Which of the following may be cause by pyelonephritis?

   A Pyonephrosis
   B Uric acid calculi
   C PUJ obstruction
   D Paraphimosis

12. Which of the following is most likely to lead to end-stage renal failure?

   A Chronic pelvic pain syndrome
   B Glomerulonephritis
   C Low-pressure chronic retention
   D Finasteride usage

13. Which of the following is not a treatment for prostate cancer?

   A Brachytherapy
   B External beam radiotherapy
   C Radical prostatectomy
   D Phytotherapy

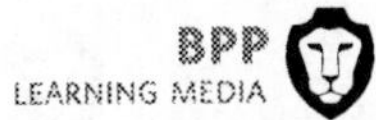

14. In which of these conditions is a sickle cell blood test most useful?

    A Priapism
    B Phimosis
    C Recurrent UTI
    D Pyelonephritis

15. Which of the following can be used to treat phimosis?

    A Alpha blocker
    B Topical methotrexate
    C Topical emollient
    D Topical steroid

Extended Matching Questions

Choose the most appropriate treatment for prostate cancer.

A LHRH analogue
B Palliative radiotherapy to bone
C Active surveillance
D Radical prostatectomy

1. A 77-year-old man with a small focus in a single biopsy core of Gleason 6 (3+3) prostate cancer.

2. A 68-year-old man with known metastatic prostate cancer, already on androgen deprivation therapy, who has new severe bone pain.

3. An 88-year-old man with a new diagnosis of asymptomatic metastatic prostate cancer.

Choose the most appropriate radiological imaging.

A CTKUB (non-contrast)
B DMSA scan
C MAG3 renogram
D Triple phase CT urogram

4. A 55-year-old man with haematuria and a suspicious mass in the right kidney on USS.

5. A 31-year-old lady with acute severe left loin to groin pain and microscopic haematuria.

6. A 40-year-old man with longstanding right loin pain and CT suggestive of pelvi-ureteric junction obstruction.

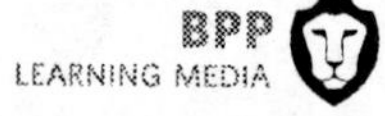

Choose the most appropriate treatment for bladder cancer.

A Radical cystectomy
B Intravesical Mitomycin C
C Regular check cystoscopies
D Intravesical BCG

7. A 76-year-old man with previous G1Ta (low grade, superficial) bladder cancer with occasional single recurrences.

8. A 60-year-old lady with G3T2 (high grade, muscle invasive) bladder cancer.

9. A 72-year-old man with G3T1 (high grade, non-muscle invasive) bladder cancer with CIS.

Choose the most appropriate treatment for the following.

A Alpha blocker (eg tamsulosin)
B 5-alpha reductase inhibitor (eg finasteride)
C Transurethral resection of the prostate (TURP)
D Prostatic urethral stent

10. A 70-year-old man who presents in retention with a two litre residual and a creatinine of 400 which improves after catheterisation.

11. A 67-year-old man with bothersome LUTS, a Qmax of 10ml/s and a post void residual of 120ml.

12. A 76-year-old man with marked COPD and IHD, who has been taking tamsulosin for years but has deteriorating LUTS and a large prostate on DRE.

What is the most likely diagnosis for these inguinoscrotal lesions?

A Hydrocele
B Testicular cancer
C Inguinal hernia
D Varicocele

13. A hard painless mass in the body of the testis.

14. A transilluminable swelling in the scrotum which you can get above.

15. A swelling in the scrotum which you cannot get above and has a cough impulse.

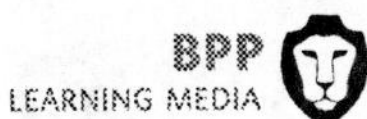

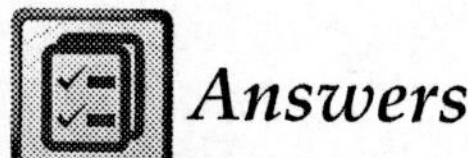

Answers

SBAs		EMQs	
1	C	1	C
2	A	2	B
3	B	3	A
4	B	4	D
5	D	5	A
6	A	6	C
7	D	7	C
8	B	8	A
9	A	9	D
10	C	10	C
11	A	11	A
12	B	12	B
13	D	13	B
14	A	14	A
15	D	15	C

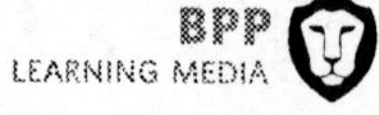

Chapter 17

Neurosurgery

Mr Dermot Mallon

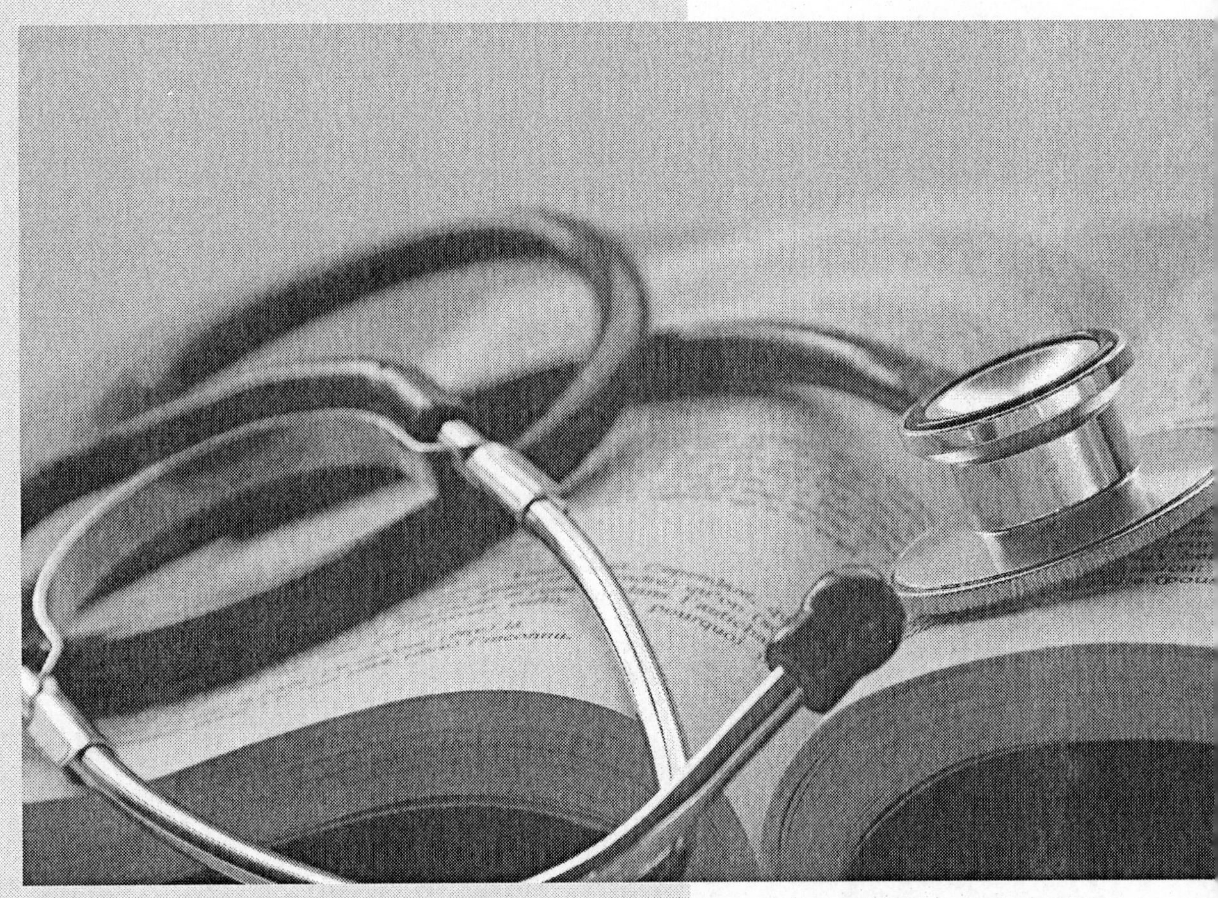

Trauma

Glasgow coma scale (GCS)

The Glasgow coma score is method of assessing patients with altered consciousness. Coma is arbitrarily defined as a GCS<8 at which point intubation is often mandated. Change in GCS is often more informative than the absolute figure.

	Eyes	Verbal	Motor
6			Obeys commands
5		Oriented, appropriate speech	Localises to pain
4	Eyes open spontaneously	Confused, disoriented speech	Withdrawal in response to pain
3	Eyes open in response to voice	Uses inappropriate words	Abnormal flexion in response to pain
2	Eyes open in response to pain	Makes incomprehensible sounds	Extension in response to pain
1	Unable to open eyes	Unable to make sound	Unable to move

Table 17.1: Glasgow coma scale

Cerebral persusion and Cushing's reflex

Cerebral perfusion pressure (CPP) = Mean arterial pressure (MAP) – Intracranial pressure

The Monro-Kellie Doctrine states that a change in one component of the intracranium (blood, parenchyma, CSF) must be compensated for a change in another.

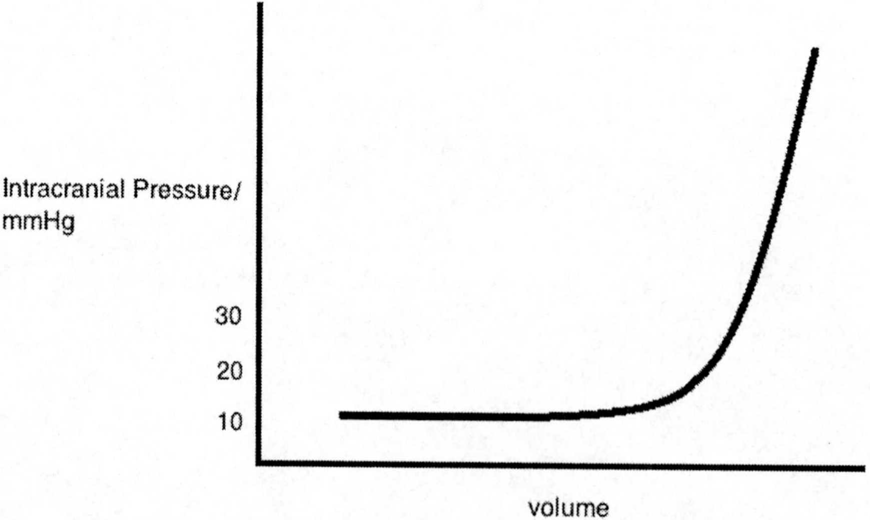

Figure 17.1: Volume-pressure relationship for intercranial pressure

Normal ICP is 7–15mmHg and the brain is capable of compensating for a change in volume up to a pressure of ~20mmHg. Symptoms of rasied ICP occur above 25mmHg.

Cushing's reflex: elevated ICP causes mixed vagal and sympathetic stimulation leading to hypertension, bradycardia and irregular respiration.

Head injury

P Symptoms caused through a combination of direct parenchymal damage, hypoxia and mass effect.

S Altered level of consciousness, focal neurology, racoon eyes / Battle's sign (mastoid ecchymosis) suggestive of base of skull fracture, Cushing's reflex: bradycardia (early), irregular breathing (late) and hypertension (late).

Sx Pain, altered level of consciousness (be aware of possible 'lucid interval' seen in EDH), amnesia, concomitant injury eg cervical spine fracture.

I CT head, ICP monitoring.

T Expedient diagnosis, prevent hypotension, consider antiepileptics if parenchyma injury, evacuation of haematoma, monitor ICP and treat accordingly (eg mannitol, hyperventilation).

C Seizures, permanent loss of function.

Pr Dependent on nature of injury and rapidity of treatment.

- GCS less than 13 at initial assessment
- GCS less than 15 two hours after injury
- Suspected open or depressed skull fracture
- Any sign of basal skull fracture (hematotympanum, 'racoon' eyes, Battle's sign, cerebrospinal flbuid leakage from the ear or nose)
- Two or more episodes of vomiting in adults; more than two episodes of vomiting in children
- Post-traumatic seizure
- Coagulopathy (bleeding diathesis, warfarin therapy) with amnesia or loss of consciousness
- Focal neurological deficit

Box 17.1: Indications for CT head within one hour of admission

Skull fracture

P Disruption of cranial bones, classified as linear, basal and depressed.

A Trauma, most commonly occur at areas of thin bone namely temporal, parietal and skull base (sphenoid bone).

S Soft tissue haematoma, neurological deficient, reduced GCS, CSF rhinorrhoea, ears, Battle's sign, racoon eyes.

Sx Pain, neurological deficit, altered GCS.

I Meticulous neurological examination followed by CT head. Tissue paper can be used to look for 'halo' sign when dabbed with suspected CSF.

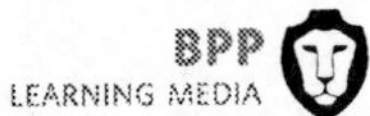

T Small linear fractures do not require inpatient stay in adults. Children should be admitted for observation.

Surgery may be required for depressed skull fractures, or when there is a vascular injury or raised ICP.

C Fracture may cause dural tear or affect inner ear.

Antibiotic prophylaxis should be given for meningitis in open / skull base fractures, intracranial bleeding / haematomas. Prophylactic anticonvulsant therapy may be considered especially if depressed skull fracture.

Pr Dependent degree of trauma.

Excellent recover expected if no parenchymal damage and fractures, and therefore their potential complications, are diagnosed early.

Coma

P A state of prolonged deep unconsciousness where normal neurological responses are absent.

A Trauma or metabolic disturbance eg hypoglycaemia, intoxication.

S Asymmetrical pupils, may have decerebrate (elbows, wrists, knees extended) or decorticate (flexed elbows, wrists, extended legs).

Sx Unconsciousness which may mask other physical signs of underlying cause.

I Dependent on suspected cause of coma, serum electrolytes and glucose. Toxicology screen, CT head, EEG.

T Medical emergency and initial concern must be over maintenance of definitive airway (intubation) and ventilation. Pressure sores must be prevented and nutritional support given. Advanced investigations eg ICP monitoring must be directed as per cause of coma.

Pr Greatly variable depending on cause of coma however is universally improved through active avoidance of pneumonia and pressure sores.

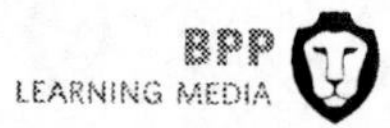

Intracranial haemorrhage

Subarachnoid haemorrhage

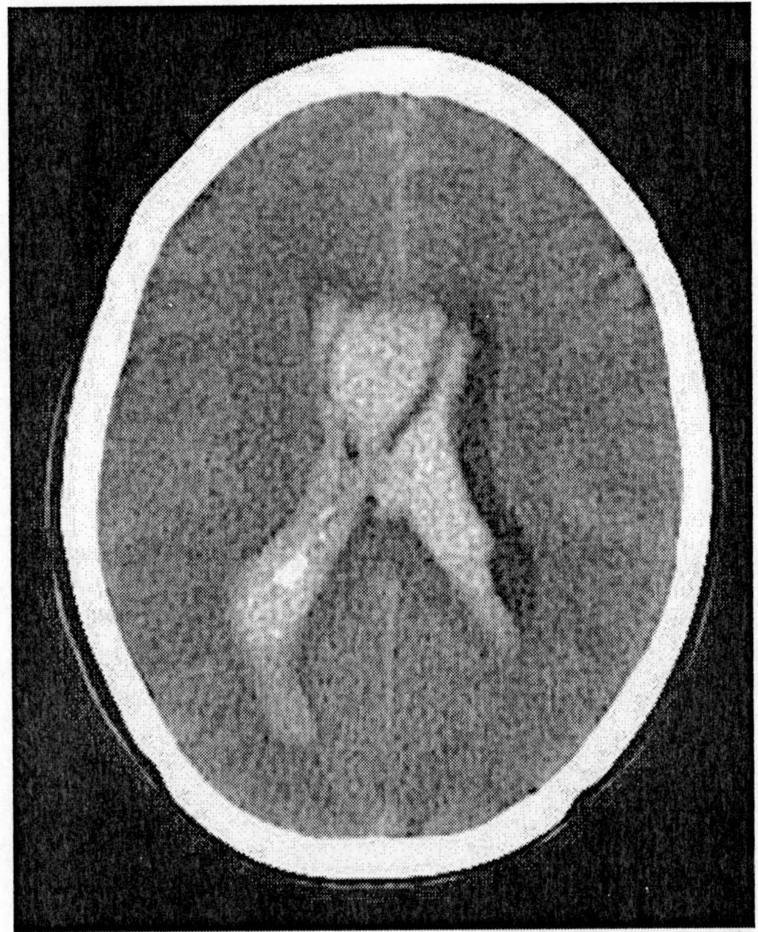

Figure 17.2: SAH from ruptured anterior communicating artery berry aneurysm. (Reproduced with permission from SW Deanery.)

P Haemorrhage into the CSF-containing subarachnoid space.

A 85% are from rupture of berry aneurysms; remainder includes arteriovenous malformations and trauma.

S Meningism (neck stiffness, Kernig's sign), reduced level of consciousness, neurological signs secondary to decreased perfusion and vasospasm.

Sx Headache classically described as 'thunder clap', decreased consciousness.

I CT head showing hyperdense (white) areas in subarachnoid space, angiography looking for bleeding point and AVM, lumbar puncture looking for raised RBCs, xanthochromia (caused by degradation of haemoglobin) and raised pressure.

T Fluid resuscitation to avoid cerebral hypotension, nimodipine to prevent vasospasm, interventional neuroradiologists or neurosurgeons to coil / clip aneurysm. Failing this open surgery to control bleed.

C Hypernatremia (secondary to SIADH), obstructive hydrocephalus, persistent neurological deficit.

Pr Proportional to severity of initial symptoms, significant mortality of >30% in first few days.

Rate of re-bleed with conservative management is reported between 4–25% in first month.

- 90% of congenital cerebral aneurysms
- Located at branches of large arteries
- Rupture causes SAH
- May present more insidiously with mass effect (eg 3rd CN nerve palsy with Posterior inferior cerebellar artery aneurysm), seizures or headache
- Mortality of 60%
- Management may be conservative (low risk of rupture if <10mm), surgical clipping or neuro-radiological coiling

Box 17.2: Berry aneurysms

Extradural haemorrhage

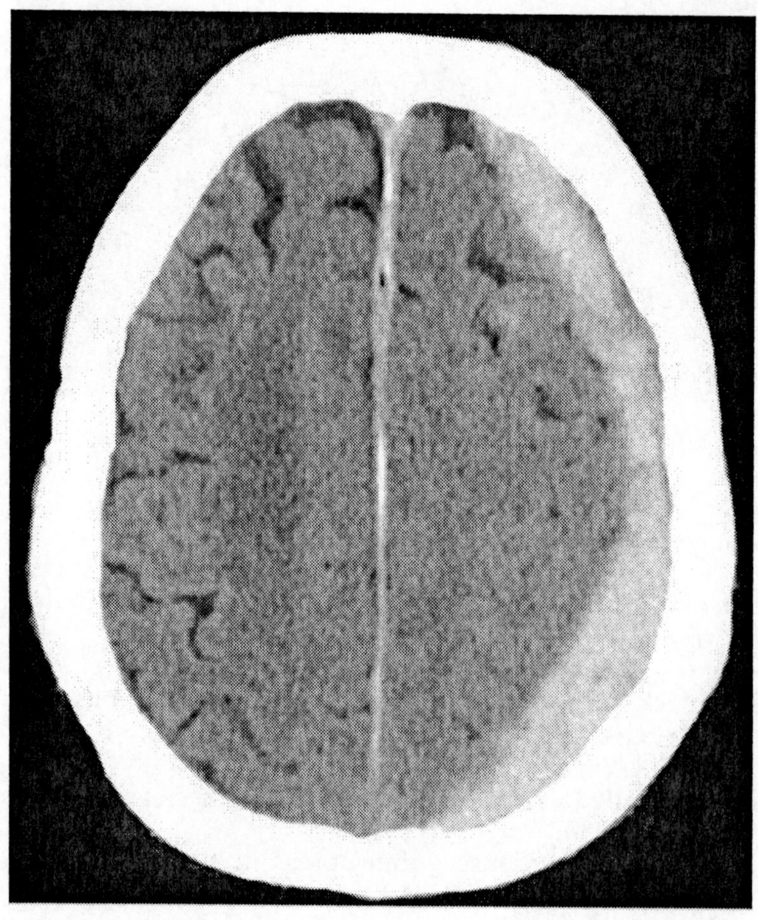

Figure 17.3: Left extradural haemorrhage. (Reproduced with permission from SW Deanery.)

P Bleeding into space between the dura and skull most commonly originating from the middle meningeal artery.

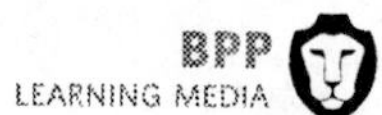

A Trauma to temporal bone causing rupture of middle meningeal artery.

S Classic progression of post-traumatic loss of consciousness, lucid interval and then decrease in level of consciousness as haematoma expands.

Examine for signs of raised ICP.

Sx Loss of consciousness, vomiting.

I CT head showing a biconvex area of high density, limited by suture lines.

T Surgical evacuation / cautery of bleeding vessel.

C Herniation and death if not resolved.

Pr Dependent on degree of trauma and GCS at presentation (0% if GCS 15 at presentation, >40% if GCS <8 at presentation).

Subdural haemorrhage

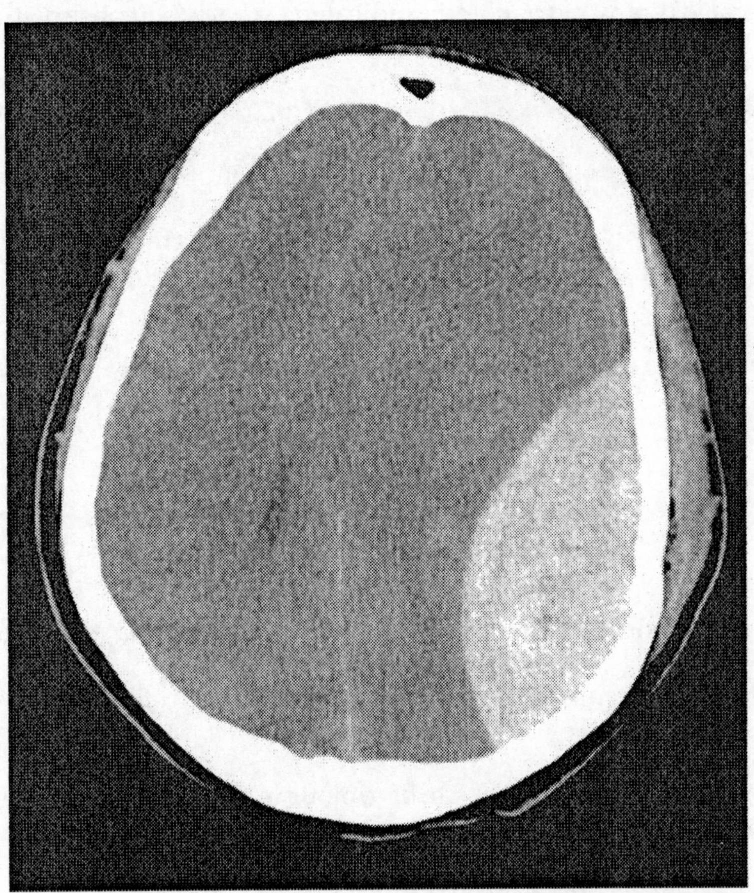

Figure 17.4: Left subdural haemorrhage. (Reproduced with permission from SW Deanery.)

P Haematoma forms between arachnoid and dura mater May be acute (<72 hours), sub-acute (3–20 days) or chronic (>20 days) depending time between injury and onset of symptoms.

A Tearing of bridging veins in subarachnoid space, which are stretched by cerebral atrophy and alcohol abuse.

S *Acute:* decreased GCS, dilated pupil due to compression of parasympathetic supply on circumference of IIIrd nerve, Cushing's response.

Chronic: may be normal, may have 3rd or 4th nerve palsy, papilloedema, asymmetrical reflexes, hemiparesis.

Sx Dependent on level of trauma, neurological deficit, chronic may be asymptomatic. May have signs of raised ICP (nausea, vomiting, papilloedema).

I CT head: crescentic lesion on inner surface of skull. May cause obliteration of ventricles and midline shift. Colour of lesion progresses from hyperdense (white) acutely, to isodense (grey) to hypodense (black) when chronic.

T *Acute:* management of head trauma with immobilisation of cervical spine, and intubation if GCS <8, surgical evacuation of haematoma may be considered.

Chronic: if symptomatic or considerable mass effect on CT (midline shift >5mm or haematoma >10mm) burr hole is indicated, otherwise conservative approach with serial CT scans may be considered.

C Parenchymal damage, herniation, seizures (>20%).

Monitor ICP: lower with mannitol and nurse in upright position.

Pr Mortality of 75% if cisterns effaced on CT, depends greatly on degree of underlying parenchymal damage.

Space occupying lesions

Meningioma

P Neoplasia of the arachnoid mater covering of the brain. May be intracranial or within the spinal canal.

Tumour causes cortical irritation, compression of nerves and, rarely, vascular occlusion.

A Most are idiopathic, however may be familial as in neurofibromatosis 2. More common in women than men.

S Focal neurology depending on site of tumour in CNS. Spinal cord tumours may result in Brown-Séquard syndrome due to unilateral compression.

Sx Seizures, headaches, paresis, apathy, symptoms of raised ICP.

I CT (more sensitive for bone involvement) and MRI (more sensitive for tumour and oedema), angiography for preoperative planning.

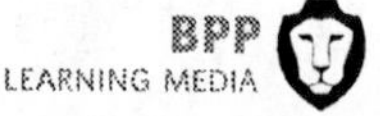

T Corticosteroids and antiepileptic drugs are routinely given preoperatively. Preoperative embolisation may be used in vascular lesions prior to definitive management through surgical resection.

Radiotherapy may be used as adjuvant therapy or for inaccessible tumours.

Meningiomas are relatively chemotherapy-resistant.

C Neurological deficient either from primary pathology or secondary to surgery / radiotherapy.

Pr Excellent prognosis if completely resected. >90% five-year survival expected.

Glioma

P Arises from glial cells (heterogeneous group of support cells for neurons).

A Most common tumour within CNS. Idiopathic although some associated with neurofibromatosis and tuberous sclerosis complex.

S Dependent on location of the lesion, tends to give focal neurological deficits, raised ICP.

Sx Nausea, vomiting, neurological symptoms depending on location.

I CT/MRI head.

T Treatment is dependent on the grade of tumour, may be a combination of surgery, radiation and chemotherapy.

C May have neurological deficit due to primary parenchymal damage from tumour invasion or secondary to surgical intervention.

Pr High-grade gliomas and glioblastoma multiforme 50% mortality at one-year.

Low-grade gliomas such as oligodenroglioma has a median survival of around 15 years.

Pituitary tumour

P Classified by size (macroadenomas >1cm, microadenomas <1cm), histology and on the hormone(s) they secrete.

A Mainly idiopathic however may be associated with MEN Type I.

S May be asymptomatic.

Mass effect: half present with visual field defects due to optic chiasm compression; classically this is bi-temporal hemianopia. Extension into cavernous sinus may give rise to optic symptoms (IV, VI).

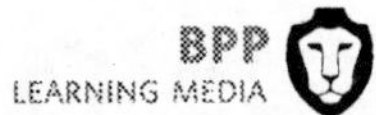

Hormonal: hyperprolactinaemia is the most common (infertility, amenorrhea, galactorrhoea).

Pituitary apoplexy: phenomenon similar to a subarachnoid haemorrhage.

Sx Rhinorrhoea, bitemporal hemianopia, obstructive hydrocephalus.

I Blood levels of pituitary hormones in descending order of frequency (prolactin, GH, ACTH, TSH, FSH and LH), CT / MRI, visual field evaluation.

T For prolactinomas bromocriptine, a dopamine agonist, inhibits prolactin release.

Acromegaly from GH hypersecretion may respond to somatostatin analogues such as octreotide.

Pituitary apoplexy often necessitates surgery. Surgery is usually using a transphenoidal endoscopy.

C Post-operative diabetes insipidus, post-operative panhypopituitarism, visual field defect loss may be permanent, obstructive hydrocephalus.

Pr Transphenoidal resection is 60–80% successful. Recurrence is approximately 15% after 10 year.

Vestibular schwannoma

P Benign intracranial tumour of schwann cells in the vestibular portion of the 8th nerve.

A Idiopathic although may be associated with neurofibromatosis 1 (unilateral) or neurofibromatosis 2 (bilateral).

S Sensorineural hearing loss, vestibular dysfunction, if large may report mass effect causing other cranial nerve deficits.

Sx Hearing loss, vertigo, nausea, vomiting, pressure sensation in ear, tinnitus.

I Audiogram, CT head, MRI more sensitive for tumours <1.5cm.

T Slow growing therefore may opt for conservative management in older patients with annual imaging.

If symptomatic, young or faster growing then radiotherapy can be used to retard growth. Definitive treatment is with surgical resection.

C Surgery risks facial nerve damage and vascular injury may cause catastrophic hindbrain compression

Pr Excellent, recurrence <0.1% if completely excised.

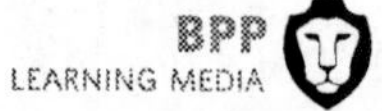

Hydrocephalus

P Hydrocephalus is an increase in the volume of CSF in the CNS. It may be due to increased production / decreased absorption (communicating) or from impaired flow from the choroid plexus to the subarachnoid space (non-communicating). The raised ICP causes dilation of ventricular system.

A *Obstructive:* may be due to congenital malformation (Arnold-Chiari and Dandy-Walker congenital malformations), post-haemorrhagic, post-meningitic.

Communicating: choroid plexus papilloma, post-haemorrhagic.

S Papilloedema, false localising sign of 6th CN palsy, gait disturbance.

In addition children may have: enlarged head, dilated scalp veins, tense fontanelle and 'setting sun' sign.

Sx Depends greatly speed of onset and age of patient.

Infants / children: headaches, nausea, vomiting, delayed milestones, drowsiness.

Adults: headaches, cognitive decline, gait disturbance, urinary incontinence.

I Culture of CSF if infective aetiology suspected.

CT and MRI head to evaluate ventricle and parenchymal changes, obstructing tumours or bony malformations.

T Medical treatment using furosemide and acetazolamide to reduce CSF production has limited effectiveness.

Repeated therapeutic LPs to drain excess CSF can be effective although the mainstay of treatment is shunting to either the peritoneum (ventriculoperitoneal) or to the cardiac atrium. Congenital malformations may be treated with surgical resection of inferior occipital bone to restore normal CSF flow.

C Permanent neurological deficit despite restoration of normal pressures, cosmetic consequences of enlarged head, shunt infection and meningitis.

Pr Largely dependent on cause of hydrocephalus. 20% of children with congenital hydrocephalus.

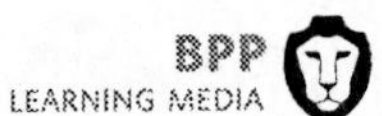

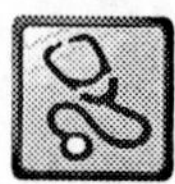

Practice Questions

Single Best Answers

1. An 80-year-old man who localises to pain, opens his eyes to voice and has confused speech has a GCS of:

   A 12
   B 9
   C 15
   D 11

2. Normal ICP is:

   A 15–20mmHg
   B 7–15mmHg
   C 5–10mmHg
   D 15–20mmHg

3. Over 80% of SAHs are due to:

   A Trauma
   B Hypertension
   C Rupture of berry aneurysm
   D Arteriovenous malformation

4. The following presents with a lucid interval after head injury:

   A SAH
   B SDH
   C EDH
   D CVE

5. Battle's sign is indicative of:

   A Communicating hydrocephalus
   B Vestibular schwannoma
   C Coma
   D Basal skull fracture

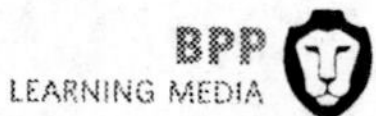

Extended Matching Questions

Head injuries

A Subdural haemorrhage
B Extradural haemorrhage
C Subarachnoid haemorrhage
D CVE
E TIA
F GCS 6
G GCS 8

For each of the following scenarios choose the **single** most likely diagnosis from the above list of options. Each option may be used once, more than once or not at all.

1. A 27-year-old man presents after being hit in the side of the head while playing rugby. His GCS is 8/15 though his rugby coach states that he was fine for a few hours after the injury.

2. A 78-year-old alcoholic gentleman presents with a reduced GCS and no history of head injury. He is known to be a falls risk.

3. A 30-year-old lady presents with a severe head ache which feels like she was 'kicked in the back of the head' and photophobia.

4. A 65-year-old man opens his eyes to pain, makes incomprehensible sounds and withdraws in response to pain. What is his GCS?

5. A 70-year-old woman is unable to open her eyes, makes incomprehensible sounds and produces abnormal flexion in response to pain. What is her GCS?

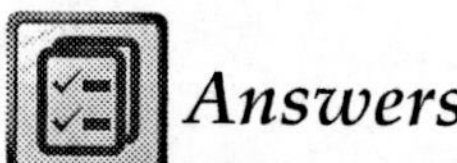

Answers

SBAs		EMQs	
1	A	1	B
2	B	2	A
3	C	3	C
4	C	4	G
5	D	5	F

Chapter 18

ENT

Mr Joseph G Manjaly and
Mr Peter J Kullar

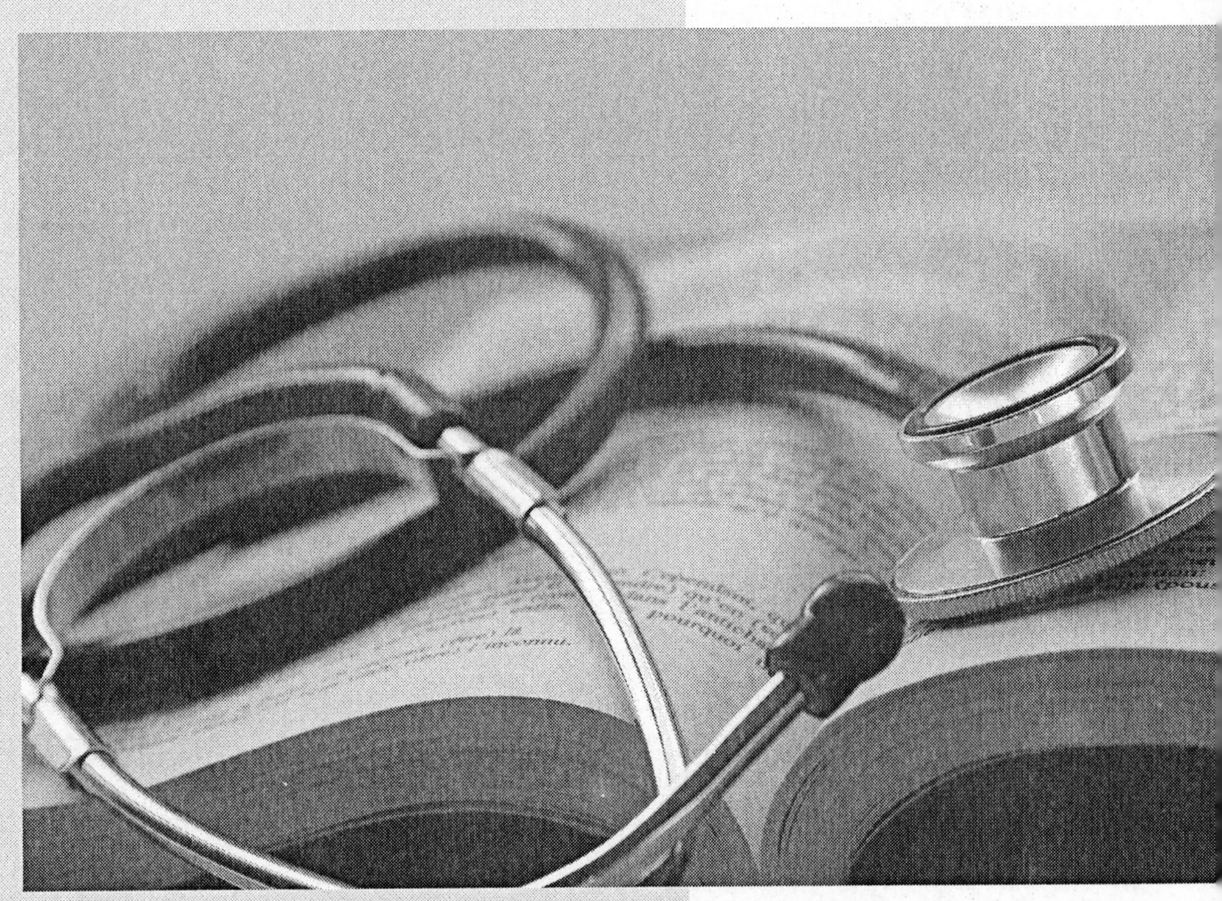

Key investigations

- **Otoscopy**: to visualise the external ear canal and tympanic membrane
- **Flexible nasendoscopy**: fibreoptic camera used to visualise the nasal cavity, pharynx and larynx
- **Pure tone audiogram (PTA)**: determines hearing thresholds at different frequencies for air and bone conduction
- **Tympanogram**: uses pressure in the external ear to record impedance of the tympanic membrane as an indirect way of measuring pressure in the middle ear. Useful for detecting middle ear effusion and Eustachian tube dysfunction
- **Rinne test**: tuning fork test to compare air and bone conduction
- **Weber test**: tuning fork test of bone conduction which tests lateralisation of sound

	Weber lateralises left	Weber lateralises right
Rinne +ve both ears AC>BC	Sensorineural loss in right	Sensorineural loss in left
Rinne -ve left BC>AC	Conductive loss in left	Sensorineural loss in left
Rinne –ve right BC>AC	Sensorineural loss in right	Conductive loss in right

Table 18.1: Rinne & Weber Test Results

- **Lateral neck X-ray**: to detect foreign body in throat or free air
- **Barium swallow**: to investigate dysphagia
- **US / CT / MRI**: all used for imaging of the head and neck

The ear

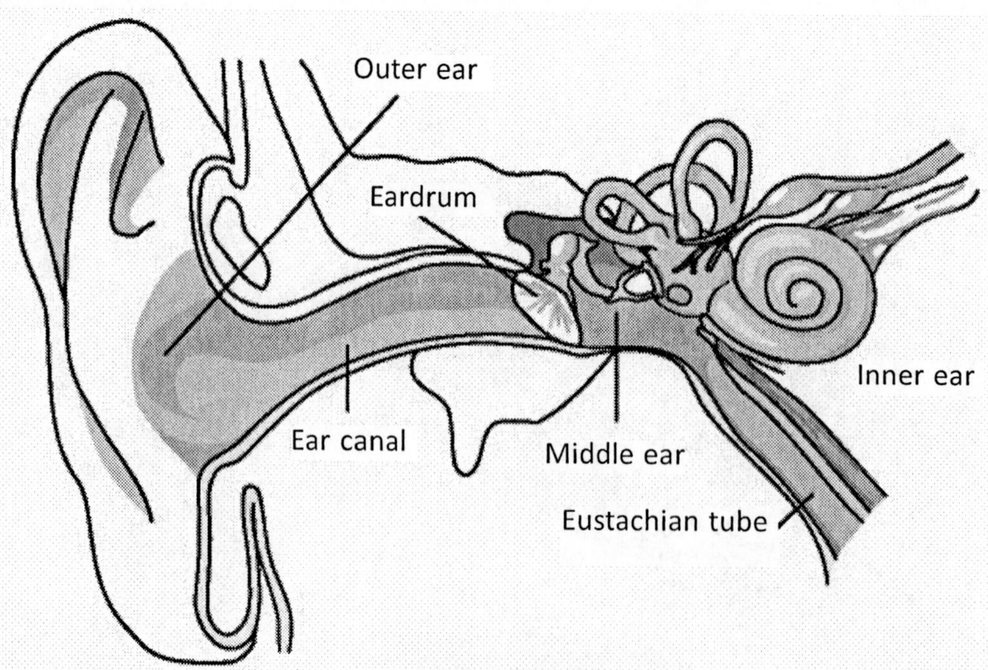

Figure 18.1: Cross-section of the ear

External ear

Otitis externa

P Inflammation of the skin of the external auditory meatus.

A Most commonly bacterial (staph or pseudomonas) or fungal.

S Ear canal debris, ear canal oedema, ear canal erythema.

Sx Otalgia, deafness, discharge.

I Swab for MC&S.

T Aural toilet, antibiotic-steroid drops, keep ear dry.

C Malignant otitis externa, mastoiditis.

Pr Usually resolves but can become chronic.

Pinna haematoma

P Collection of blood between the pinna perichondrium and cartilage.

A Traumatic.

S Fluid-filled swelling disturbing the normal pinna architecture.

Sx Swelling, pain.

I None.

T Aspiration, incision and drainage.

C 'Cauliflower ear' if left untreated.

Pr Compressive bandage required to prevent re-accumulation.

Middle ear

Acute otitis media

P Inflammation of the middle ear.

A Viral, bacterial (strep pneumoniae, haemophilus influenza, moraxella catarrhalis), commonest age 3–7, Eustachian tube dysfunction, primary or following URTI.

S Dull, hyperaemic, bulging tympanic membrane, fluid level behind tympanic membrane, fever.

Sx Otalgia, deafness.

I Otoscope visualise, FBC.

T Rest (two-thirds will resolve without treatment), oral abx if not recovering, analgesia.

C Meningitis, mastoiditis, intracranial infection, facial nerve palsy, lateral sinus thrombosis.

Pr Infection lasting >3 months is known as chronic suppurative otitis media (CSOM).

Otitis media with effusion

P Middle ear inflammation leading to fluid collection also known as 'glue ear' or 'secretory otitis media'.

A Eustachian tube dysfunction, associated with recurrent upper respiratory tract infection, commonly children aged 3–6 years.

S Dull tympanic membrane, bulging or retracted.

Sx Deafness, learning difficulty, speech delay, otalgia.

I Audiogram: conductive hearing loss. Tympanogram: flat.

T *Medical:* watchful waiting (analgesia ± abx), hearing aid.

Surgical: indication for grommets = 30db conductive hearing loss lasting three months.

C Tympanosclerosis, cholesteatoma, tympanic membrane perforation.

Pr 50% will resolve in three months, 95% in one year.

Cholesteatoma

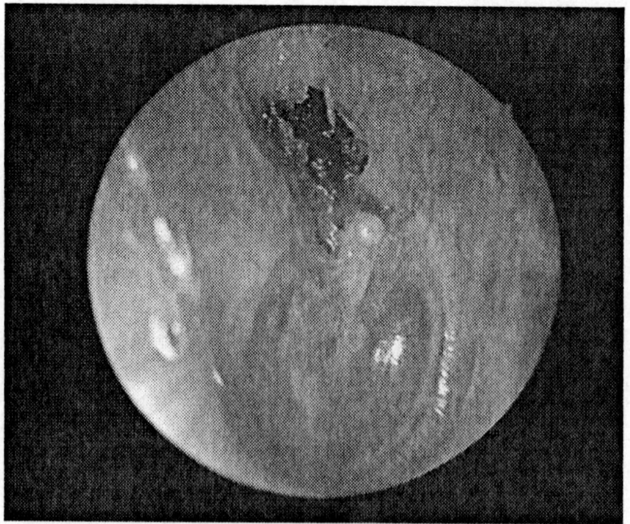

Figure 18.2: Cholesteatoma.
(Reproduced with permission fron SW Deanery.)

P Abnormal growth of skin in the middle ear (squamous epithelial cells). Behaves like a tumour resorbing bone and can recur after removal.

A Acquired (evolves from TM retraction pockets and perforations) or congenital.

S Attic crust, otoscope: pearly-white mass (Figure 18.2).

Sx Discharge (often foul-smelling), deafness, dizziness.

I Audiometry: conductive or sensorineural deafness, CT / MRI.

T Aural toilet, mastoidectomy / tympanoplasty.

C Intracranial infection, facial nerve palsy, destruction of the ossicles and labyrinth.

Pr Life-threatening complications may occur if left untreated, risk of recurrence.

Otosclerosis

P Osseous dyscrasia of the temporal bone affecting the otic capsule and ossicles.

A Autosomal dominant inheritance, F>M.

S Normal tympanic membrane, 'Schwartze sign' in 10% (flamingo pink blush in tympanic membrane).

Sx Slow progressive conductive hearing loss, tinnitus, dizziness, paracusis of Willis (improved hearing in the presence of background noise).

I Pure tone audiogram: conductive deafness with Carhart notch at 2kHz. Speech audiometry: to determine benefit of surgery, CT.

T Observation, hearing aid, stapedotomy. Bone-anchored hearing aid (BAHA).

C Operative risks.

Pr Excellent with surgery.

Inner ear

Vestibular neuronitis

P Acute vestibular failure.

A Suspected viral, predisposed by recent URTI.

S Nystagmus, positive Romberg's and Unterberger's tests.

Sx Sudden onset vertigo lasting days.

I PTA: may be normal, MRI to rule out central cause or vestibular schwannoma.

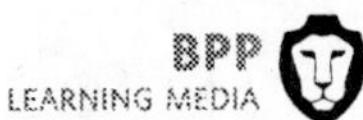

T Bed rest, vestibular sedatives acutely, vestibular exercises.

C None if diagnosis is correct.

Pr Symptoms usually subside within a few days.

Benign paroxysmal positional vertigo (BPPV)

P Particles floating in the endolymph causing positional vertigo.

A Semicircular canal lithiasis.

S Nystagmus.

S Acute positional rotatory vertigo.

I PTA, Dix-Hallpike manoeuvre.

T Epley manoeuvre, vestibular exercises.

C None.

Pr Good.

Meniere's disease

P Endolymphatic hydrops (dilated labyrinth in inner ear).

A Not fully understood.

S Normal ear examination, nystagmus during attacks.

Sx Fluctuating hearing loss, tinnitus, rotatory vertigo, usually unilateral.

I PTA: unilateral sensorineural hearing loss. MRI to exclude tumour.

T *Medical:* salt restriction, betahistine, prochlorperazine, diuretics, intatympanic steroid or gentamicin.

Surgical: vestibular nerve section, labyrinthectomy, endolymphatic sac decompression.

C Deafness.

Pr Episodic with some resolving and some progressing.

Mastoiditis

P Inflammation of the mastoid air cells.

A Often progression from untreated acute otitis media.

S Post-auricular swelling, erythema and tenderness, protruding pinna.

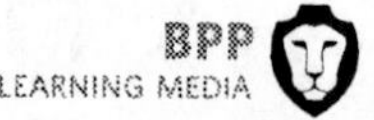

Sx Fever, pain, rarely facial weakness.

I CT head to rule out intracranial spread.

T Urgent broad-spectrum antibiotics. If it fails to resolve, may need I&D, mastoidectomy +/- grommet insertion.

C Meningitis, intracranial sepsis.

Pr Good if treated promptly.

Referred otalgia

P Referred (secondary) ear pain may arise from disease processes near sensory nerves supplying the ear.

A Depends on nerve affected (see Table 18.2).

S Normal ear examination.

Sx Otalgia, symptoms of secondary source for pain.

T Treat underlying disease / injury.

Referred from	Nerve supply
Neck soft tissues and cervical vertebrae	Great auricular nerve (C2,3)
Teeth and temporomandibular joint (TMJ)	Auriculo-temporal branch of mandibular division of trigeminal (CNVc)
Base of tongue, tonsils / throat (eg tonsillitis)	Tympanic branch of glossopharyngeal nerve (IX)
Herpes zoster infection (eg Ramsay-Hunt syndrome)	Sensory branch of facial nerve (CNVII)

Table 18.2: Referred ear pain

Ototoxic medications

P Medications that damage the cochlea, auditory nerve or vestibular system.

Sx Partial or complete hearing loss, tinnitus, vertigo.

T Immediate withdrawal of medication.

- Antibiotics:
  - Aminoglycosides (eg gentamicin, tobramycin)
  - Macrolides (eg erythromycin)
- Loop diuretics:
  - Frusemide (at high doses)
- Chemotherapeutics:
  - Platiunum based (eg cisplatin)
  - Vinca alkaloids (eg vincristine)
- Others:
  - Aspirin (at high doses)
  - Heavy metals (eg mercury, lead)
  - Quinine

Box 18.1: Ototoxic medications

The nose

Epistaxis

P Bleeding from nose, commonest ENT presentation, arbitrarily divided into anterior and posterior bleeds.

A Idiopathic, trauma, anticoagulants, bleeding disorders, infection, surgery, neoplasia.

S Blood / clot in nose and / or oropharynx.

I Rhinoscopy to visualise nose. Bloods: FBC, clotting, G&S in severe bleeds.

T Stepwise approach: 'pinch and ice', suction to remove clots and aid visualisation, cautery (with silver nitrate stick), anterior packing, posterior packing, surgery, embolisation.

C Retained clot, septal haematoma, hypotension.

Acute rhinosinusitis

P Acute inflammation of the nasal and sinus mucosa lasting <1 month.

A Viral, bacterial.

S Inflamed nasal mucosa, mucopus in middle meatus / post-nasal space.

Sx Nasal discharge, nasal congestion, facial pain, altered smell.

I Rarely indicated unless symptoms persist, pus culture.

T Oral abx, steroid nasal spray, nasal douching, nasal decongestant (eg xylometazoline), rarely surgery.

C Spread to the orbital cavity.

Pr Good.

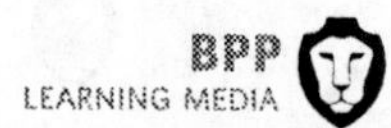

Chronic rhinosinusitis

P Chronic inflammation of the nasal and sinus mucosa lasting >3 months.

A Usually bacterial.

S Sx Similar to acute sinusitis but less severe.

I Allergy testing, ESR, ANCA, ACE (exclude granulomatous disease), CT: paranasal sinuses, Saccharin clearance test.

T Oral abx, steroid nasal spray, oral antihistamines, nasal douching, nasal decongestant, functional endoscopic sinus surgery (FESS).

C Side effects of oral steroids (nasal steroids are generally safe).

Pr Mixed dependent on extent of disease.

Nasal polyps

P Grape-like structures in the upper nasal cavity.

A Tend to occur with eosinophil-dominated chronic rhinosinusitis.

S Visualised on rhinoscopy / nasendoscopy. May be unilateral or bilateral.

Sx Nasal blockage, nasal discharge, headache, anosmia.

I Flexible nasendoscopy, CT to determine extent of disease, allergy tests, CRP may be raised if underlying infection.

T *Medical:* topical steroids, antibiotics.

Surgical: functional endoscopic sinus surgery (FESS) with polypectomy.

C Consider malignancy in unilateral disease in elderly patients.

Fractured nose

P Displacement of the nasal bones.

A Trauma.

S Asymmetrical nose.

Sx Pain, bleeding, nasal blockage.

I None.

T Manipulation under anaesthetic seven to ten days after injury.

C Epistaxis, septal haematoma: this should be ruled out / treated at initial presentation.

Pr Can recur if patient continues contact sports, some patients opt for formal rhinoplasty if unhappy with shape of nose.

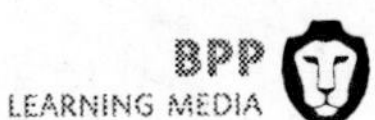

The throat

Tonsils

Tonsillitis

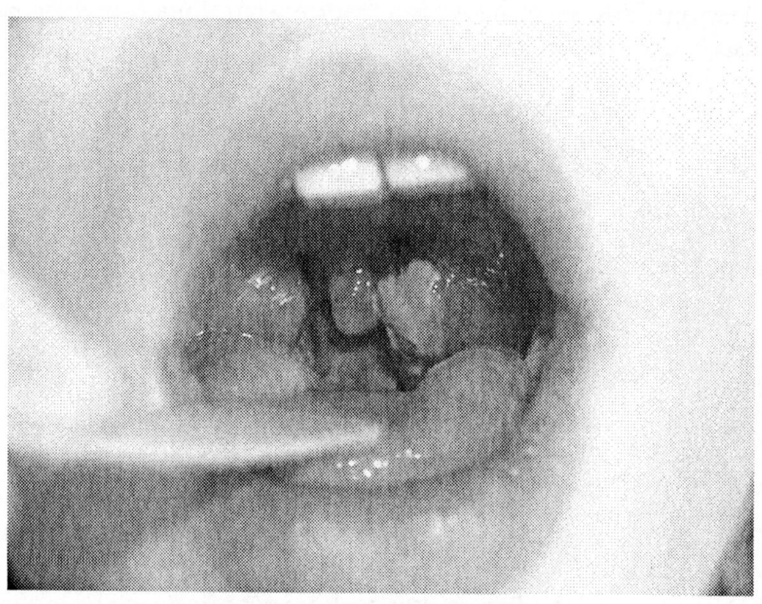

Figure 18.3: Acute tonsillitis.
(Reproduced with permission from SW Deanery.)

P Inflammation of the tonsils.

A Viral: EBV. Bacterial: beta-haemolytic strep.

S Bilaterally inflamed tonsils, cervical lymphadenopathy.

Sx Pyrexia, malaise, sore throat, otalgia, odynophagia, trismus (lock-jaw).

I FBC: ↑ WCC, infectious mononucleosis screen to exclude glandular fever.

T *Medical:* abx: IV penicillin and admission if unable to swallow, analgesia, dexamethasone if very swollen or airway concern.

Never give ampicillin-containing antibiotics if the patient has glandular fever as this will cause a generalised maculopapular rash.

Surgical: tonsillectomy (see Box 18.2).

C Airway obstruction, Quinsy (peritonsillar abscess), parapharyngeal abscess.

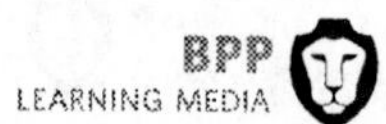

Indications:

- >5 episodes of tonsillitis per year
- Symptoms for at least one year
- Disabling and prevents normal functioning
- Two or more quinsies
- Airway obstruction eg obstructive sleep apnoea
- Suspicion of malignancy

Complications:

- Primary bleeding (<24 hours after surgery)
- Secondary bleeding (typically 5–10 days and usually due to infection)
- Retroperitoneal abscess
- Peritonsillar abscess (quinsy)

Box 18.2: Tonsillectomy

Quinsy

P Peritonsillar abscess.

A As tonsiliitis.

S Abscess formation over tonsil, usually unilateral, halitosis.

Sx As for tonsillitis but more severe.

I As for tonsillitis.

T Incision and drainage under LA, abscess tonsillectomy under GA, abx: IV penicillin and metronidazole.

C Airway obstruction, parapharyngeal abscess.

Salivary glands

Sialadenitis

P Salivary gland inflammation.

A Infective (staph aureus), mumps, dehydration, radiation, autoimmune.

S Increased size of gland on palpation.

Sx Pain, swelling.

I US to look for an obstructive cause / alternative pathology.

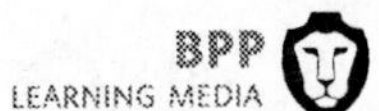

T Sialogogues, antibiotics, rehydration.

C Rare.

Pr A proportion of cases become chronic.

Sialolithiasis

P Likely due to disturbance of salivary electrolyte secretion leading to increased viscosity and obstruction.

80% submandibular gland.

10% parotid gland.

10% sublingual gland.

A Calculi often composed of hydroxyapatite.

80% of submandibular stones are radio opaque.

S Palpable stone in floor of mouth or cheek.

Sx Pain, swelling particularly before eating.

I Floor of mouth X-ray may reveal submandibular stone, US / CT for parotid gland.

T Sialogogues, antibiotics if inflammation, surgery (lithotripsy, sialendoscopy, sialadenectomy).

Salivary gland tumours

P Benign or malignant, primary or secondary, main glands are parotid (80%), submandibular (10%) and sublingual (10%).

A 80% of salivary tumours are parotid.

80% of parotid tumours are benign.

80% of benign parotid tumours are pleomorphic adenomas.

Facial nerve involvement suggests malignancy.

Most are slow-growing even if malignant.

Commonest malignant tumour is adenoid cystic carcinoma.

S Neck mass, if malignant: nerve palsy, skin ulceration, lymphadenopathy.

Sx Pain.

I FNA (85% accuracy benign v malignant), CT / MRI.

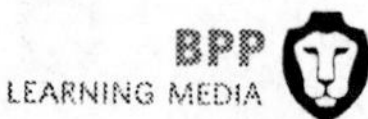

T *Surgical:* partial or complete excision +/- radiotherapy or neck dissection in malignant tumours with nodal involvement.

C Due to surgery.

Early: haematoma, trismus, nerve palsy, infection.

Late: tumour recurrence, hyperaesthesia of skin, Frey's syndrome (up to 50% patients post-parotidectomy, involves gustatory sweating of face sweat glands due to regeneration of secretomotor parasympathetic nerve fibres).

Pr Malignant tumours have 50% five-year survival.

Benign	Intermediate	Malignant
Pleomorphic adenoma (mixed parotid tumour)	Mucoepidermoid tumour	Adenoid cystic carcinoma
Adenolymphoma (Warthin's tumour)	Acinic cell carcinoma	Adenocarcinoma
Haemangioma	Oncocytoma	Squamous cell carcinoma
Lymphangioma		

Table 18.3: Salivary gland tumours

Larynx

Laryngitis

P Inflammation of the larynx.

A URTI.

S Dysphonia, pain, malaise.

Sx Sore throat, loss of voice.

I Flexible nasendoscopy: vocal cords may appear normal or slightly erythematous.

T Voice rest, analgesia, steam inhalation.

C Rare.

Pr Usually self-limiting.

Epiglottitis / supraglotittis

P Bacterial infection of the supraglottis, including, most significantly, the epiglottis.

Though rare, this is a life-threatening condition, particularly in children for whom the epiglottis easily obstructs a smaller-diameter airway.

A Most commonly haemophilus influenza B (reduced since HIB vaccine).

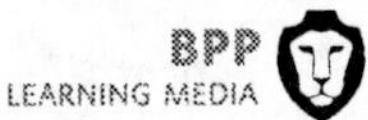

S **Sx** History of URTI rapidly progressing to severe sore throat and dysphagia → stridor, drooling and leaning forward, toxic → quiet and floppy.

I None.

In children, do **not** examine throat due to risk of airway obstruction.

T Humidified oxygen, reassurance with parents, contact senior anaesthetist and ENT surgeon urgently, secure airway in theatre (intubation or surgical).

C Airway obstruction, death.

Pr Good if treated quickly.

Oropharyngeal malignancy

P 85% SCC, 10% Non-Hodgkin's lymphoma.

A Smoking, chewing tobacco, alcohol, HPV.

S Neck lump, lymphadenopathy.

Sx Sore throat, otalgia, dysphonia, dysphagia, odynophagia, weight loss, cough.

I CT, MRI, panendoscopy and biopsy.

T Radiotherapy, chemotherapy, surgery, swallowing frequently requires significant rehabilitation, nutrition needs to be addressed during this time.

Pr Dependent on patient age and disease stage.

Laryngeal malignancy

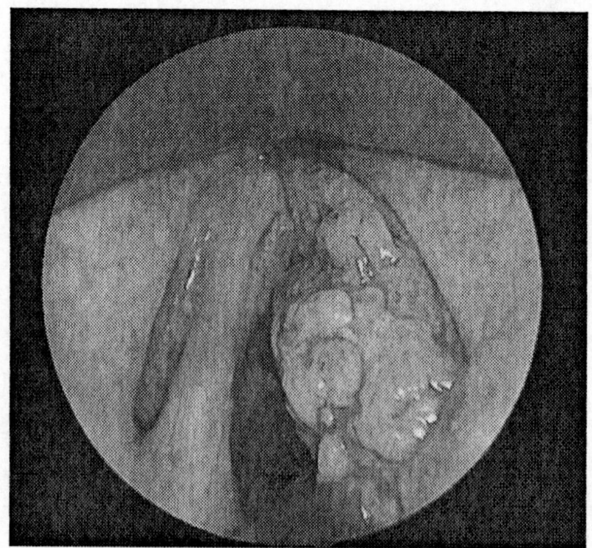

Figure 18.4: Laryngeal malignancy.
(Reproduced with permission from SW Deanery.)

P Commonest head and neck malignancy, 95% treatable, ~33% mortality. Supraglottic, glottic and subglottic.

A Smoking, alcohol, HPV, GORD, low socioeconomic status, previous radiotherapy.

S Persistent hoarse voice (often the only sign), dyspnoea and stridor (late), lymphadenopathy.

Sx Sore throat, otalgia, dysphagia, neck swelling, cough, haemoptysis, weight loss.

I Laryngoscopy and biopsy, panendoscopy (to look for second tumour), CXR, CT / MRI.

T Surgery (laser surgery, partial / total laryngectomy, neck dissection), radiotherapy.

Pr 50–60% five-year survival.

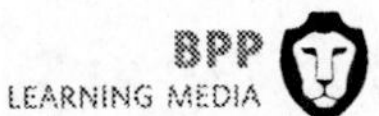

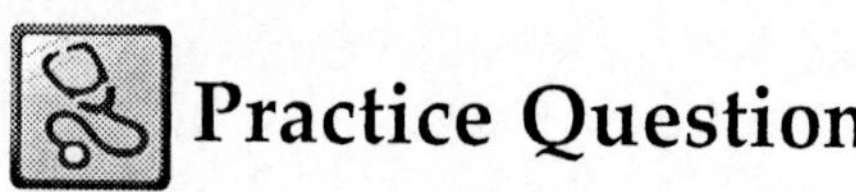

Practice Questions

Single Best Answers

1. Which of these is a common presentation of a vestibular schwannoma (acoustic neuroma)?

   A Unilateral deafness
   B Upper motor neurone signs in the arms
   C Loss of visual acuity
   D Ear pain

2. Which of these operations is most often used in the treatment of otosclerosis?

   A Myomectomy
   B Myringoplasty
   C Stapedectomy
   D Myringotomy

3. Which of these blood tests is routinely requested for a patient about to undergo a tonsillectomy?

   A FBC
   B LFTs
   C Coagulation studies
   D No blood tests

4. What is the most common complication of a tonsillectomy?

   A Damage to the facial nerve
   B Perioribital haematoma
   C Sinusitis
   D Bleeding

5. Which of these is a common treatment for Meniere's disease?

   A Dietary salt restriction
   B Beta blockers
   C Propofol
   D Radiotherapy

6. What is the most common indication for grommets?

   A Sinusitis
   B Pinna haematoma
   C Otitis media with effusion
   D Nasal obstruction

7. Which of these is a recognised complication of a cholesteatoma?

   A Meningitis
   B Nasal discharge
   C Epistaxis
   D Foetal malformations

8. Which is the most common genetic cause of deafness?

   A Connexin 34 mutation
   B Connexin 26 mutation
   C Sodium / potassium / chloride cotransporter mutation
   D PTEN mutation

9. What is the most common type of thyroid cancer?

   A Follicular
   B Papillary
   C Medullary
   D Anaplastic

10. What is the most common type of laryngeal cancer?

   A Adenocarcinoma
   B Lymphoma
   C Squamous cell
   D Sarcoma

11. Which virus is associated with glandular fever?

   A Cytomegalovirus
   B HIV
   C Epstein-Barr virus
   D Adenovirus

12. Which bacteria is associated with malignant otitis externa?

   A Staph. aureus
   B Staph. epidermidis
   C Haemophilus influenzae
   D Pseudomonas

13. Which of these arteries is commonly associated with nosebleeds?

   A Middle cerebral artery
   B Inferior thyroid artery
   C Anterior ethmoidal artery
   D Posterior auricular artery

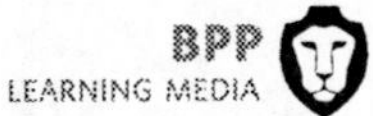

14. Which of these viruses is associated with oropharyngeal cancer?

    A Picornavirus
    B Polio virus
    C Human papilloma virus
    D Rotavirus

15. What is another name of a pharyngeal pouch?

    A Zenker's diverticulum
    B Thomas' diverticulum
    C The pouch of Douglas
    D Posterior pouch of Tröltsch

Extended Matching Questions

Hearing loss

A Presbyacusis
B Vestibular schwannoma
C Otosclerosis
D Meniere's disease
E Glue ear

For each of the following scenarios choose the **single** most likely diagnosis from the above list of options. Each option may be used once, more than once or not at all.

1. A 35-year-old woman presenting with unilateral sensorineural hearing loss, tinnitus and a feeling of ear blockage.

2. A 75-year-old man presenting with a symmetrical gradual decline in his hearing.

3. A 5-year-old child with poor speech development.

Sore throat

A Glandular fever
B Bacterial tonsillitis
C Squamous cell carcinoma
D Lymphoma
E Dental abscess

For each of the following scenarios choose the **single** most likely diagnosis from the above list of options. Each option may be used once, more than once or not at all.

4. A 21-year-old university student with a sore throat and a positive monospot test.

5. A 50-year-old male smoker with unilateral otalgia.

6. A 34-year-old female with a neck lump and night sweats.

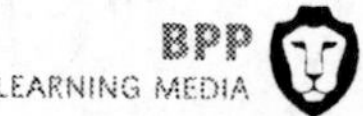

Microbiology in ENT

A Haemophilus influenza
B Staph. aureus
C Pseudomonas
D Strep. pneumoniae
E Mycobacteria

For each of the following scenarios choose the **single** most likely diagnosis from the above list of options. Each option may be used once, more than once or not at all.

7. A 5-year-old child with a sore throat, drooling and stridor.

8. A 43-year-old diabetic with a discharging ear.

9. A 76-year-old man with a chronically deep neck space infection.

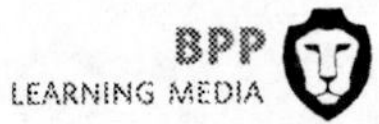

Answers

SBAs		EMQs	
1	A	1	D
2	C	2	A
3	D	3	E
4	D	4	A
5	A	5	C
6	C	6	D
7	A	7	A
8	B	8	C
9	B	9	B
10	C		
11	C		
12	D		
13	C		
14	C		
15	A		

Chapter 19

Plastic surgery

Mr Jonathan A Dunne and
Mr Jeremy M Rawlins

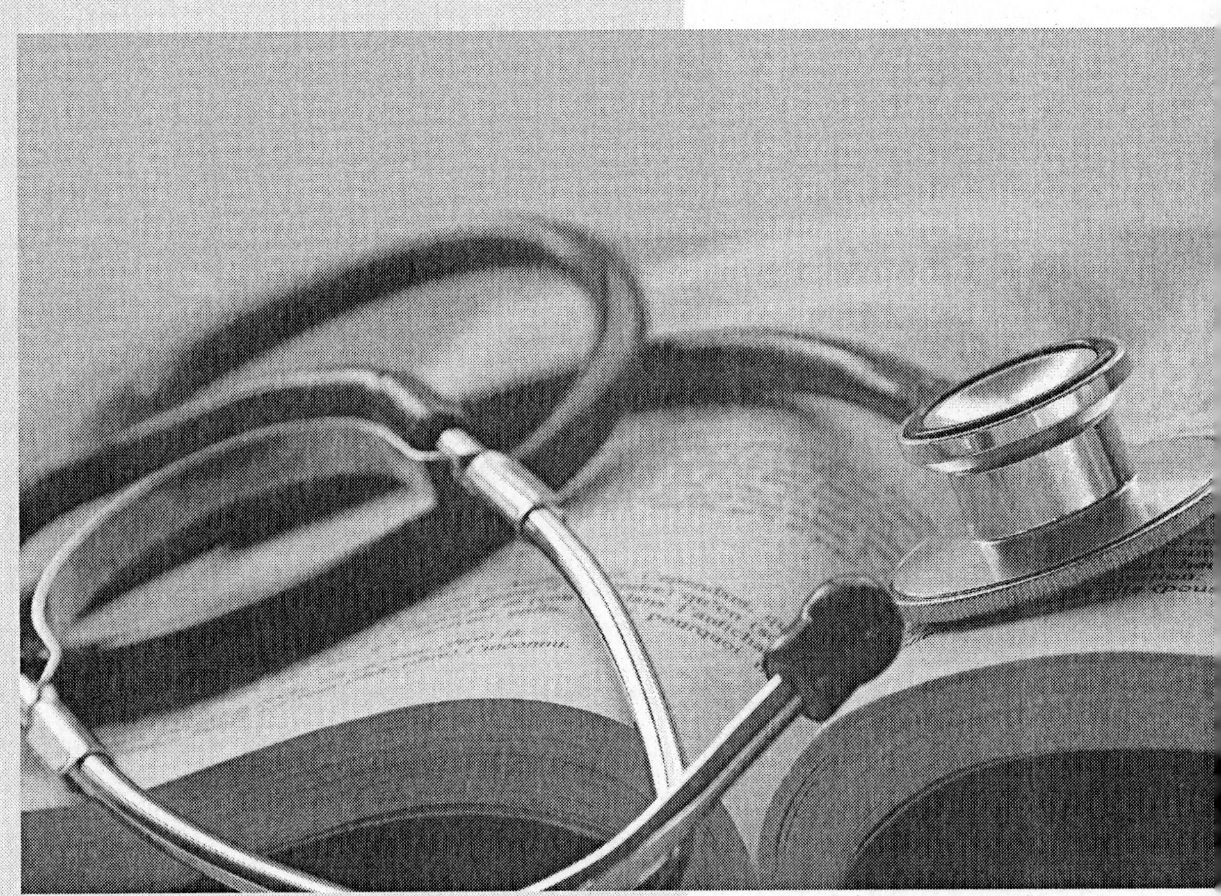

Burns

Calculating burn surface area

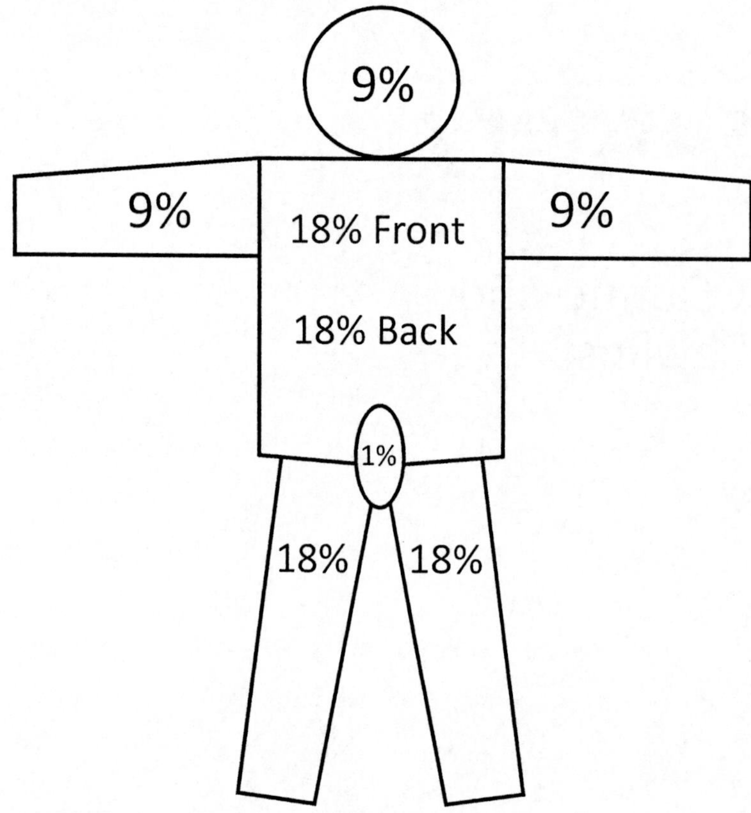

Figure 19.1: Wallace rule of 9s chart

The 'Rule of 9s': Head and each arm = 9%
Back and chest each = 18%
Each leg = 18%
Perineum = 1%

Lund-Browder charts are more accurate and should always be used to calculate BSA in children.

Burn injuries

P *Local:* loss of skin continuity leads to altered capillary permeability and fluid loss.

Systemic: release of inflammatory mediators from damaged tissue (leukotrienes, prostaglandins).

A *Adult:* flame and scald burns most common.

Children: scalds commonest, then contact burns, electrical, chemical, friction and sunburn.

S *Cutaneous:* see signs according to depth (Box 19.1).

Inhalation: singed nasal hair, soot in mouth, blistered palate, stridor, hoarse voice, respiratory distress, decreased conscious level.

Electrical: entry and exit points.

Depth	Colour	Blisters	Capillary refill	Sensation
Epidermal	Red	No	Present	Present
Superficial dermal	Pink	Yes	Present	Present
Deep dermal	Dark pink, mottled	Sometimes	Slow	May be present
Full-thickness	White	No	Absent	Absent

Box 19.1: Burn depth

S Pain, breathless, confusion, cardiac arrhythmia.

I Bloods: FBC, U+E, clotting, amylase, albumin, calcium, carboxyhaemoglobin.

Other: ECG / cardiac monitoring, ABG, BP, pulse, respiratory rate, pulse oximetry, catheter and measurement of urinary output.

Electrical: cardiac monitoring, U+E (myoglobinuria secondary to trauma – renal failure).

Chemical: pH measurement of burn, calcium level (hydrofluoric acid causes hypocalcaemia).

T *Trauma:* ATLS protocol.

First aid: remove clothing, irrigate burn with cool (15°C) running water for 20 minutes up to three hours post-injury, wrap burn in cling film / cover with dry cloth, analgesia.

Resuscitation: See Box 19.2.

Referral: See Box 19.3.

Chemical: Hydrofluoric acid – calcium gluconate (topical, wound injection, IV).

Escharotomy: division of skin to level of fascia. Used in circumferential burns which may cause limb iscahemia and respiratory distress.

Fasciotomy: division of skin and fascia. Used in high voltage electrical burns and other trauma.

Coverage: excision of burn and covering with skin grafting (Box 19.4).

C *Early:* immunosuppression and infection, fluid loss, loss of airway, hypoxia, (<3 weeks) cardiac dyrshythmias, myocardial depression, renal failure.

Late: scarring and deformity, contractures, impaired function (>3 weeks)

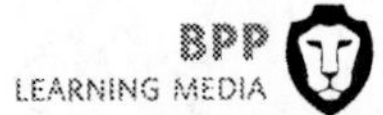

- For burns >15% BSA in adults and >10% in children
- Insert urinary catheter

Parkland formula:

Adults: **3–4 ml/kg/% burn of Hartmann's solution**

- 50% of volume in first 8 hours and 50% in the next 16 hours
- 1st 50% of volume is given within 8 hours from time of burn
- Above is a guide – titrate to ≥ 0.5ml/kg/hour urine output

Children: As above but add maintenance fluids.

Example*:*

A 26-year-old male (80kg) sustains 20% burns at 12.00 and arrives at hospital at 15.00.

- 4ml × 80kg × 20 = 6,400ml
- 3,200ml in 1st 8 hours; 3,200ml in next 16 hours
- 1st 3,200ml must be given by 20.00

Box 19.2: Calculating fluid replacement

- Total burn >10% in adults and >5% in children
- Burns to special areas – face, hands, feet, genitalia, perineum
- Full thickness >1%
- Electrical and chemical burns
- Circumferential burns
- Inhalational injury
- Burns in the very young, elderly or patients with multiple co-morbidities
- Burns associated with major trauma
- Non-accidental injury

Box 19.3: When to refer to burns unit

A skin graft is a sheet of skin harvested from one part of the body and grafted to another.

	Split-thickness	**Full-thickness**
Graft anatomy	Epidermis and part of dermis	Epidermis and entire dermis
Harvest	Dermatome, knife +/- mesh	Scalpel excision
Donor site management	Dressings	Sutured
Securing graft	Glue, sutures	Sutures
Contra-indications	Inadequate bed, infected bed, cosmetic importance	Inadequate bed (eg exposed tendon), large area

Box 19.4: Skin grafts

Cleft lip and palate

P Failure of fusion of palatal shelves of maxillary processes.

A Genetic and environmental factors.

Associated with many congenital syndromes (eg Pierre Robin) and infections (eg rubella) and teratogens (eg steroids) in the first trimester.

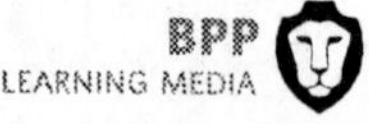

S Facial deformity, nasal or poorly understood speech, dental problems.

Sx Poor feeding, shortness of breath, developmental delay (hearing impairment).

I Antenatal ultrasound.

T Surgery: orthodontics, lip repair, muscle repair to restore function, bone grafts.

Other: speech therapy, dental care, parental counselling.

C Psychosocial problems.

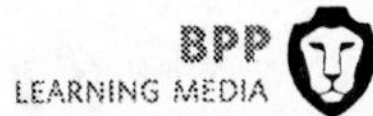

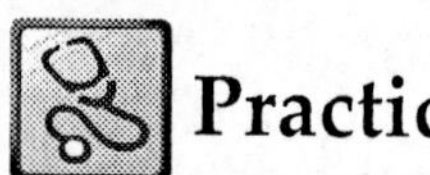

Practice Questions

Single Best Answers

1. What is the most common cause of burn in children?

   A Flame
   B Contact
   C Electrical
   D Scald

2. First aid should be administered within what time frame to reduce the deepening of the burn?

   A 1 hour
   B 3 hours
   C 4 hours
   D 8 hours

3. Which one of the following warrants referral to a burns unit?

   A 7% flame burns in an adult
   B 4% scald burn to thigh in an 8-year-old child
   C 2% electrical burn to arm in a 60-year-old man
   D 8% contact burn to a 21-year-old man

4. Which of the following would be a poor recipient of a skin graft?

   A Exposed tendon
   B Fascia
   C Muscle
   D Bone

5. A 70kg lady was rescued from a house fire at 9pm. She has partial-thickness burns covering 30% BSA. Using the Parkland formula what fluid volume should she receive within 24 hours?

   A 4,200ml colloid solution
   B 2,100ml Hartmann's
   C 8,400ml Hartmann's
   D 4,200ml 0.9% sodium chloride

6. You are called to A&E to assess a patient with cutaneous burns. To calculate the extent of burn injury which of the following do you require?

   A Parkland chart
   B Muir and Barclay chart
   C Lund and Browder chart
   D Snellen chart

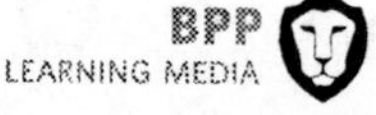

Extended Matching Questions

Burns resuscitation

A 4,800 ml
B 2,400 ml
C 1,600 ml
D 9,600 ml
E 3,200 ml

For each of the following scenarios choose the **single** most likely diagnosis from the above list of options. Each option may be used once, more than once or not at all.

1. A 40-year-old woman (60kg) sustains 20% burns. How much fluid resuscitation should she receive in the first 8 hours?

2. A 65-year-old man (120kg) sustains 20% burns. How much fluid resuscitation should he receive in the first 8 hours?

3. A 36-year-old man (100kg) sustains 24% burns. How much fluid resuscitation should he receive in the first 24 hours?

Burn depth

A Epidermal
B Mid-dermal
C Full-thickness

For each of the following scenarios choose the **single** most likely diagnosis from the above list of options. Each option may be used once, more than once or not at all.

4. A 31-year-old man suffers flame burns to his right hand. The skin is blistered with sluggish capillary refill and sensation is in tact.

5. An 87-year-old woman collapses and sustains contact burns to her left thigh from an electric heater. The skin is white and insensate.

6. A 15-year-old boy sustains a flame burn to his face when petrol is poured on a bonfire. His skin has peeled, capillary refill is <2 seconds and sensation is in tact.

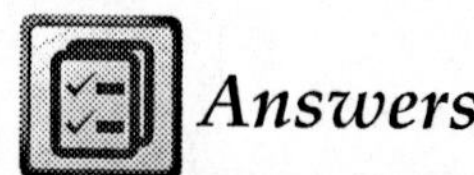

Answers

SBAs		EMQs	
1	D	1	B
2	B	2	A
3	C	3	D
4	A	4	B
5	C	5	C
6	C	6	A

Chapter 20

Trauma and orthopaedic surgery

Mr Alexander Young and
Mr Samuel Carter Jonas

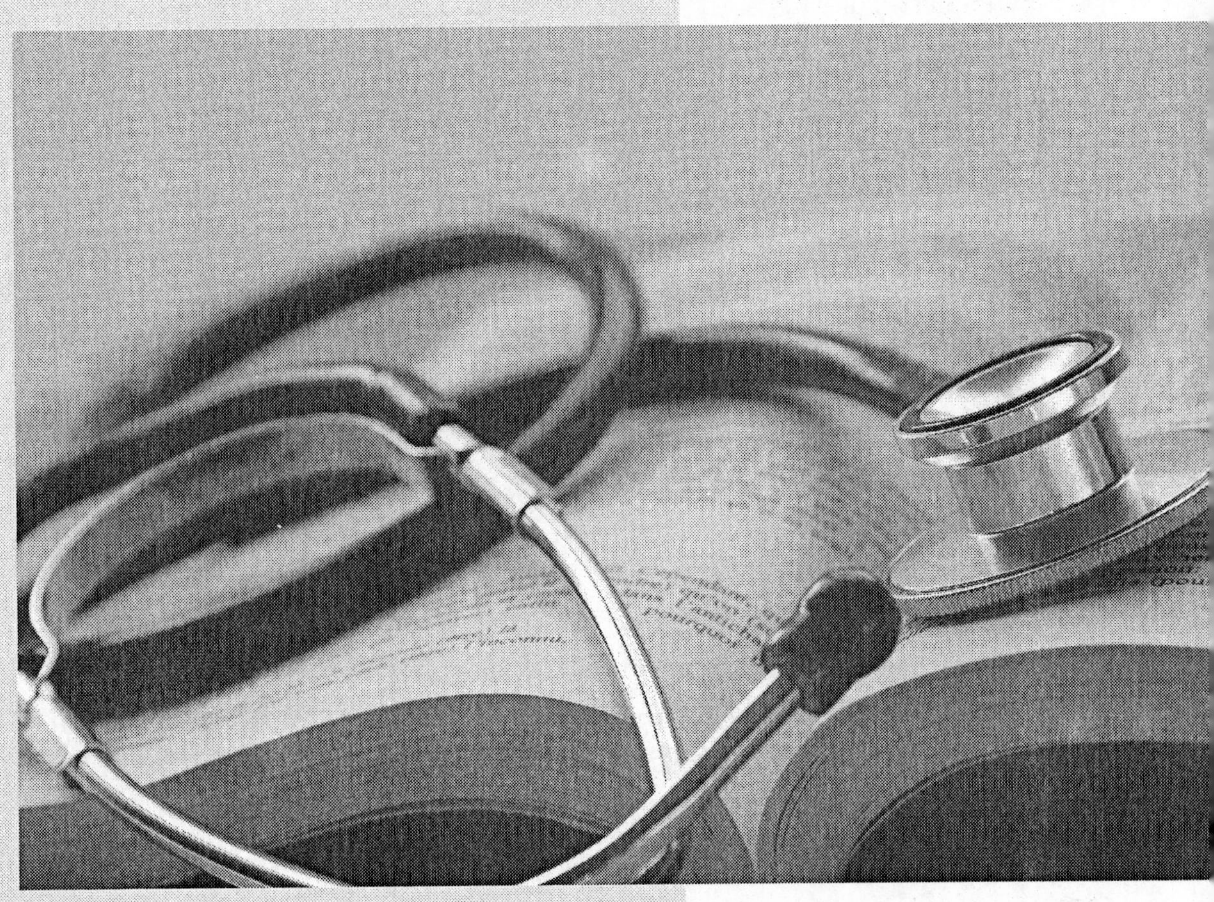

 Key investigations

- **Arthroscopy**: minimally invasive, direct visualisation of joint with arthroscope used for diagnosis and treatment
- **CT**: used for preoperative planning or where diagnosis is unclear on XR
- **Joint aspiration**: sample of joint fluid is aspirated from a joint, used to diagnose joint effusion and can be therapeutic
- **MRI**: used to identify spinal pathology and soft tissue injuries
- **X-ray**: AP and lateral views, including the joint above and below, are standard

 Terminology

- **Arthrodesis**: fusion of a joint
- **Arthroplasty**: surgery of a joint
- **AVN**: avascular necrosis (loss of blood supply causing bone death)
- **CHS**: compression hip screw
- **Delayed union**: failure of a fracture to heal within its expected time period
- **Kyphosis**: outward curvature of the spine in saggital plane
- **Lordosis**: inward curvature of the spine in saggital plane
- **Malunion**: healing of bone in an abnormal position
- **MUA**: manipulation under anaesthetic
- **Non-union**: the cessation of bony healing without bony union (typically after three to six months)
- **ORIF**: open reduction and internal fixation
- **POP**: plaster of paris
- **Scoliosis**: spinal deformity with curvature in the coronal plane
- **Screw**: converts rotational movement into vertical movement
- **Traction**: application of a pulling force to straighten broken bone

Principles of fracture management

A fracture is a break in the continuity of the bone. Fractures may be classified by:

- Their communication with the skin: open / compound or closed / simple fractures
- Their radiological appearance: transverse, oblique, spiral, comminuted
- Their anatomical position: metaphyseal, epiphyseal, diaphyseal, intra-articular
- Specific classification systems relating to bone involved: Neer, Danis-Weber etc

Resuscitation

For all trauma injuries ATLS guidelines should be followed (ABCDE – Airway, Breathing, Circulation, Disability, Exposure).

Reduction

Displaced fractures should be reduced to their anatomical position. Reduction can be achieved by open or closed methods or through traction.

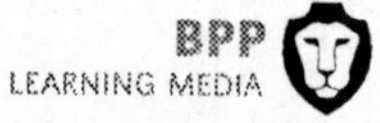

Restriction

Having been reduced to an anatomical position fractures should be restricted to limit movement and allow bone healing to take place in a controlled manner.

- *Non-operative:* simple splinting (neighbouring strap, sling), plaster of paris, functional bracing, fibreglass cast, continuous traction
- *Operative*: internal fixation: intramedullary nail, screws / plates, Kirschner (K) wires. External fixation: Ex-Fix, Ilizarov frame

Indication for operative treatment: polytrauma, displaced intra-articular fractures, open fracture, associated vascular injury or compartment syndrome, pathological fractures, non-unions.

Rehabilitation

Having successfully repaired a fracture patients may need ongoing rehabilitation to regain function in the affected area.

Methods of rehabilitation include physiotherapy, occupational therapy, walking aids.

Emergencies

Open fractures

P Fracture associated with a break in the skin.

A Trauma transferring energy into bones and soft tissue.

Type I	Laceration <1cm Simple fracture with minimal soft tissue disruption
Type II	Laceration >1cm Minimally comminuted fracture without extensive soft tissue damage and minimal to moderate crushing
Type III	Extensive damage to soft tissues, including muscles, skin, and neurovascular structures with a high degree of contamination Any high-energy trauma or gunshot wounds
III A	Soft tissue coverage of the fractured bone is adequate
III B	Soft tissue coverage not possible, flap / graft required Commonly massive contamination
III C	Vascular injury requiring repair

Box 20.1: Gustilo Anderson classification of open fractures

S **Sx** Fracture associated with an open wound. May have associated vascular or neurological injury.

I Plain XR.

T Managed as per BOAST / BAPRAS guidelines (www.boa.ac.uk).

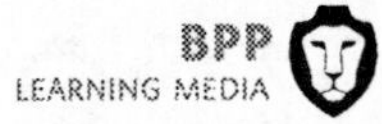

- ATLS resuscitation
- Early broad-spectrum IV antibiotics and tetanus, continue antibiotics until 72 hours or skin coverage
- Assess neurovascular status and for compartment syndrome, correct vascular impairment within 3–4 hours (6 maximum)
- Photograph wound then clean and dress with saline soaked gauze
- Splint fracture
- Early transfer to a specialist centre if severe injury unless unsafe to transfer
- Involve Plastic Surgeons for definite wound coverage

Box 20.2: BOAST / BAPRAS guidelines for open fractures

C All complications of closed fractures increased due to high-energy nature of injury and infection.

Pr Dependent on severity of injury.

Compartment syndrome

P Occurs when pressure in a muscle compartment exceeds that of the capillary blood supply.

Compartmental pressure >30mmHg or within 30mmHg of diastolic BP.

It is progressive leading to muscle oedema and ischaemia.

A Anterior compartment of leg commonest site (after tibial fracture) can occur in any fascial compartment.

- *Trauma:* open / closed fractures (most common cause), crush injury, burns, penetrating injury, vascular injury
- *Iatrogenic:* plaster and dressings, traction table, IM injection

Box 20.3: Causes of compartment syndrome

S Sx Pain out of proportion with the injury is the most important symptom, pain on passive stretch of the muscle compartment.

Paraesthesia and diminished distal pulses are late signs due to compartment pressure exceeding that of arterial flow.

I Diagnosis should be made on clinical grounds but compartment pressures can be measured using an external probe (useful when patient has low GCS).

T Remove dressings / cast, immediate fasciotomy and decompression of the compartment.

C Loss of limb, sensory / motor dysfunction, chronic pain, Volkmann's ischaemic contracture.

Pr Good if early diagnosis and intervention (fasciotomy) <6 hours.

Poor if delayed >12 hours.

Septic joint

P Purulent invasion of a joint by an infectious organism.

A Through direct penetration of the joint (traumatic or iatrogenic) or indirect spread haematologically / locally from another source of infection (staphylococcus aureus is the most common pathogen).

S Hot, red, swollen joint with effusion.

Sx Rapid onset joint pain, worse on movement, fever.

I XR to exclude other pathology.

Bloods: ↑ WCC, ↑ CRP, uric acid (to exclude gout).

Joint aspiration to be sent for M,C&S and crystals (NB prosthetic joints must only be aspirated in theatre).

T IV antibiotics (after joint aspiration).

Washout in theatre within 48 hours to prevent destruction of articular cartilage.

Prosthetic implants may need to be removed.

C Avascular necrosis of epiphysis, joint subluxation / dislocation, growth disturbance, secondary osteoarthritis.

Pr Good if diagnosis and treatment is prompt.

Cauda equina syndrome

P The spinal cord terminates at L1 / L2 level in adults.

The cauda equina ('horse tail') extends below and is compressed leading to neurological dysfunction.

A *Lesion:* central disc prolapse, tumour.

Trauma: spinal anaesthesia, burst fractures, penetrating injury.

Other: spinal stenosis, spinal inflammatory conditions.

S Reduced lower limb power, reduced anal tone, reduced / absent reflexes, saddle anaesthesia.

Sx Weakness of the lower limbs, disturbance of bladder / bowels (in particular urinary retention), bilateral leg pain.

I Urgent MRI lumbar spine.

T Surgical decompression within 48 hours of symptom onset if indicated.

Palliative radiotherapy for non-operative tumours.

C Temporary / permanent neurological dysfunction.

Pr Dependent on severity and duration of compression.

Post-op complications

Immediate (mins–hours)	Early (24–72 hours)	Late (7–14 days)
Haemorrhage	Haematoma	Chronic wound sinus
Shock	Wound dehiscence	Reduced mobility
Low urine output	Wound infection	Deep prosthetic infection
Acute renal failure	Confusion	Osteomyelitis
Basal atelectasis	Compartment syndrome	DVT / PE
Stroke	Fat embolism syndrome: SoB, hypoxia, agitation, coma, petechial rash, anaemia	Sudeck's atrophy: pain, swelling, stiffness, skin changes due to overactive sympathetic action
MI	Pneumonia	Complex regional pain syndrome
Pain	UTI	Malunion, delayed union, non-union
	Paralytic ileus	

Table 20.1: Common post-op complications

Trauma

Nerve injuries

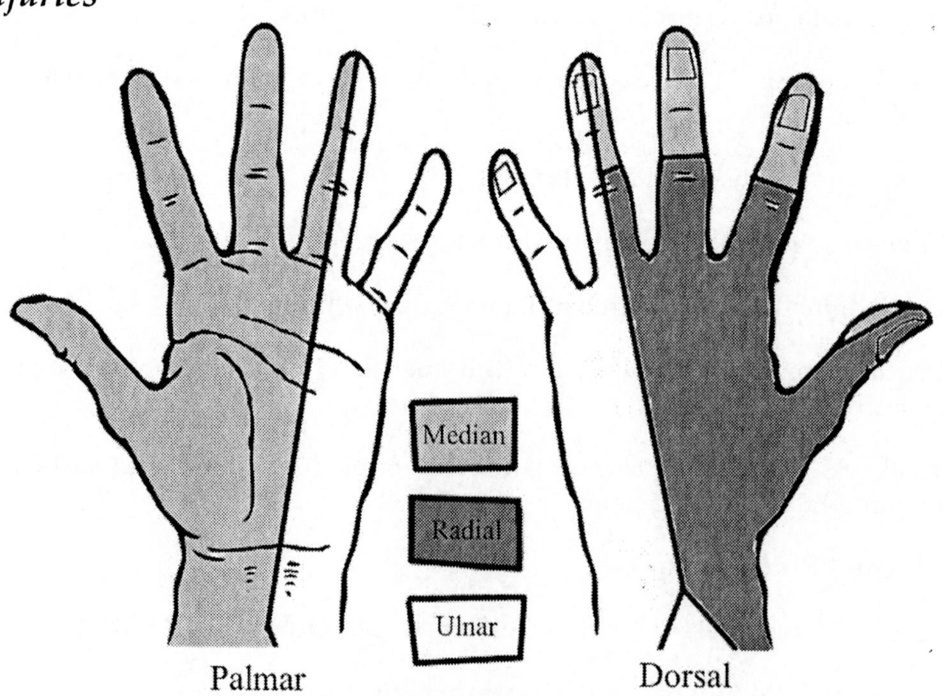

Figure 20.1: Nerve sensory distribution of the left hand

Median nerve

P Formed by medial and lateral cords of the brachial plexus from roots C5-T1.

Motor supply: all the flexors of the forearm **except** flexor carpi ulnaris and medial two digits of flexor digitorum profundus. Supplies LOAF muscles of the hand: lateral two **L**umbicals, **O**pponens Pollicis Brevis, **A**bductor Pollicis Brevis and **F**lexor Pollicis Brevis.

Sensory supply: thumb, index finger, middle finger and radial aspect of ring finger (above).

A Compression of nerve at carpal tunnel (or elbow). CTS more common in pregnancy, hypothyroid, acromegaly, obesity.

S Loss of thumb abduction and opposition.

Sx Loss of sensation in thumb, index finger, middle finger and radial aspect of ring finger.

I Phalen test, Tinel's sign, nerve conduction studies.

T *Non-operative:* rest, splinting.

Operative: steroid injection, carpal tunnel decompression.

Ulna nerve

P Formed by the medial cord of the brachial plexus from roots C8-T1.

Motor supply: small muscles of the hand excluding the LOAF muscles.

Sensory supply: little finger and the medial half of the ring finger, and the corresponding part of the palm (above).

A Most commonly damaged at the medial epicondyle as it passes the elbow. Can also be compressed at Guyon's canal at the wrist.

S Ulna claw hand (claw hand is worse in Guyon's canal compression due to ulna paradox).

Sx Altered / loss of sensation in little finger and the medial half of the ring finger, and the corresponding part of the palm.

I Froment's sign.

T *Non-operative:* rest, fix fracture.

Operative: decompression.

Radial nerve

P Formed by the posterior cord of the brachial plexus by roots C5-T1.

Motor supply: posterior muscles of the arm and extrinsic extensors of the hand and wrist.

Sensory supply: dorsum of the hand (above).

A Most commonly damaged in mid-shaft humeral fractures as it travels in the radial groove.

S Wrist drop.

Sx Loss / altered sensation over the anatomical snuff box area.

I Nerve conduction studies.

T Splinting, physio / OT.

Brachial plexus

P C5-T1 nerve roots carry nerve fibres from spinal cord to upper limb. Injuries divided into upper, lower and whole brachial plexus lesions.

Upper lesion: occurs from excessive lateral neck flexion away from the shoulder principally affecting C5-6 producing an Erb's Palsy. Commonly arising from shoulder dystocia during a difficult birth.

Lower lesion: sudden upward pulling on an abducted arm principally affecting C8-T1 producing a Klumpke's paralysis mechanism of injury produced by catching arm on a tree branch while falling.

A Commonly injured in shoulder trauma (birth injuries commonest), tumours and inflammation.

S Upper limb weakness, sensory deficit and reduced reflexes.

Sx *Erb's Palsy:* paralysis and atrophy of the deltoid, biceps, and brachialis muscles producing 'waiter's tip' position.

Klumpke's paralysis: claw hand, paralysis of intrinsic hand muscles.

I Nerve conduction studies.

T Physiotherapy / OT, nerve transfer in severe injury.

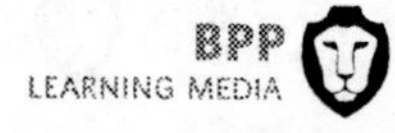

Lateral cutaneous nerve of the thigh

P Arises from the dorsal divisions of L2-3 in the lumbar plexus. Injured by entrapment or compression as it passes between the ilium and inguinal ligament near the ASIS.

Known as meralgia paraesthetica.

A Compressed by seatbelts, tight clothing, obesity.

S Sx Pain, altered sensation / loss of sensation over dermatome (outer thigh).

I Nerve conduction studies.

T Analgesia, weight loss, nerve decompression if severe.

Sciatic nerve

P Arises from L4-S3 in the lumbar and sacral plexus.

Supplies sensation to most of the leg, motor to posterior thigh and leg.

A Compression of the nerve or nerve roots by lumbar spinal disc herniation, lumbar spinal stenosis, piriformis syndrome.

S Lasègue test (straight leg raise) +ve if produces sciatic pain between 30–70 degrees.

Sx Pain, altered sensation, weakness in lower back radiating down buttocks posterior thigh and leg.

I MRI lumbar spine.

T Of underlying cause, analgesia, discectomy.

Pr 90% of pain caused by disc prolapse resolves without surgical intervention.

Common peroneal nerve

P Arises from dorsal branches of L4-5 and S1-2.

A Damaged as it winds around the neck of the fibula.

S Sx Foot drop, sensory loss to dorsal surface of foot (1st web space sensory loss if deep peroneal nerve only).

I Clinical.

T Rest, fix fracture.

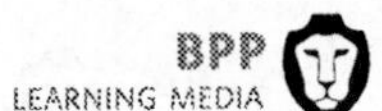

Chapter 20

Upper limb

Clavicle fracture

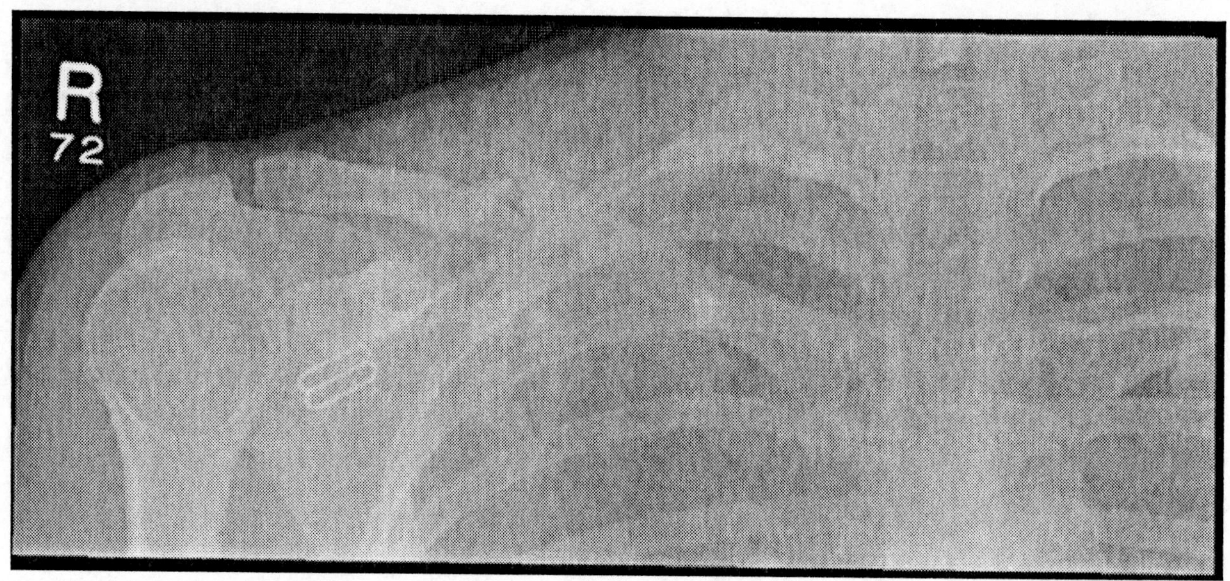

Figure 20.2: Right clavicle fracture. (Reproduced with permission from SW Deanery.)

P 80% of fractures are middle third.

A Fall onto shoulder (majority), direct impact, falls onto outstretched hand.

S Sx Pain, deformity of the clavicle and / or damage to the overlying tissue, reduced shoulder movement.

I XR, CT if complex fracture or soft tissue complication.

T Vast majority conservative with broad arm sling.

Indications for ORIF (controversial): non-union, open fractures, skin tenting, neurovascular compromise, significantly displaced and shortened fractures, ipsilateral proximal humerus fracture (floating shoulder).

C Associated rib fractures, damage to pleura, vessels and brachial plexus, proximal 1/3 fractures, malunion, non-union and post-traumatic AC joint arthritis.

Pr In adults minimum three to four weeks' immobilisation required for bone and soft tissue healing.

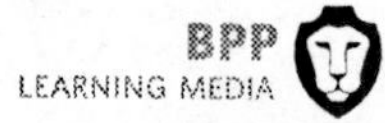

Shoulder dislocation

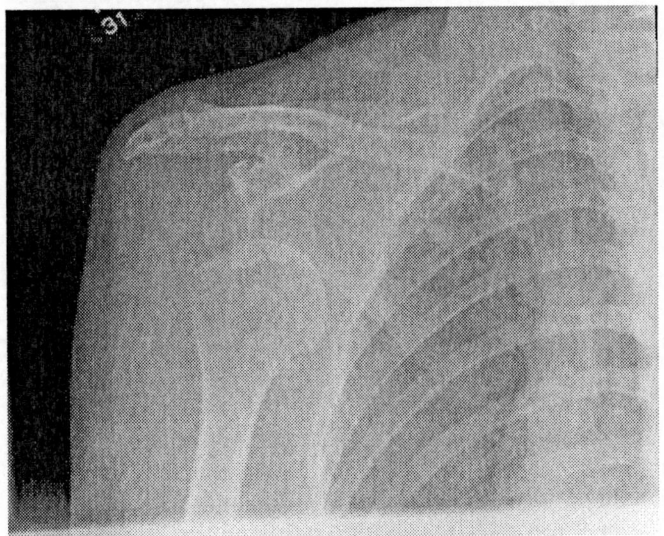

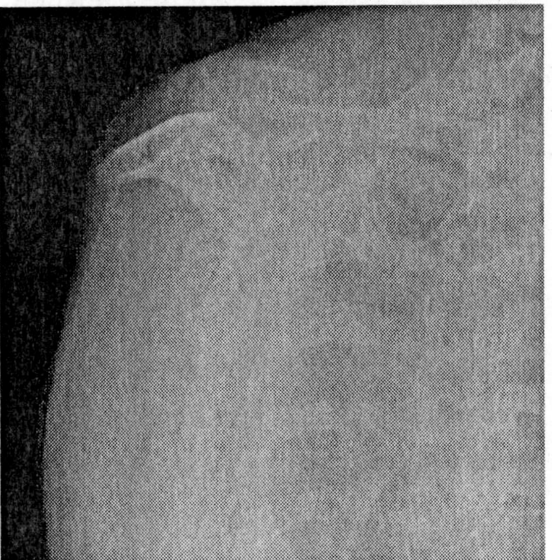

Figure 20.3: Right shoulder dislocation AP and scapular-Y views. (Reproduced with permission from SW Deanery.)

P Most commonly dislocated joint in the body.

Incidence peaks 21–30 years and 61–80 years.

90% anterior. Posterior accounts for the majority of the rest.

A *Anterior:* most commonly indirect trauma to upper limb in abduction, extension and external rotation, direct posterior trauma.

Posterior: epilepsy, electric shock, direct anterior trauma.

S Sx *Anterior*: shoulder held in slight abduction and external rotation. The shoulder may be squared.

Posterior: shoulder held in sling position, adducted and internally rotated. Limited external rotation on examination.

I Careful neurovascular examination should be carried out and should be documented before attempted relocation.

XR AP, scapular-Y and axillary views.

CT may be indicated if associated fracture.

MRI / MRI arthrography may be used for evaluation of rotator cuff and glenoid labrum respectively.

T Closed reduction with adequate analgesia / sedation: Kocher's, Milch, Hippocratic methods.

Open reduction: if unable to reduce closed.

Post reduction the arm should be immobilised in a sling for two to five weeks.

Check axillary nerve function post-reduction: sensation over 'regimental badge' area.

C Associated fracture of glenoid or humerus, rotator cuff tear, glenoid labrum tear, capsular damage and neurovascular injury (axillary and musculocutaneous nerves in particular).

Pr Recurrence (50% in all ages, up to 89% in 14–21 years group).

Rotator cuff disorders

P Tears in the four muscles that make up the shoulder girdle.

Can either be chronic or acute and partial or full.

NB must exclude other causes of pain and weakness about the shoulder girdle.

A Trauma 10%, impingement syndrome 75%, multi-directional instability 10–15%.

S Pain, weakness of the specific rotator cuff muscles when compared to the contralateral shoulder.

Sx Pain and weakness.

I MRI.

T *Conservative:* physiotherapy generally reserved for older, non-operative patients.

Operative: arthroscopic / open rotator cuff repair +/- sub acromial decompression / biceps tenolysis / stabilisation surgery.

C Failed repair, captured shoulder, re-tears.

Pr Good in both surgical and conservative groups.

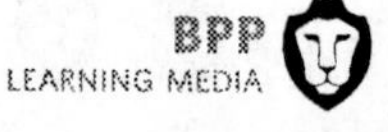

Proximal humerus fractures

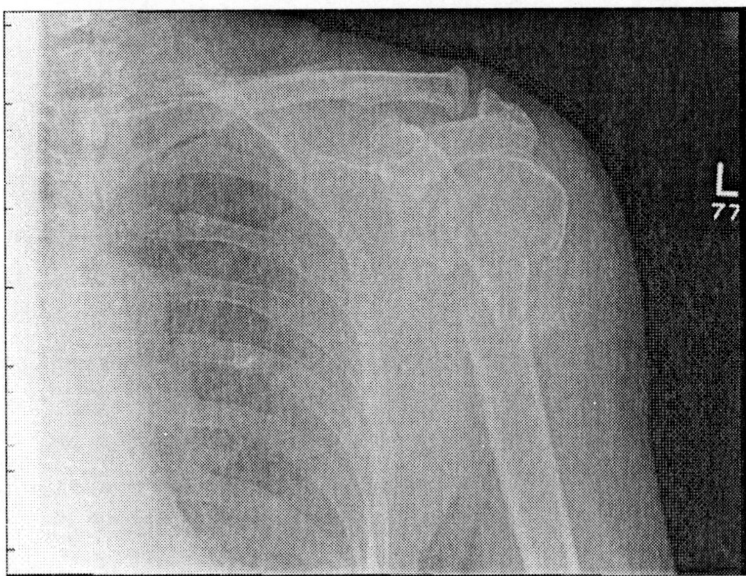

Figure 20.4: Left proximal humerus fracture. (Reproduced with permission from SW Deanery.)

P Most common humeral fracture.

Incidence associated with increasing age and female sex.

85% undisplaced.

A Most commonly caused by falling onto an outstretched upper limb from standing height in the osteoporotic population.

S **Sx** Painful and tender upper limb with bruising around site.

Neurovascular damage, in particular axillary nerve.

I XR shoulder AP, scapular-Y and axillary views.

T 85% minimally displaced and can be managed conservatively.

- *One-part fractures:* majority are minimally displaced and can be treated conservatively in collar and cuff with early passive motion to prevent stiffness
- *Two-part fractures:* generally require ORIF but some may be reduced closed and stabilised percutaneously. In anatomical neck fractures some may require hemi-arthroplasty due to the risk of avascular necrosis
- *Three- and four-part fractures:* unstable due to distracting muscle forces. Require either ORIF or hemi-arthroplasty unless patient cannot tolerate surgery. Decision is dependant on patient age and functional demands

Box 20.4: Abbreviated Neer classification proximal humeral fractures

C Avascular necrosis (particularly in three- and four-part fractures), neurovascular injury, myositis ossificans, shoulder stiffness, non-union, malunion.

Pr Greater comminution is associated with greater complication in conservatively managed and ORIF population.

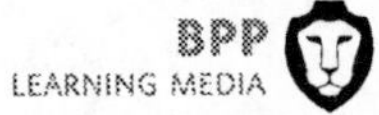

Biceps tendon rupture

P Can occur proximally (long-head of biceps) or distally.

A Higher incidence in men >30 years, smokers and those using cortico-steroids.

Proximal tears usually secondary to chronic attrition.

Distal tears usually secondary to a forced load against active arm flexion.

S *Proximal*: bunching of the fibres in typical 'pop-eye' appearance.

Distal: tendon still palpable in ante-cubital fossa, may cause median nerve symptoms.

Sx *Proximal*: minimal loss of power.

Distal: 30% decrease in flexion strength, 40% decrease in supination strength.

I MRI if diagnosis in question.

T *Proximal:* conservative generally, operative for cosmesis or shoulder reconstruction in younger patients.

Distal: early surgical intervention to prevent weakness, either surgical re-attachment or tenodesis with substantial post-operative physiotherapy.

C Long-term weakness, re-rupture.

Pr *Proximal:* good results either conservative or surgical.

Distal: good results if early surgical intervention and compliance to post-operative care.

Forearm

- *Colles' fracture:* extra-articular distal radius fracture with dorsal displacement / angulation of distal fragment
- *Smith's fracture:* extra-articular distal radius fracture with volar displacement / angulation of distal fragment (reverse Colles')
- *Barton's fracture:* intra-articular distal third radius fracture with dislocation of radiocarpal joint
- *Galleazzi fracture:* middle to distal third radius fracture with disruption of the distal radio-ulna joint ('ZZ' = distal end radius)
- *Monteggia fracture:* proximal third ulna fracture with associated dislocation of the radial head ('GG' = proximal end ulna)

Box 20.5: Summary of eponymous forearm fractures

Colles' fracture

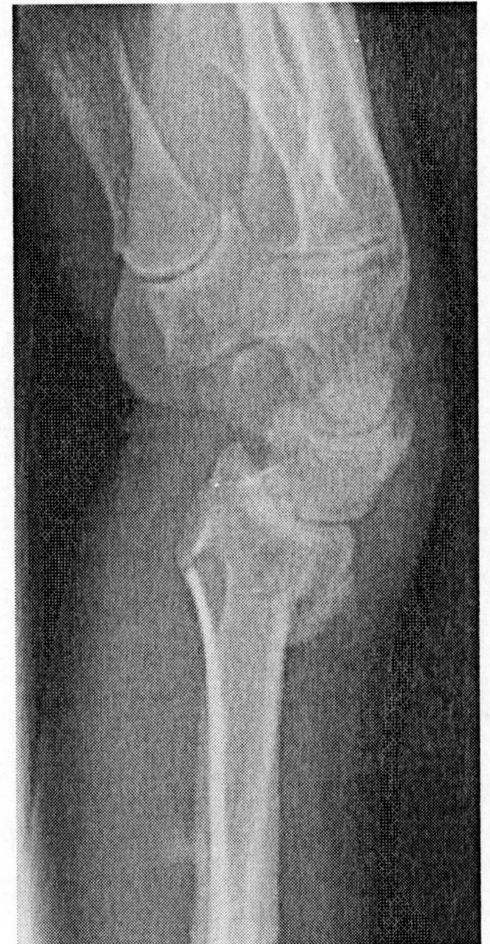

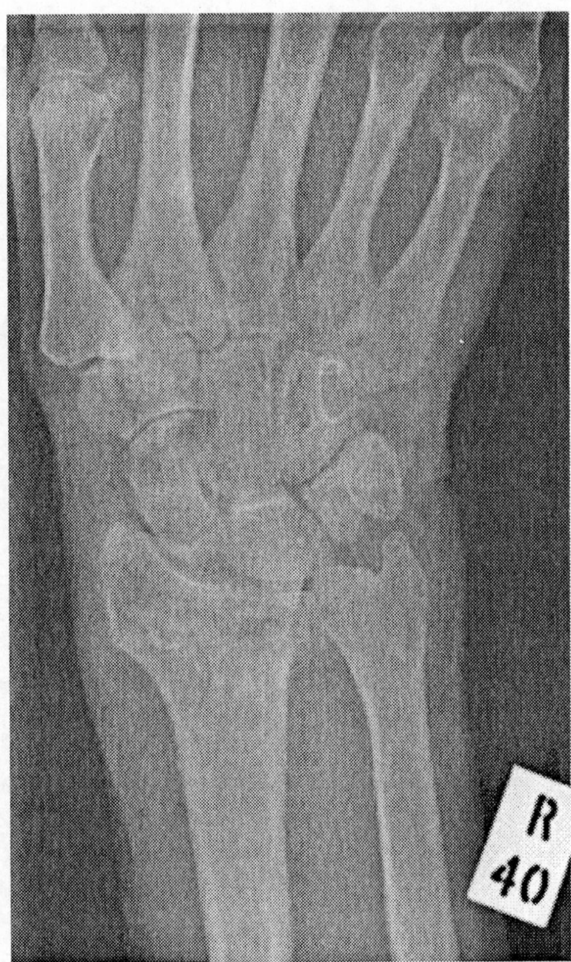

Figure 20.5: Right Colles' fracture.
(Reproduced with permission from SW Deanery.)

P Extra-articular distal third radius fracture with dorsal displacement / angulation of distal fragment.

A Fall onto outstretched hand, elderly population.

S **Sx** Pain, 'dinner-fork' deformity.

I XR AP + lateral.

T Closed reduction in A&E with application of backslab.

ORIF: K-wires, volar locking plate.

C Ulnar styloid fracture, neurovascular injury, compartment syndrome, non-union, arthritis, Sudeck's atrophy.

Pr Good if anatomical reduction.

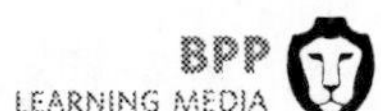

Smith's fracture

P Extra-articular distal third radius fracture with volar displacement / angulation of distal fragment.

A Fall onto flexed wrist, elderly population.

S Sx Pain, 'reverse dinner fork' deformity.

I XR AP + lateral.

T Closed reduction in A&E with application of backslab.

ORIF if unstable.

C Neurovascular injury, compartment syndrome, non-union, arthritis.

Pr Good if anatomical reduction.

Barton's fracture

P Intra-articular distal third radius fracture with dislocation of radiocarpal joint. Displacement / angulation of distal fragment may be volar or dorsal.

A Fall onto outstretched hand, elderly population.

S Sx Pain, deformity.

I XR AP + lateral.

T ORIF: locking plate as intra-articular.

C Neurovascular injury, compartment syndrome, non-union, arthritis.

Pr Good if anatomical reduction.

Galleazzi fracture

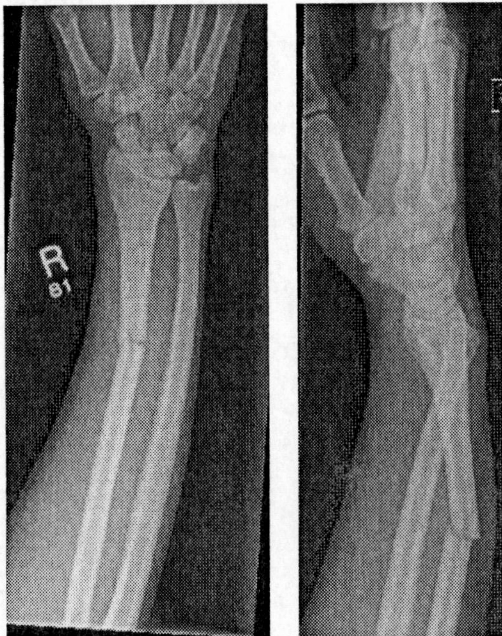

Figure 20.6: Right Galleazzi fracture. (Reproduced with permission from SW Deanery.)

P Middle to distal third radius fracture associated with an intact ulna and disruption of the distal radio-ulna joint.

A Fall onto outstretched hand, peak incidence 9–12 years.

S **Sx** Swelling about distal third of ulna.

I Plain X-ray.

T Closed reduction with arm held in supination by long arm cast.

If closed reduction not possible ORIF indicated.

C Neurovascular injury (anterior interosseus and radial nerves), compartment syndrome, non-union and persistent ulna subluxation.

Pr Good if anatomical reduction.

Monteggia fracture

P Proximal third ulna fracture or plastic deformation with associated dislocation of the radial head.

A Peak incidence 4–10 years.

Either direct blow on back of upper forearm or fall onto outstretched hand in the hyperpronated position.

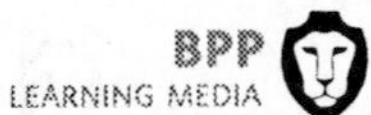

S Sx Elbow swelling and deformity, painful range of movement especially pronation / supination and crepitus.

I Plain X-ray.

T Conservative, ORIF.

C Non-union, malunion, nerve palsy and radial head instability.

Pr Good if radial head is stable after reduction of the ulna fracture.

Hand

Scaphoid fracture

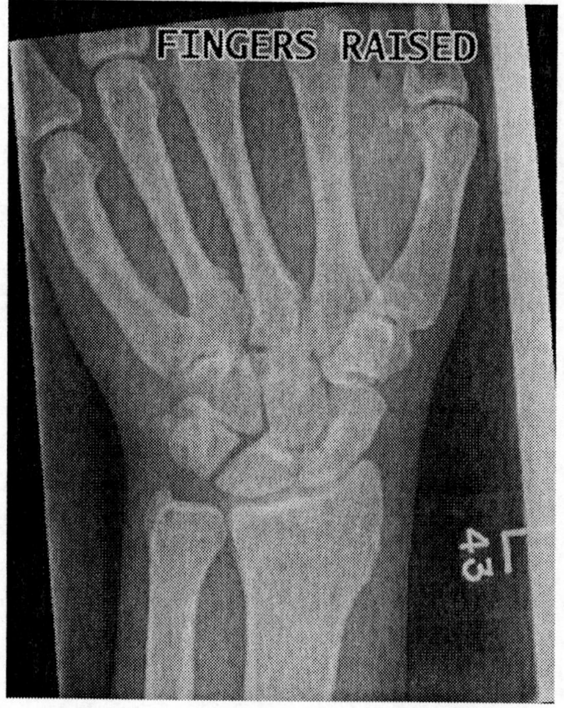

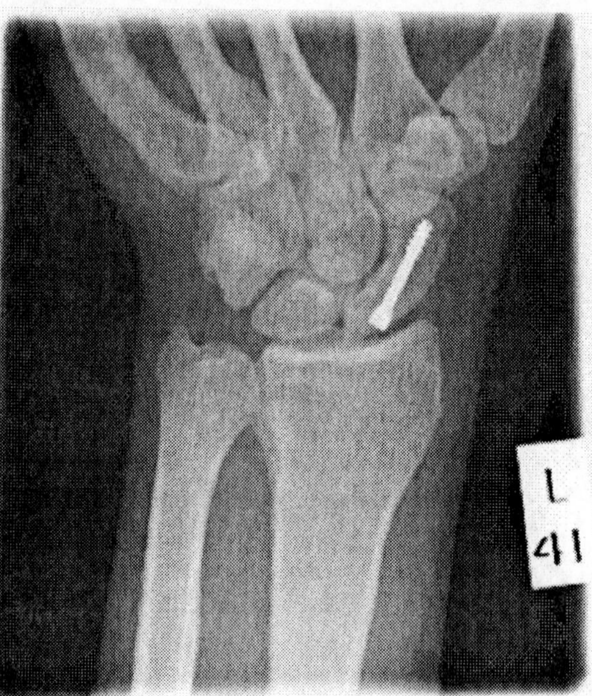

Figure 20.7: Left scaphoid fracture before and after Herbert screw. (Reproduced with permission from SW Deanery.)

P Common fractures.

Scaphoid blood supply is derived from branches of radial artery supplying the distal bone end.

Fractures of the scaphoid waist or proximal third depend on union for revascularisation therefore risk avascular necrosis.

A Most common mechanism is fall onto an outstretched hand with forced dorsiflexion, ulnar deviation and intercarpal supination.

S Sx Tenderness over the anatomical snuffbox region, positive scaphoid shift test, pain and swelling at the base of the thumb.

I Plain XR (scaphoid views) initially non-diagnostic in 25% of fractures.

If clinically tender but X-ray non-diagnostic a trial of immobilisation with follow up and repeat XR in one to two weeks.

MRI or CT may be used to diagnose scaphoid fractures if XR non-conclusive.

T *Non-operative*: (non-displaced distal 1/3 or tuberosity fractures) immobilisation in a thumb spica cast.

Operative: ORIF with Herbert screw fixation and immobisation in a thumb spica for six weeks. Operative management is indicated in proximal pole fractures (as prone to AVN), fracture displacement >1mm, radiolunate angle >15 degrees, scapholunate angle >60 degrees and non-union.

C Delayed union, non-union, malunion and avascular necrosis.

Pr Conservative treatment gives varying rates of union.

Tuberosity and distal third 100%, waist 80–90% and proximal pole 60–70%.

Bennett's fracture

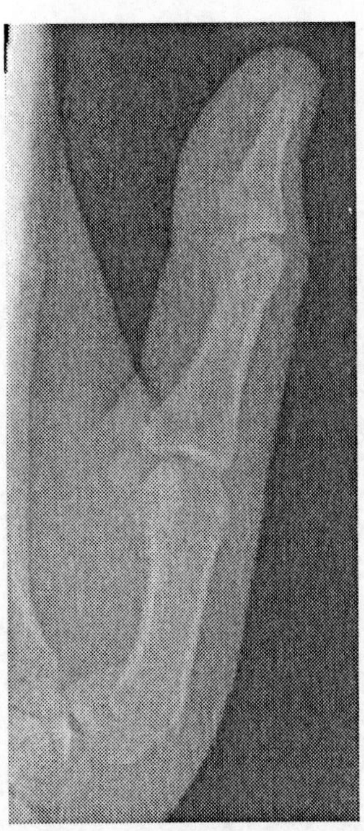

Figure 20.8: Left Bennett's fracture.
(Reproduced with permission from SW Deanery.)

P Fracture of the base of the first meta-carpal extending into the carpo-meta-carpal joint.

Commonly associated with joint sublaxation / dislocation.

A Caused by an axial load on the thumb either from punching a hard object or as a result of a fall onto the thumb.

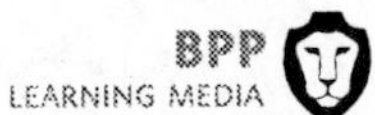

S Tenderness, swelling and bruising over the base of the thumb.

Sx Instability of the CMC joint of the thumb accompanied by weakness of the pinch grip.

I Plain X-ray.

T All need to be immobilised in a thumb spica cast for four to six weeks.

Conservative: minimally displaced <1mm.

Operative: closed reduction and K-wire fixation (metacarpal to trapezium): 1–3mm displacement at trapezio-metacarpal joint.

ORIF: >3mm displacement at trapezio-metacarpal joint.

C Thumb weakness and osteoarthritis.

Pr Dependent on accuracy of reduction.

Boxer's fracture

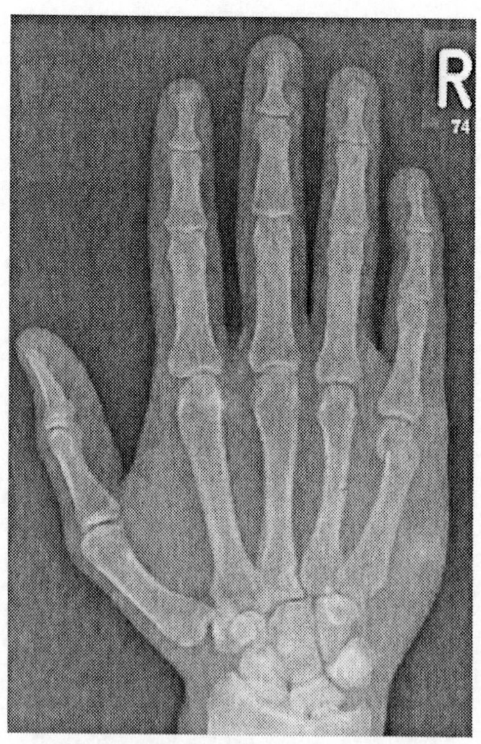

Figure 20.9: Right boxer's fracture.
(Reproduced with permission from SW Deanery.)

P Transverse neck fracture of the 5th metacarpal.

A Typically sustained when an inexperienced fighter throws a punch and sustains the majority of the force through the 5th knuckle.

S Localised swelling, loss of the 5th knuckle contour.

Sx Pain, swelling and loss of function.

I Plain X-ray including AP and true lateral views to assess displacement and angulation.

T *Conservative:* if minimal angulation may be managed by splinting with a pop in the Edinburgh position.

Operative: closed reduction under LA / GA and insertion of K-wires.

C Malunion, non-union.

Pr Full functional recovery in three to four months.

Hip and pelvis

Fractured neck of femur

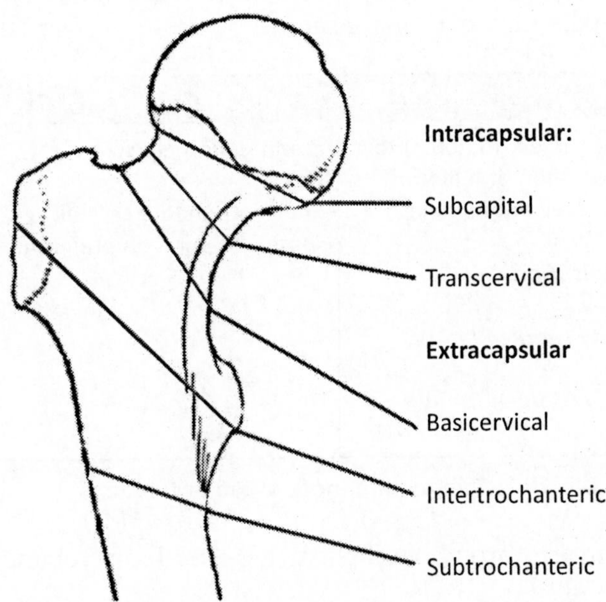

Figure 20.10: Anatomical classification of femoral neck fractures

P >70,000 admissions per year in UK.

Femoral head blood supply: circumflex and retinacular arteries – compromised in displaced, intracapsular fractures leading to AVN of femoral head.

A 80% low energy falls in elderly with osteoporosis, high energy in young.

S Sx *Displaced fracture:* painful, shortened, externally rotated leg, unable to weight bear.

Undisplaced / impacted fracture: groin pain only.

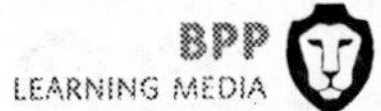

I XR hip AP + lateral: look for break in continuity of the trabeculae.

Bloods: FBC, U&Es, G&S, INR.

Investigate fall eg ECG, CXR.

Assess NV status, assess mobility level.

Classified on XR by anatomical position (above) and displacement (Garden I–IV).

Based on valgus displacement on AP radiograph Type I: Incomplete fracture or impacted Type II: Undisplaced complete fracture Type III: Partial displacement / angulation Type IV: Complete displacement	Garden I + II: Screw Garden III + IV: Austin Moore (Hemiarthroplasty)

Box 20.6: Garden classification of intracapsular NOFs

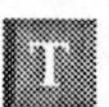

Based on patient age, level of mobility, fracture position and fracture pattern.

Elderly: early surgery (48 hours), involve orthogeriatric team, bone protection, analgesia: regional block, oral analgesics.

Intracapsular	Extracapsular
Fractures pts <50 years: urgent surgery (6 hours) to restore blood supply and preservation of femoral head with cancellous screws to prevent multiple THRs in the future *Undisplaced / impacted fractures (Garden I / II):* fixation with ×3 cancellous screws *Displaced fracture good mobility (Garden III / IV):* total hip replacement *Displaced fracture poor mobility (Garden III / IV):* hemiarthroplasty (cemented or uncemented)	Compression hip screw Or Short intramedullary nail (Based on surgeon preference and fracture pattern)

Box 20.7: Treatment of neck of femur fractures

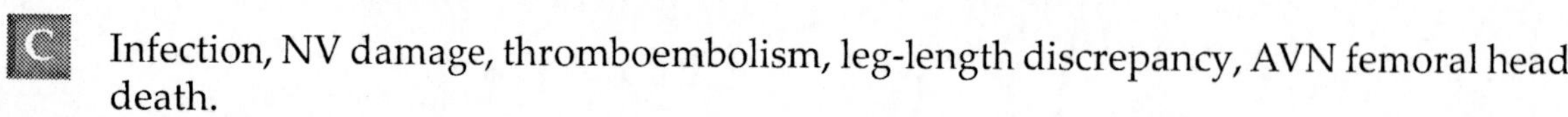

Infection, NV damage, thromboembolism, leg-length discrepancy, AVN femoral head, death.

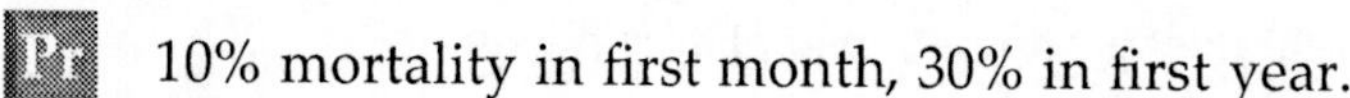

10% mortality in first month, 30% in first year.

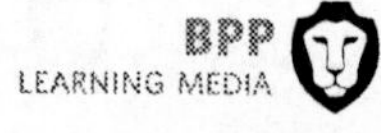

Intracapsular

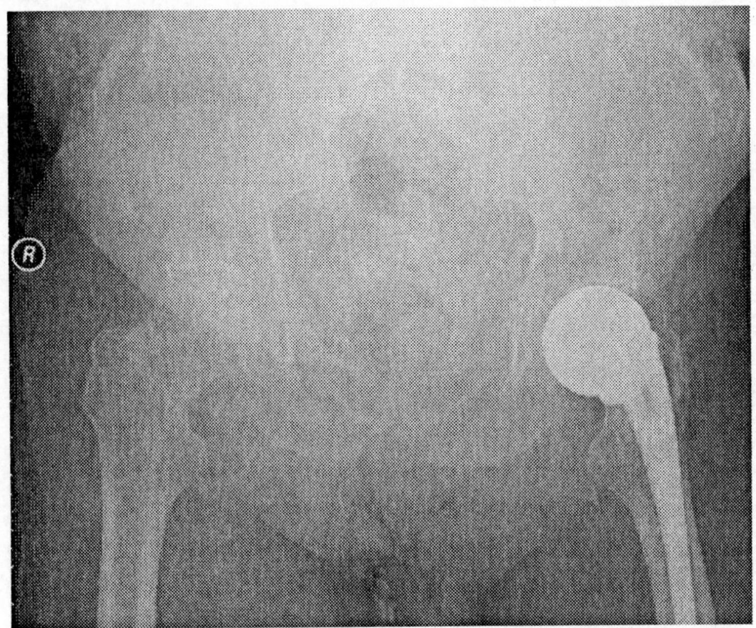

Figure 20.11: Right transcervical fractured NOF.
(Reproduced with permission from SW Deanery.)

Extracapsular

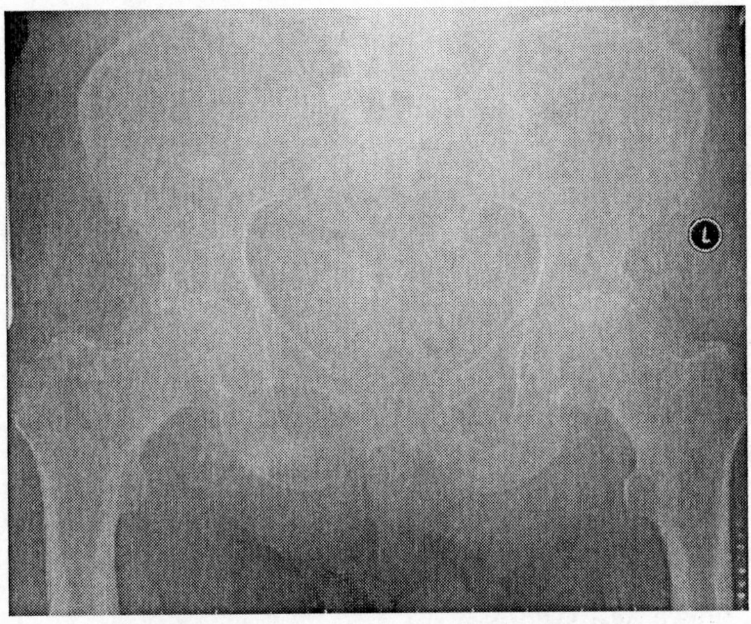

Figure 20.12: Right intertrochanteric fractured NOF.
(Reproduced with permission from SW Deanery.)

Pelvic fracture

P Fracture of pelvic ring, high mortality due to haemorrhage from pelvic venous plexus.

A High-energy trauma eg RTC, fall from height or fall in elderly.

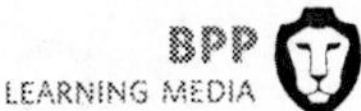

S Sx Pain, unable to weight bare, flank / buttock contusions, hypovolaemic shock, haematuria, urethral / perineal bruising.

I AP pelvis, judet views (for acetabular fractures), CT. Young and Burgess classification (based on mechanism of injury): anteroposterior compression, lateral compression, vertical Shear and combined.

T ATLS resusciation, pelvic binder or Ex-Fix to provide immediate stabilisation and haemorrhage control.

Referral to pelvic surgeon for ORIF.

C Damage to bladder (20%) or urethra (10%), vascular injury.

Knee

Anterior cruciate ligament tear (ACL)

P Complete or partial tear of the anterior cruciate ligament due to trauma. ACL stabilises the knee when in extension.

A Deceleration followed by sudden change in direction, twisting the knee on landing.

S Anterior drawer test +ve, Lachman test +ve, pivot shift test +ve.

Sx Sudden pop, sudden haemarthrosis, pain on bending knee, knee locks or buckles.

I MRI.

T *Conservative*: RICE, knee brace, rehab.

Surgery: arthroscopic ACL reconstruction.

C Haemarthrosis, infection, ongoing pain or instability.

Posterior cruciate ligament (PCL)

P PCL prevents posterior translation at knee joint.

A Direct blow to the flexed knee displacing the tibia posterior to the femur eg knee hitting the dashboard.

Sx Posterior drawer test +ve.

S Pain, instability.

I MRI.

T Arthroscopic PCL repair.

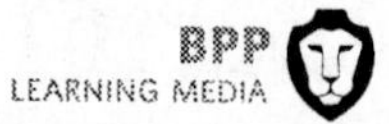

Meniscal tear

P Medial and lateral menisci are C-shaped pads of fibrocartilage between the femoral condyles and tibial plateau.

A Trauma due to twisting of a flexed knee.

S Tender over joint line, McMurray's test +ve, Thessaly's test +ve.

Sx Pain on loading, swelling, mechanical symptoms eg locking, clicking, catching or 'giving way'.

I MRI.

T Conservative: analgesia, quadriceps strengthening exercises. Surgery: arthroscopic meniscal repair, partial removal or total menisectomy.

C Total menisectomy increases risk of developing OA.

Tibial plateau fracture

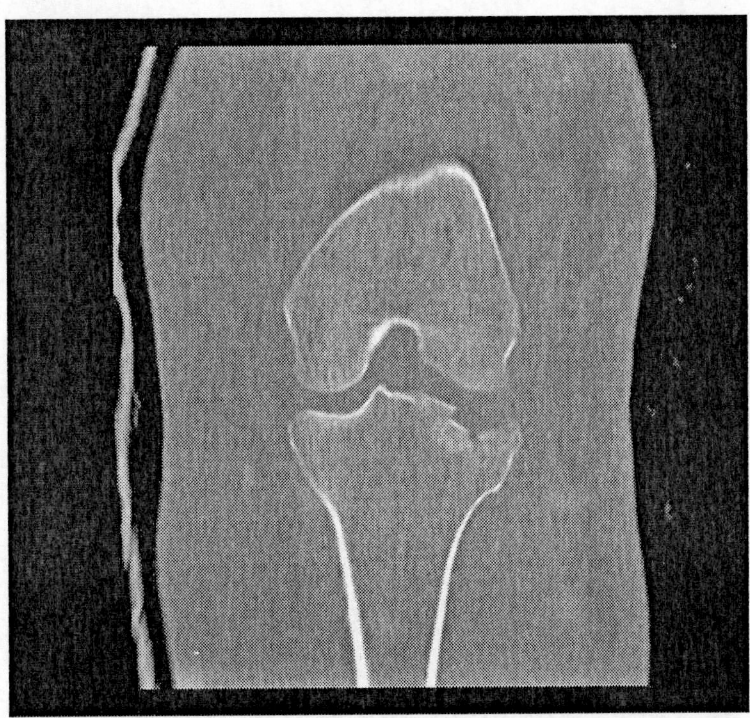

Figure 20.13: CT tibial plateau Schatzker II. (Reproduced with permission from SW Deanery.)

P Varus or valgus force to a weight-bearing knee.

Classically a car bumper hitting a pedestrian's fixed knee.

A High energy trauma eg RTA or low energy in osteoporotic bone. 70% lateral plateau, 20% medial, 10% bicondylar.

S Sx Knee pain, effusion, bruising.

I XR knee Ap + lateral; CT; MRI: useful for meniscal and ligamentous injuries.

Type I: lateral plateau split
Type II: lateral plateau split / depressed
Type III: lateral plateau depressed
Type IV: medial plateau
Type V: bicondylar
Type VI: plateau fracture with metaphyseal / diaphyseal dissociation

Box 20.8: Schatzker classification tibial plateau fractures

T *Non-operative:* minimally displaced (<2mm) fractures, stable fractures, patients unsuitable for operative intervention – NWB 4-8 / 52 then hinged knee brace.

Operative: displaced (>2mm), unstable / open fractures – ORIF or Ex-Fix.

C Compartment syndrome, infection, knee stiffness, malunion / non-union, peroneal nerve injury, popliteal artery injury, knee arthritis.

Lower limb

Tibial fracture

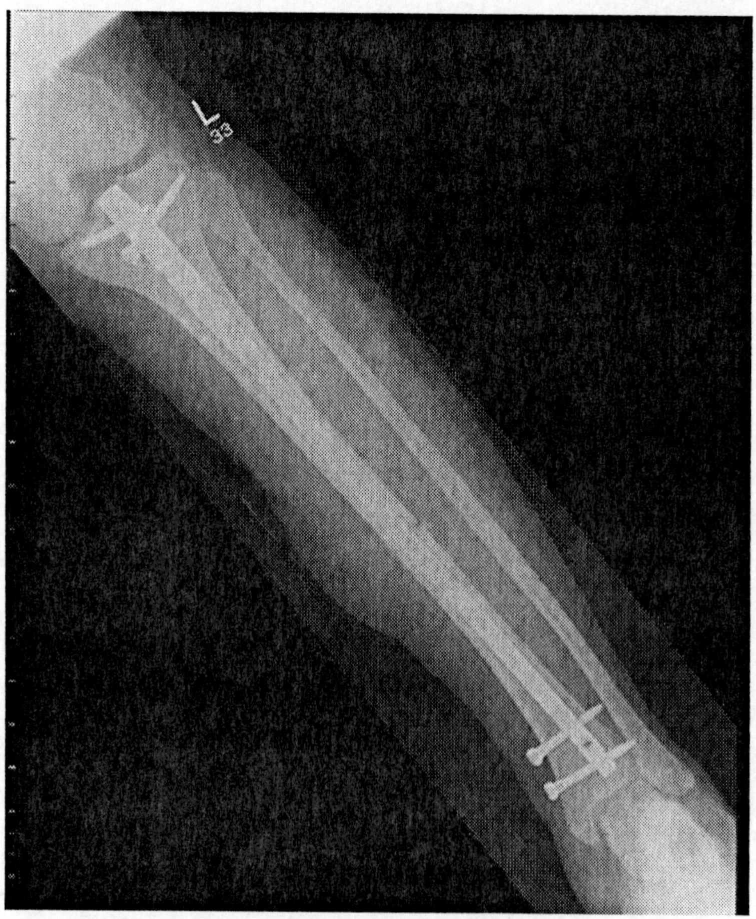

Figure 20.14: Left tibial fracture fixated with an IM nail. (Reproduced with permission from SW Deanery.)

P RTC or sport in young, falls in elderly.

A Commonest long bone fracture, up to 20% are open fractures.

S **Sx** Pain, deformity, swelling.

I XR AP + lateral tibia.

T *Non-operative:* for low-energy mechanisms with acceptable alignment (<5 varus / valgus, <1cm shortened) – above knee cast.

Operative: high-energy fracture, unacceptable alignment, open fracture – Ex-Fix, ORIF (IM Nail).

C Compartment syndrome (8%), non-union, infection, knee / ankle stiffness, knee pain (>50% in IM Nail), NV injury.

Achilles tendon rupture

P Achilles tendon connects gastrocnemius and soleus to calcaneum enabling plantar flexion.

A Commonest tendon rupture, occurs during sudden plantar flexion eg sprinting, jumping.

Risk factors: steroids, recreational athletes, previous tears.

S Simmonds' test +ve (absence of plantar flexion on squeezing calf with patient prone), palpable gap at tendon insertion.

Sx Loud 'pop', feeling of being 'kicked in the back of leg', pain, swelling, unable to plantar flex (foot drop).

I Clinical, USS achilles can help confirm, MRI if still doubt.

T *Non-operative:* full equinus cast / boot (foot points down) for six to eight weeks.

Operative: tendon repair.

C Re-rupture.

Ankle

Ankle fracture

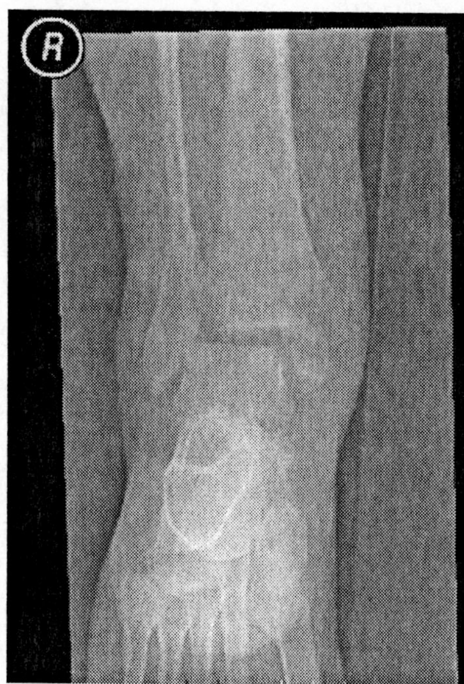

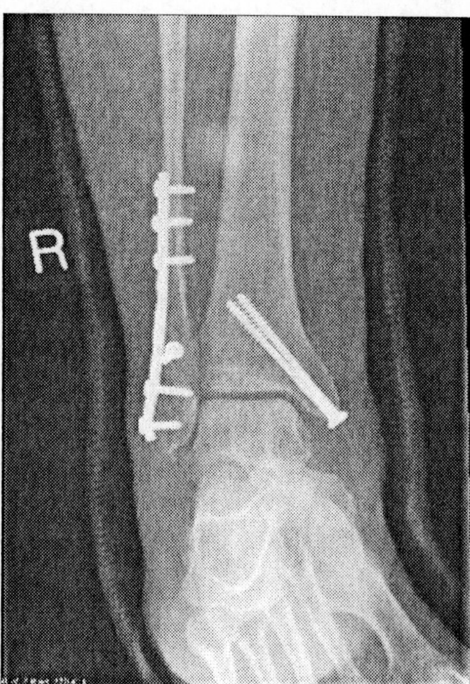

Figure 20.15: Right bimalleolar ankle fracture before and after ORIF. (Reproduced with permission from SW Deanery.)

P Fractures of medial / lateral malleoli due to rotation, commonly external rotation with foot supinated.

A Syndesmosis between distal tibia and fibula provides stability.

S Sx Ankle pain, swelling, bruising.

I Ottowa ankle rules for XR.

XR AP, lateral, mortise views of ankle, CT for complex fractures.

- *Type A:* below level of the syndesmosis, syndesmosis intact (stable)
- *Type B:* at the level of the syndesmosis, syndesmosis may be intact (stable or unstable)
- *Type C:* above the level of the syndesmosis, syndesmosis disrupted (unstable)

Box 20.9: Danis-Weber classification ankle fracture

T Weber A: non-operative.

Weber B: non-operative unless talar shift, medial malleolar fracture or deltoid ligament injury.

Weber C: ORIF.

C Ankle stiffness, infection, malunion, non-union, arthritis, wound complications.

Pr Poor outcome in diabetics.

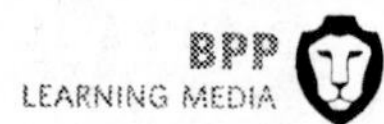

Paediatric injuries

Salter-Harris fractures

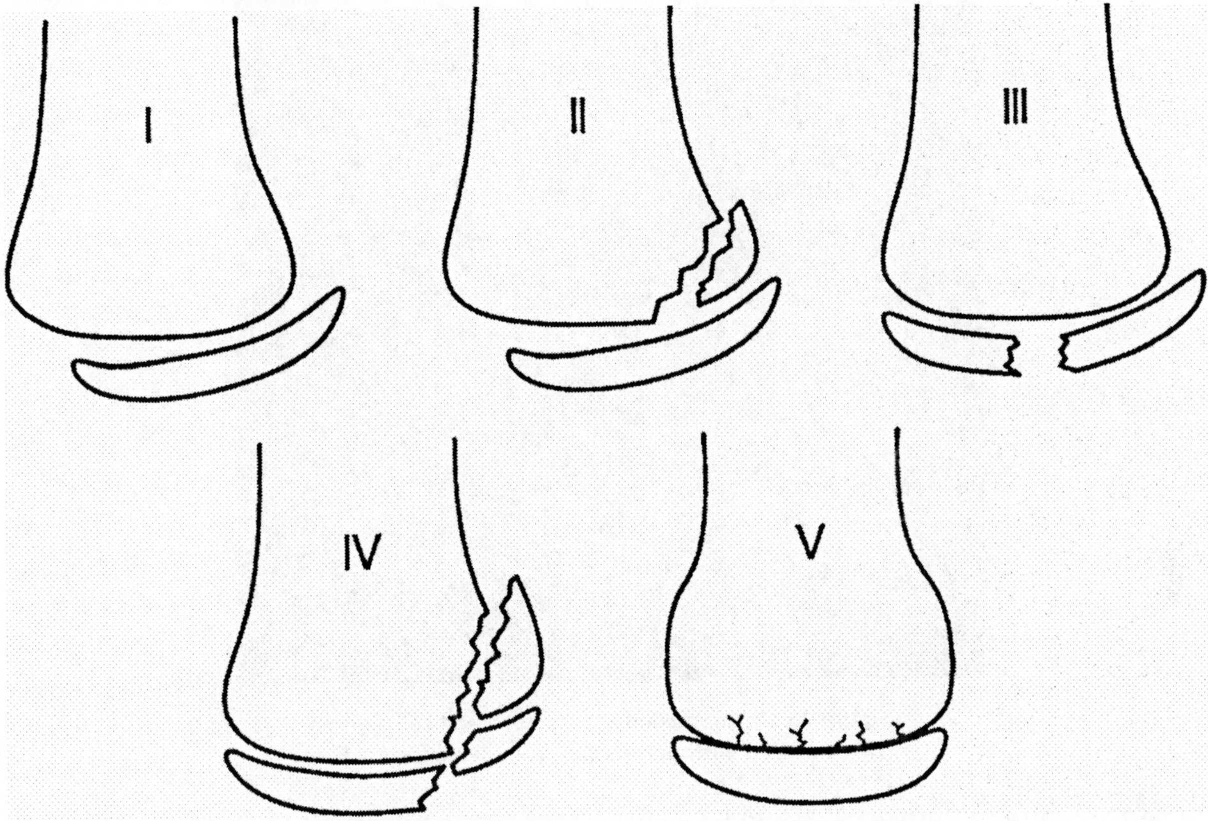

Figure 20.16: Salter-Harris epiphyseal injury classification

P Epiphyseal injuries in immature bones.

A 15% of childhood long bone fractures. 80% are type II.

I	**S** lipped: separation of physis (growth plate)
II	**A** bove: fracture lies above the physis
III	**L** ower: fracture lies below the physis in the epiphysis
IV	**T** hrough: fracture through the metaphysis physis and epiphysis
V	**R** ammed (Crushed): physis has been crushed

Box 20.10: Salter-Harris classification

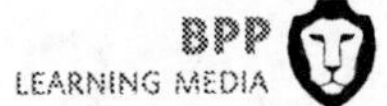

Elbow supracondylar fracture

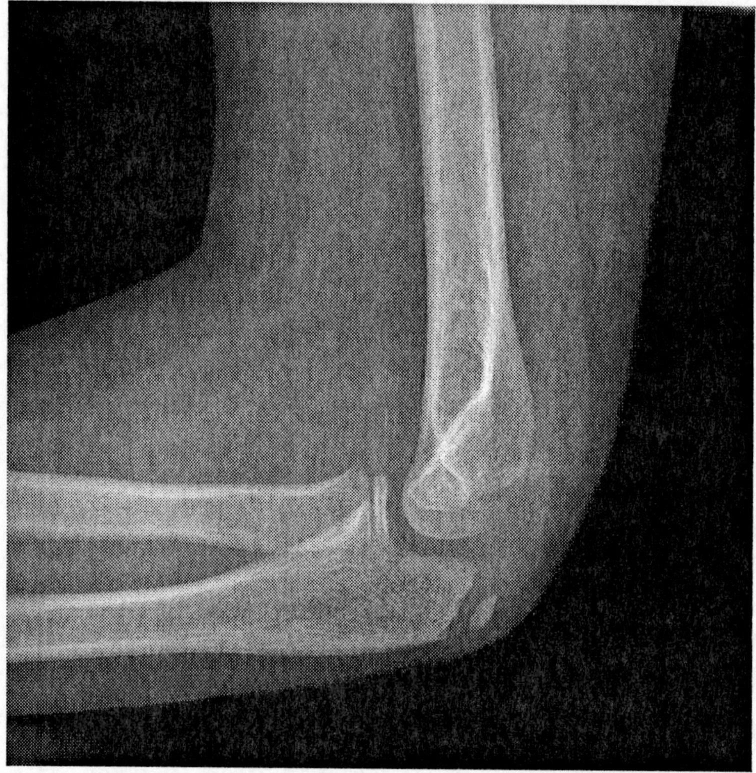

Figure 20.17: Supracondylar fracture and sail sign. (Reproduced with permission from SW Deanery.)

P Fall onto outstretched hand causing elbow hyperextension, fracture runs through distal humerus above epicondyles.

A Common in 5–15 year olds, important due to artery and nerve involvement.

Sx Pain, swelling, unable to move elbow.

I XR AP + lateral: anterior sail sign and posterior fat pad sign due to effusion suggest a fracture.

Classification:

- Gartland Type I: nondisplaced
- Type II: displaced with intact posterior or anterior cortex
- Type III: complete displacement

T Monitor neurovascular status: a poorly perfused hand with absent radial pulse warrants immediate reduction of the fracture. If the hand remains poorly perfused following reduction immediate vascular review is warranted.

- Type I: immobilise in above-elbow cast for two to three weeks
- Type II: closed reduction with above elbow cast may require K-wires if unstable
- Type III: ORIF may be necessary

C Nerve injury (7–10%) commonly ulnar nerve at medial epicondyle, vascular injury (1%), myositis ossificans, angular deformity.

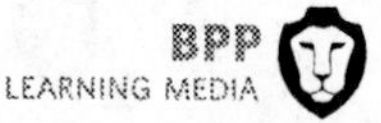

Developmental dysplasia of the hip (DDH)

P Congenital or acquired malalignment of the hip joint affecting infants.

A Females > males.

S Barlow and Ortolani tests, asymmetrical gluteal folds.

Sx Irritable hip, difficulty walking.

I USS hip (<5 months), XR AP and frog views (>5 months).

T Pavlik harness, hip spica, open reduction.

C Arthritis in later life.

Perthes' disease

P Avascular necrosis of the femoral head.

A Age 4–10 years, males > females.

S Sx Hip / groin pain, referred knee pain, reduced range of movement, antalgic gait.

I XR AP pelvis: flattening of capital femoral epiphysis.

T Self-limiting condition, conservative.

C Arthritis in later life, AVN.

Pyogenic / septic arthritis

P Infection of hip joint, usually staphlococcus.

A Children <2 years.

S Sx Hip pain, high temp, septic.

I Bloods: ↑ WCC, ↑ CRP, ↑ ESR.

USS hip, hip joint aspiration under GA.

Kocher criteria helps differentiate from transient synovitis.

T IV abx, joint washout.

C OA, recurrent infections, AVN of epiphysis.

Slipped upper femoral epiphysis (SUFE)

P Also known as slipped capital femoral epiphysis.

Slipping of the femoral growth plate due to repeated trauma.

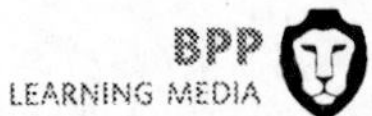

A Children 10–15 years, males > females, obesity, Afro-Carribeans. Bilateral in 20%.

S Klein's line or Trethowan's sign on XR.

Sx Limp, hip pain.

I XR AP pelvis: femoral head slipped over femoral neck.

USS hip: effusion, MRI.

T Cannulated screw.

C Avascular necrosis of the femoral head (10–15%), arthritis, leg-length discrepancy.

Osgood-Schlatter disease

P Irritation of the patella tendon at the tibial tuberosity.

A Active children 9–16 years, coincides with growth spurts.

Sx Knee pain exacerbated by exercise.

I XR knee AP + lateral: may show calcification over tibial tuberosity.

T Self-limiting resolving in two to three months, RICE.

C 10% symptoms continue into adulthood.

Spine

- Jefferson fracture: burst fracture of C1 (atlas), best seen on peg XR view. Generally stable
- Hangman's fracture: fracture of C2 (axis) due to neck hyperextension
- Chance fracture: hyperflexion injury commonest at thoracolumbar junction and classically associated with wearing a lap belt in a RTA. 50% have associated intra-abdominal injuries

Box 20.11: Eponymous spine fracture

Spinal cord compression

P Compression of the spinal cord.

A Trauma, disc prolapse, cord tumour, spinal metastasis, abscess, haematoma, myeloma.

S Hyperreflexia (absent reflexes in cauda equina), reduced power, reduced sensation.

Sx Sudden onset leg weakness, leg pain, sensory loss, urinary retention.

I MRI.

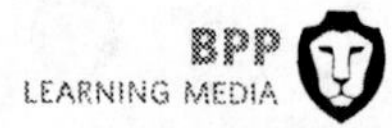

T Trauma / prolapse: decompression + / - instrumented fusion.

Abscess: IV abx and drainage.

Tumour: IV steroids, radiotherapy, surgical decompression.

C Paralysis.

Cervical spondylosis

P Degeneration of the intervertebral discs causing compression of cord and nerve roots as the neck is flexed / extended.

A Leading cause of progressive spastic quadriparesis with sensory loss below neck.

Sx Neck stiffness, crepitus on neck movement, arm / wrist pain. LMN signs at the level of nerve root compression, UMN signs below.

I MRI.

T Immobilisation in collar, laminectomy, laminoplasty.

Spondylolisthesis

P Anterior or posterior displacement of a vertebra in relation to the vertebra below.

A Congenital, degenerative, traumatic, pathological (due to tumours or mets).

S Sx Dependent on amount of displacement. Back pain, kyphotic deformity, neurological signs.

I XR spine AP + lateral, CT, MRI.

T Conservative.

Surgical: spinal fusion +/- decompression.

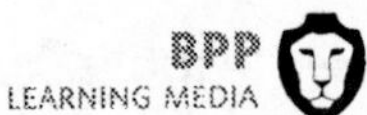

Elective orthopaedics

Osteoarthritis

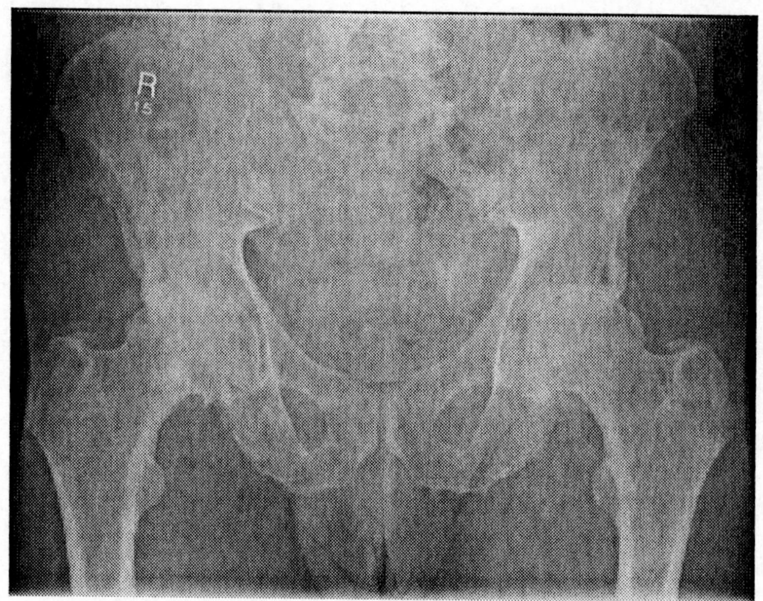

Figure 20.18: XR AP pelvis showing osteoarthritis of both hips. (Reproduced with permission from SW Deanery.)

P Degenerative wear of the articular joint with loss of articular cartilage.

A Affects weight-bearing joints, not simply due to ageing.

Risk factors: obesity, post-trauma, hypermobile joints.

Primary with no underlying cause or secondary to: trauma, avascular necrosis, malalignment of joint.

S Heberden's nodes (DIP joint), Bouchard's nodes (PIP joint), crepitus.

Sx Increasing pain over months / years, stiffness, reduced range of movement, referred pain to joint below.

I XR AP + lateral of affected joint.

- Loss of joint space (due to loss of cartilage)
- Osteophyte formation (bony spurs protrude out)
- Sclerosis (underlying bone becomes hard)
- Subchondral cyst formation (due to microfractures)

T Conservative: analgesia, joint injection (LA +/- steroid), PT / OT, lifestyle changes (weight loss).

Surgery: when conservative tx fails, joint replacement, osteotomy, joint fusion.

C Loosening of THR, THR dislocation.

Pr Hip replacement lasts around 20 years.

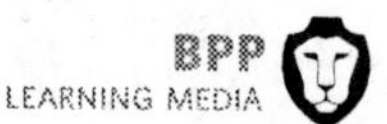

Baker's cyst

P Benign posterior bulge of knee joint capsule.

A Secondary to OA.

S Sx Painless swelling in popliteal fossa, non-pulsatile. Beware popliteal aneurysm.

I USS.

T None unless painful. Analgesia, aspiration to reduce size if necessary.

C Burst cyst can produce acute pain and calf-swelling similar to DVT.

Lumbar back pain

P Very common, due to multiple pathologies.

A *Disc:* prolapse, discitis, degeneration.

Vertebra: fracture, degeneration, tumour, myeloma, infection, spondylolisthesis, spinal stenosis, ankylosing spondylitis.

S Sx Pain, altered neurology. Beware red flags.

• Age <20 or >55 • Acute onset in elderly • Progressive pain • Nocturnal pain • Pain worse on being supine • Fever, night sweats	• Weight loss • Evidence of sepsis • History of malignancy • Abdominal mass • Immunosupression • Leg claudication or exercise-related leg weakness (spinal stenosis)

Box 20.12: Red flags for sinister causes of back pain

I Bloods: FBC, CRP, myeloma screen; XR spine AP + Lat; MRI.

T *Non-operative:* analgesia, mobilisation, posture education.

Operative: steroid +/- LA injection, discectomy, decompression, instrumented fusion.

C Unemployment, depression.

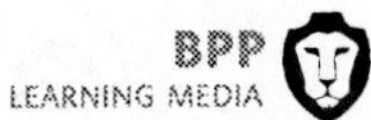

Bone tumours

Benign

Osteoma

P Benign bony outgrowth of membranous bones found most commonly on the skull and facial bones.

A Highest incidence in the sixth decade, male:female ratio of 1:3.

Sx Slow growing, usually asymptomatic.

I XR: well-delineated sclerotic lesion.

T Only necessary if symptomatic.

Osteoid osteoma

P Benign lesion, commonly occurs in long bones, especially the femur and tibia.

A Occurs most frequently in the second decade, with a peak age in the early twenties, male:female 2:1.

Sx Dull pain, worse at night, relieved by aspirin and NSAIDS.

I XR: radiolucent nidus surrounded by reactive sclerosis in the cortex of the bone.

T Usually resolve without treatment within two to three years.

Local surgery is curative.

Osteochondroma

P Benign tumour that occurs in bones developing from cartilage (enchondral ossification).

A Commonest skeletal neoplasm, most often found in long bones (40% occurring around the knee), occur in <20 years, male:female 15:1.

Sx Pain due to mechanical irritation or a painless mass.

I XR: sessile tumour.

T Usually self-limiting.

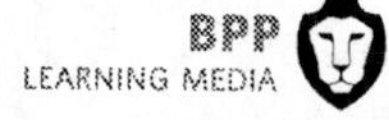

Enchondroma

P Solitary, benign, intramedullary cartilage tumour.

A Usually found in the short tubular bones of the hands and feet.

Peak incidence in 20s–30s, male = female.

Sx Pain, swelling.

I XR: long and oval with well-defined margins.

T Self-limiting, surgery if pain or fracture.

C Ollier disease (enchondromatosis): rare, multiple enchondromas throughout the body.

Malignant

Osteosarcoma

P Malignant tumour composed of spindle cells producing osteoid and bone.

A Commonest primary sarcoma of bone, peak age of incidence late teens, commonly affects metaphyses of long bones particularly around the knee and proximal humerus.

Sx Pain, worse at night and after exercise then becoming constant, swelling.

I XR: poorly defined, mixed sclerotic and lytic lesion, periosteal elevation (Codman's sign) and 'sunburst' appearance due to soft-tissue swelling, CT, MRI.

T Referral to specialist tumour centre for biopsy and work-up, surgery, chemotherapy, radiotherapy.

C Early haematogenous spread.

P 50% five-year survival.

Chondrosarcoma

P Malignant tumour producing cartilage matrix.

A Occurs in fifth to sixth decade, more common in appendicular skeleton (pelvis).

Sx Pain (can be excruciating in high-grade tumours), swelling, pelvic tumours may present as urinary frequency / retention.

I XR: fusiform, lucent defect with scalloping of the inner cortex and periosteal reaction; CT; MRI.

T Referral to specialist tumour centre for biopsy and work-up; surgery, chemotherapy, radiotherapy.

Pr Dependent on grade and location of tumour.

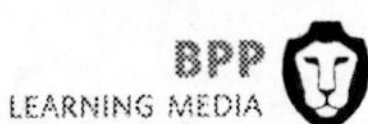

Ewing's sarcoma

- **P** Highly malignant round-cell tumour presenting in childhood or early adulthood.
- **A** Commonest between 1–20 years, commonly affecting diaphysis of long bones femur > humerus.
- **Sx** Pain and swelling over weeks / months.
- **I** XR: 'onion peel' periosteal reaction (areas new bone laid down around areas of destruction); CT; MRI.
- **T** Referral to specialist tumour centre for biopsy and work-up; surgery, chemotherapy, radiotherapy.
- **Pr** 70–80% five-year survival for localised disease treated with chemotherapy.

Secondary bone tumours

- **P** Commonest bone tumour occurring in 30% of patients with malignant disease.
- **A** **5 Bs:** **B**reast (35%), **B**rostate (30%), **B**ronchus (10%), **B**idney (5%), **B**yroid (2%).
- **S** Pathological fracture (10%), hypercalcaemia, spinal cord compression.
- **Sx** Pain, weight loss, symptoms relating to underlying primary.
- **I** CT chest, abdo, pelvis.
- **T** Management of underlying tumour, oncology referral.

Practice Questions

Single Best Answers

1. Perthes' disease

   A Is more common in girls
   B Usually presents in teens
   C Obesity is a risk factor
   D The capital femoral epiphysis is small, dense and flat on AP X-ray

2. Regarding the radial nerve

   A Is commonly injured as it crosses the wrist joint
   B Originates from nerve roots C3–C5
   C When injured sensation is lost over the anatomical snuffbox area
   D Injury produces claw hand

3. Regarding hip fractures

   A The affected limb is shortened and internally rotated
   B Extracapsular fractures may be treated with a compression hip screw
   C Subtrochanteric fractures are intracapsular
   D In the elderly population it is not appropriate to investigate the cause of the fall

4. Shoulder dislocation

   A Inferior dislocation is the commonest presentation
   B Axillary nerve function is tested by asking the patient to make the 'ok' sign
   C Posterior dislocations are seen in epileptic fits and electric shock injuries
   D Fracture dislocations are easily reduced in the emergency department

5. Bone metastases

   A Thyroid cancer is the commonest cause of metastatic spread
   B Prostate cancer may cause osteosclerotic lesions
   C 1% of patients with malignant disease develop bony metastases
   D 50% patients develop pathological fractures

6. Supracondylar fractures

   A. With loss of radial pulse and poorly perfused hand do not require urgent MUA
   B Rarely occur in children
   C Classified by the Neer classification system
   D Anterior and posterior fat pad signs are due to soft tissue swelling and indicate a fracture

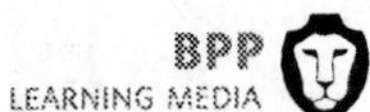

7. Ewing's sarcoma

   A Highest incidence is in the elderly population
   B Produces an 'onion-peel' sign on plain XR
   C Is a benign tumour
   D Five-year survival <10%

8. Compartment syndrome

   A Loss of pulses is the first sign
   B Fasciotomy should be delayed if the patient is in extreme pain
   C Can never occur in an open fracture
   D Characteristically features pain out of proportion to the injury

9. Which of the following is not part of the immediate management of open fractures

   A Taking a picture of the wound
   B IV antibiotics
   C Ensuring tetanus status up to date
   D Skin graft

10. Simmonds' test is diagnostic in

   A Achilles tendon rupture
   B Biceps tendon rupture
   C DVT
   D Developmental dysplasia of the hip

Extended Matching Questions

Peripheral nerve lesions

A Median nerve
B Sciatic nerve
C Radial nerve
D Common peroneal nerve
E Ulnar nerve
F Lateral cutaneous nerve of thigh

1. Supplies sensation to the little finger and medial half of ring finger

2. Elicited using Tinel's test and Phalen's test

3. Compressed as it crosses close to the inguinal ligamanent

4. Damaged in midshaft humeral fractures

5. Injury causes foot drop

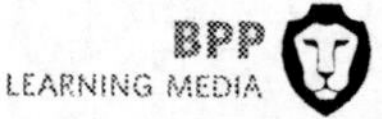

Paediatric injuries

A SUFE
B Perthes' disease
C Osgood-Schlatter disease
D DDH
E Pyogenic arthritis
F Ewing's sarcoma

Match the below scenarios to the most appropriate diagnosis.

6. An overweight 14-year-old boy presents with limp, no history of trauma.

7. Fever, crying and reduced mobility in 18-month girl. Left hip is irritable on examination.

8. Knee pain following PE sessions in a 15-year-old boy.

9. Groin pain and antalgic gait in an eight-year-old boy. XR shows flattened femoral head.

10. Barlow and Ortolani tests helpful in diagnosis.

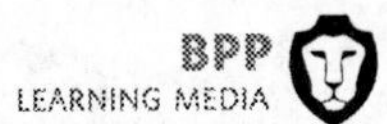

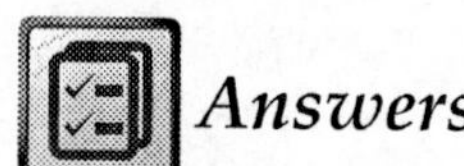

Answers

SBAs		EMQs	
1	D	1	E
2	C	2	A
3	B	3	F
4	C	4	C
5	B	5	D
6	D	6	A
7	B	7	E
8	D	8	C
9	D	9	B
10	A	10	D

Chapter 21

Fluids and electrolytes

Mr Alexander Young and
Dr Tom Teare

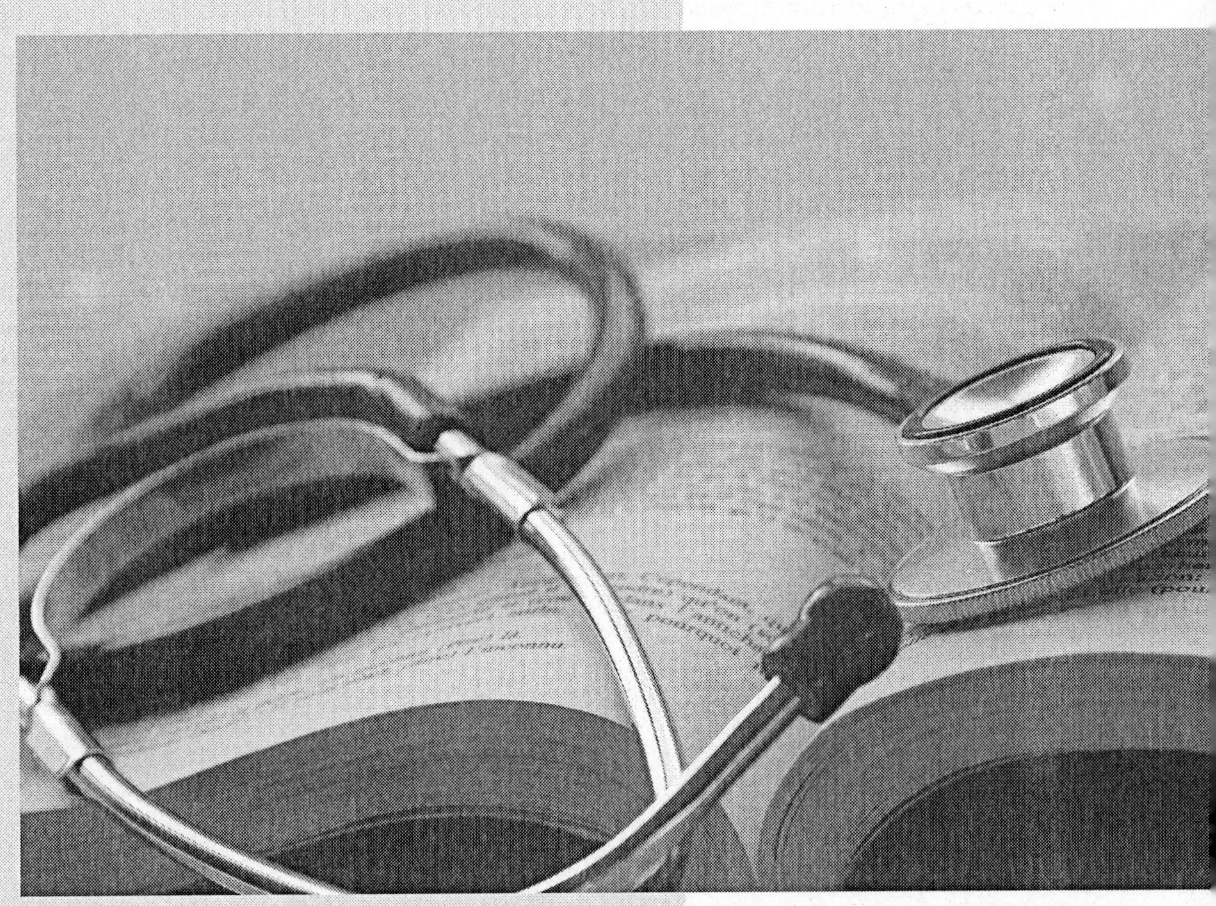

Fluid balance

Body fluid

For a 70kg man:

- Total body water is 42 L (~60% of body weight)
- 28 L (2 / 3) is intracellular
- 14 L (1 / 3) is extracellular
  Of the extracellular water:
  - 3 L is in blood plasma
  - 11 L is interstitial fluid
  - + small volume is transcellular eg CSF, intaoccular fluid

Water balance

Water is lost in the following ways:

- Urine 1,500ml
- Respiratory (evaporation) 500ml
- Skin (insensible) 400ml
- Faeces 100ml
- Total = 2,500ml

Normal daily requirement:

- 3L water, 100mmol sodium, 60mmol potassium in 24 hours
- Can be significantly increased in fever, diarrhea, vomiting, high-output stoma etc.

Standard replacement regime:

- 1L 0.9% saline + 20mmol KCl over 8 hours
- 1L 0.9% saline + 20mmol KCl over 8 hours
- 1L 5% dextrose + 20mmol KCl over 8 hours

Clinical note: there is increasing evidence that this regimen is outdated and does not consider the large chloride load received by the patients. So-called 'normal' saline is significantly acidic and consequently many hospitals are moving to the use of Hartmann's as their default crystalloid. However, for revision purposes the 'two salt, one sweet' method is fine (and easy to remember).

- Crystalloids: salt ions in water
  Of volume infused 1/3 stays in intravascular compartment, 2/3 pass into ECF; therefore risk of oedema. Good for rapidly correcting ECF deficit in shock.
- Colloids: osmotically-active particles in solution
  Remain in circulation for longer and exert oncotic effect drawing interstitial fluid into plasma. Good for acute replacement of plasma deficit.

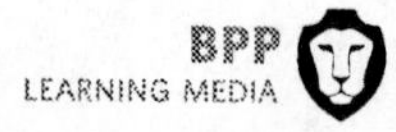

	0.9% saline	Hartmann's solution	Dextrose saline	5% dextrose
Sodium (mmol/L)	150	131	30	0
Chloride (mmol/L)	150	111	30	0
Potassium (mmol/L)	0	5	0	0
Lactate (mmol/L)	0	29	0	0
Calcium (mmol/L)	0	2	0	0
Osmolality (mosmol/L)	308	280	284	278

Table 21.1: Composition of common crystalloids

Electrolytes

Sodium

Total body Na is 4,200mmol (50% in ECF).

- Major cation of ECF
- 100–150mmol Na normal daily requirement
- Excretion is renal and in sweat
- Excess loss with D&V or sweating
- Excess loss with third space loss eg obstruction, peritonitis

Hypernatraemia

P Usually due to water loss in excess of sodium loss.

A See Box 21.1.

Water depletion	Sodium excess
• Reduced intake • Renal: osmotic diuresis, ARF, diabetes insipidus • Other: burns, fever, diarrhoea	• Conn's syndrome • Cushing's syndrome • Excess IV saline • Liver cirrhosis

Box 21.1: Causes of hypernatraemia

S Sx Dehydration, thirst, lethargy, confusion, coma, fits.

I ↑Na, ↑PCV, ↑U&Es.

T Oral water replacement if possible or slow IV dextrose.

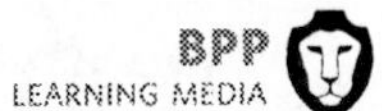

Hyponatraemia

P Due to water retention and / or sodium depletion.

A See Box 21.2.

Water retention	Sodium depletion
Water retention • CCF • Liver cirrhosis • Water overload • Nephrotic syndrome • SIADH Low intake • Reduced intake • Saline-free IV replacement	Sodium depletion • Excess GI loss: diarrhoea, fistula, ileus, obstruction • Excess sweating • Burns • Addison's disease • Diuretics

Box 21.2: Causes of hyponatraemia

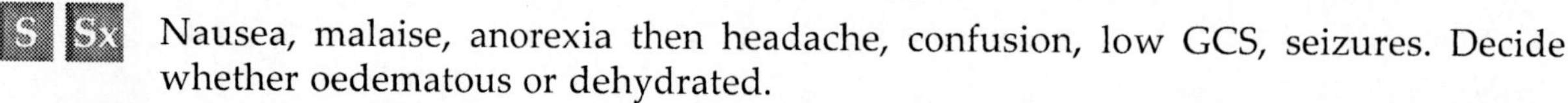

S Sx Nausea, malaise, anorexia then headache, confusion, low GCS, seizures. Decide whether oedematous or dehydrated.

I Serum and urinary Na and osmolalities. See Box 21.2.

T *Hypervolaemic (oedematous):* slowly correct, fluid restriction, demeclocycline (ADH antagonist), treat underlying cause.

Hypovolaemic (dehydrated): slow rehydration with 0.9% saline, at sodium levels <110mmol/L hypertonic (18%) saline may be used.

Aim is to gradually increase serum Na by 1mmol/L per hour.

C Rapid changes to Na can result in central pontine myelinolysis.

Potassium

- 97% intracellular
- 60mmol normally required per day
- Replace as 20mmol/litre ×3 per 24 hours
- Excess loss in D&V, alkalosis (eg pyloric stenosis)
- Serum levels significantly affected by:
  - pH – acidosis leads to hyperkalaemia
  - Insulin – forces potassium into cells causing hypokalaemia
- Trauma and transfusion release potassium
- Low K associated with long PR interval, ST depression, inverted T waves
- Total body K^+ is 3,500mmol (only about 50–60mmol in ECF)

Hyperkalaemia

See Chapter 1 *Cardiology*.

Hypokalaemia

P Potassium <2.5mmol/L.

A See Box 21.3.

- Drugs: diuretics, steroids
- Gastointestinal: vomiting and diarrhoea, pyloric stenosis, intestinal fistula
- Endocrine: Conn's syndrome (hypotension with hypokalaemic alkalosis), Cushing's syndrome
- Surgery (low K^+ is a common cause of post-op AF or arrhythmia)
- Renal failure

Box 21.3: Causes of hypokalaemia

S Hypotonia, hyporeflexia, tetany.

Sx Muscle weakness, cramps, palpitations.

I U&Es, Mg^{2+}, ABG, ECG: AF, long PR interval, small / inverted T waves, prominent U waves (follow T waves).

T Asymptomatic: oral K^+ supplements eg Sando-K, hold diuretics, IV in IVI fluids if NBM, correct MG^{2+} if low (hypokalaemia difficult to correct till magnesium corrected).

Symptomatic: cautious administration of IV K^+, not faster than 20mmol/hr and not more concentrated than 40mmol/L.

C Hypokalaemia exacerbates digoxin toxicity, arrhythmias.

Acid-base balance

Respiratory acidosis

P CO_2 retention due to inadequate alveolar ventilation.

$\downarrow$pH $\uparrow$$PCo_2$ chronic compensation occurs by $\uparrow$$HCO_3^-$ (bicarbonate buffer system) and $\downarrow$$H^+$ (kidneys).

A Any cause of hypoventilation (type 2 resp failure).

S **Sx** Of type 2 respiratory failure (see Chapter 2).

I ABG.

T Treat underlying cause, may require BIPAP or ITU to aid ventilation.

Respiratory alkalosis

P CO_2 lost via hyperventilation.

$\uparrow$pH $\downarrow$$PCo_2$ chronic compensation occurs by $\downarrow$$HCO_3^-$ (bicarbonate buffer system) and $\uparrow$$H^+$ (kidneys).

A Any cause of hyperventilation: anxiety, hysteria, pain, stimulation of respiratory centre (altitude, pneumonia, PE, fever, head injury).

S Sx Lightheadedness, paraesthesia.

I ABG.

T Treat underlying cause.

Metabolic acidosis

P ↓pH, ↓HCO_3^-

A Normal anion gap: loss of bicarbonate or increase in H^+.

Increased anion gap: due to increased production / decreased excretion of organic acids.

Normal anion gap	Increased anion gap
• Diarrhoea • Addison's disease • Renal tubular acidosis • Pancreatic fistula • Drugs: acetazolamoide	• Lactic acid: shock, infection, ischaemia • Ketones: diabetes, alcohol • Urate: renal failure • Drugs / toxins: ethylene glycol, salicylates

Box 21.4: Causes of metabolic acidosis

S Sx Of underlying cause.

I ABG.

T Treat underlying cause.

Metabolic alkalsosis

P ↑pH, ↑HCO_3^-

A Vomiting, diuretics (↓K^+), burns, ingestion of base.

I ABG.

T Of underlying cause.

Practice Questions

Single Best Answers

1. For a 70kg man with total body water of 42L what volume of this is intracellular.

   A 28L
   B 14L
   C 7L
   D 32L

2. For the man in question 1 what volume is held in the interstitial compartment?

   A 3L
   B 500ml
   C 14L
   D 11L

3. What is the normal daily requirement for water and electrolytes?

   A 5L water, 150mmol sodium, 30mmol potassium in 24 hours
   B 3L water, 100mmol sodium, 60mmol potassium in 24 hours
   C 3L water, 150mmol sodium, 40mmol potassium in 24 hours
   D 3L water, 100mmol sodium, 30mmol potassium in 24 hours

4. The major extracellular cation is

   A Sodium
   B Potassium
   C Magnesium
   D Calcium

5. 'U' waves are an ECG finding in which electrochemical distrurbance?

   A Hyperkalaemia
   B Hypokalaemia
   C Hypercalcaemia
   D Hyponatraemia

Extended Matching Questions

Complete the crystalloids table by matching the letters to their correct values.

Composition of common crystalloids				
	0.9% saline	**C**	**D**	5% dextrose
Sodium (mmol/L)	150	A	30	0
Chloride (mmol/L)	**B**	111	30	0
Potassium (mmol/L)	0	E	0	0
Lactate (mmol/L)	0	29	0	0
Calcium (mmol/L)	0	2	0	0
Osmolality (mosmol/L)	308	280	284	278

1. Hartmann's solution
2. Dextrose saline
3. 150mmol/L
4. 131mmol/L
5. 5mmol/L

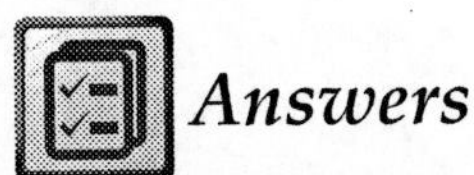

SBAs		EMQs	
1	A	1	C
2	D	2	D
3	B	3	B
4	A	4	A
5	B	5	E

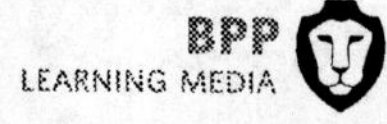

Chapter 22

Ophthalmology

Dr Tara Bader

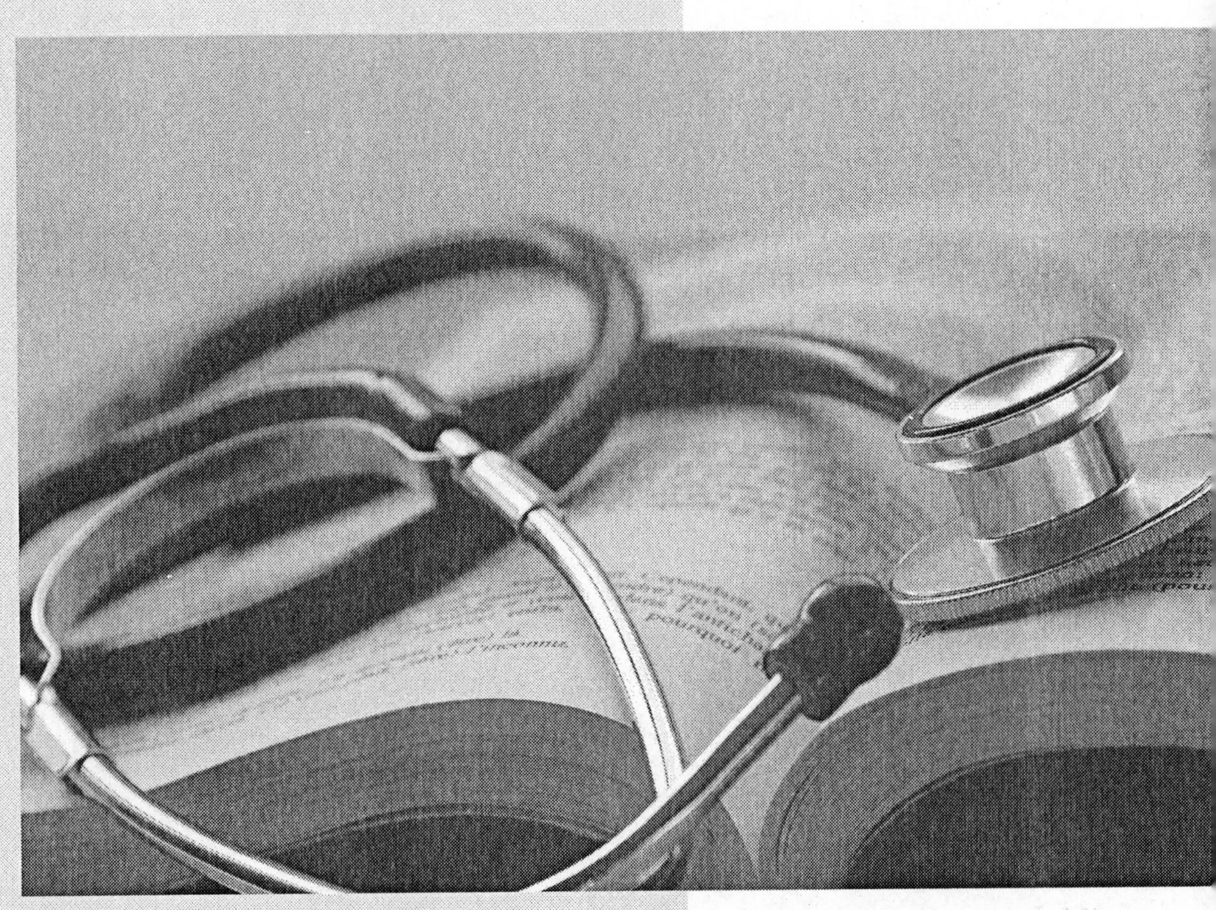

Drugs and the eye

- Mydriatics:
  - Tropicamide, cyclopentolate, atropine, phenylephrine
- Miotics:
  - Pilocarpine, carbachol
- Topical Anaesthetics:
  - Proxym etacaine, tetracaine, lidocaine, oxybuprocaine
- Steroids:
  - Fluorometholone, dexamethasone, prednisolone
- Topical antimicrobials:
  - Chloramphenicol, ciprofloxacin, fusidic acid, gentamicin, ofloxacin

Box 22.1: Drugs and the eye

The external eye

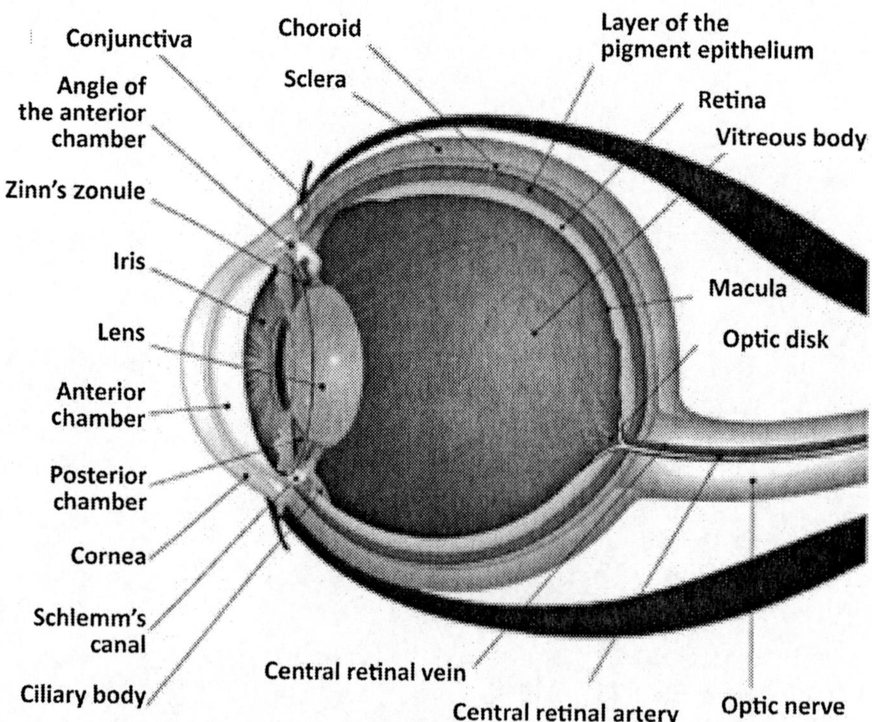

Figure 22.1: Cross-section of the external eye

Entropion

P Inversion of the eyelid margin.

A Involutional change, mostly associated with ageing, occasionally congenital.

S Inverted lid, usually lower.

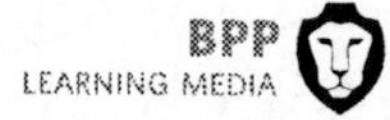

Sx Irritation, blepharospasm.

I Check for lid laxity, inferior retractor weakness.

T Taping, botulinum-toxin injection, surgery to evert the lid margin.

C Corneal abrasion and secondary infection.

Ectropion

P Eversion of the eyelid margin.

A Involutional change, ageing tissue laxity, occasionally congential, CN VII palsy.

S Everted lid, usually lower, dry eye.

Sx Irritation, epiphora.

I Check for lid laxity.

T Surgery, commonly horizontal tightening.

C Corneal erosions due to exposure and dryness, infection.

Chalazion

P Lipogranulomatous inflammation.

A Blocked meibomian gland.

S Eyelid lump.

Sx Tender lump.

I Warm compress, lid hygiene, if persistent, surgical incision and curettage.

Stye (external hordeolum)

P Infection around eyelash follicle.

A Staphylococcal infection.

S Eyelid lump, around eyelashes.

Sx Tender lump.

T Eyelash epilation, warm compress, antibiotics.

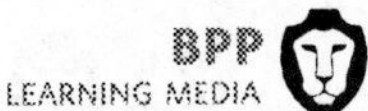

Blepharitis

- **P** Lid margin inflammation.
- **A** Bacterial, meibomian, seborrhoeic.
- **S** Crusty lids, thickened lid margins.
- **Sx** Irritation, redness at lid margins.
- **T** Lid hygiene is key, plus possible topical antibiotics / steroids / lubrication.

Keratoconjunctivitis sicca (dry eye)

- **P** Tear film dysfunction.
- **A** Deficient tear production, excess evaporation.
- **S** Reduced tear quantity / quality, conjunctival injection.
- **Sx** Irritation, redness, compensatory watering.
- **I** Schirmer test shows reduced wetting, reduced tear break up time.
- **T** Artifical tears, lubricating ointment, if more severe consider punctual occlusion.

Orbital and preseptal cellulitis

- **P** The fibrous orbital septum can limit infection spread around the eye. If infection involves the orbit, this is a medical emergency.

  Infection commonly spreads from skin, meibominan glands, sinuses, nasolacrimal duct or trauma.
- **A** Streptococcus pneumoniae, staphylococcus aureus, streptococcus pyogenes, haemophilus influenzae.

  Preseptal infection can progress to orbital (postseptal) infection.
- **S** Orbital cellulitis: fever, pain, lid swelling / erythema, proptosis, restricted eye movements, diplopia, optic nerve dysfunction.

  Preseptal cellulitis: fever, pain, lid swelling / erythema, no proptosis, normal eye movements, white conjunctiva, no optic nerve dysfunction.
- **Sx** Fever, pain, lid swelling, sometimes recent sinus infection.
- **I** Observations including temperature, FBC, CRP, CT if suspected orbital / sinus disease (CT orbit, sinus, brain).
- **T** It is important to differentiate orbital from preseptal disease. Involve ophthalmology and ENT early to assist with diagnosis. If orbital, admit and start IV antibiotics, may need surgical drainage. If preseptal and systemically well, oral antibiotics and daily review.
- **C** Loss of vision, mortality.

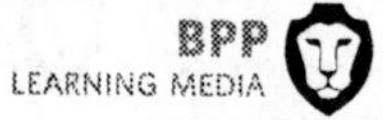

Herpes zoster ophthalmicus (ophthalmic shingles)

- **P** Viral infection resulting in rash, neuralgia in dermatome of the ophthalmic branch of trigeminal nerve.
- **A** Varicella zoster virus reactivation.
- **S** Rash affecting area of ophthalmic division of trigeminal nerve, Hutchinson's sign.
- **Sx** Neuralgia, rash.
- **T** Systemic antivirals (aciclovir). If associated keratitis: topical lubrication, topical steroids.
- **C** Corneal involvement.

Refractive errors

Myopia

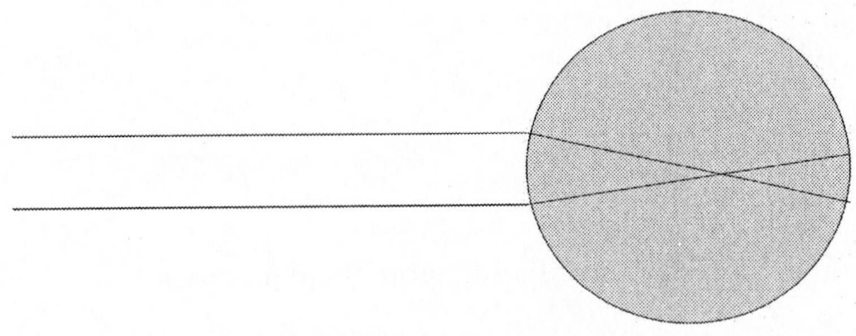

Figure 22.2 Myopic refraction

- **P** Short sightedness. Light focuses in front of the retina.
- **A** Long eye (axial myopia) or increased dioptric power (refractive myopia).
- **Sx** Blurred vision.
- **I** Refraction.
- **T** Spectacle / contact lens correction.

Hypermetropia

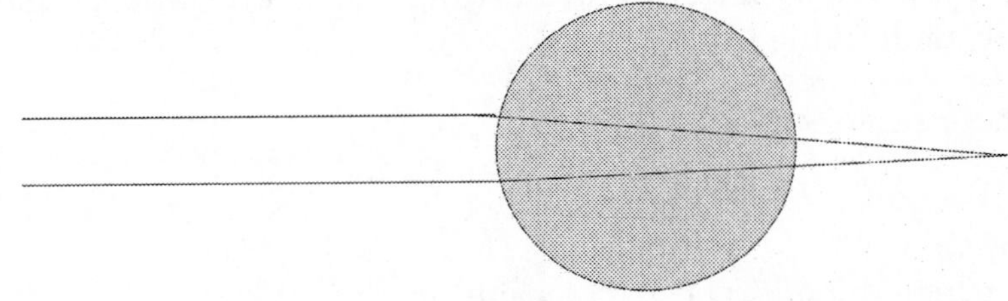

Figure 22 3: Hypermetropic refraction

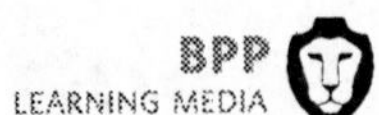

P Long sightedness. Light focuses behind the retina.

A Short eye (axial hypermetropia) or reduced dioptric power (refractive hypermetropia).

Sx Blurred vision.

I Refraction.

T Spectacle / contact lens correction.

Presbyopia

P Reduction in ability of accommodation with age.

A Ageing.

Sx Reduced ability to focus, reduced near vision.

I Refraction.

T Spectacles / reading lenses for converging power.

The red eye

Conjunctivitis

P Infective and non infective inflammation of conjunctiva.

A Bacterial, viral, chlamydia, allergic, toxic / drops.

S Red eye, purulent or watery discharge.

Sx Itchy, gritty, red, sticky eye.

I If severe / recurrent: conjunctival swab.

T Dependent on cause: topical antibiotics if bacterial.

Subconjunctival haemorrhage

P Blood under conjunctiva.

A Trauma, valsalva, hypertension, bleeding disorder, anticoagulation medication, idiopathic, underlying orbital mass.

S Blood under conjunctiva.

Sx Red eye.

I BP. If recurrent: bloods, check for coagulopathy.

If other orbital signs: CT head.

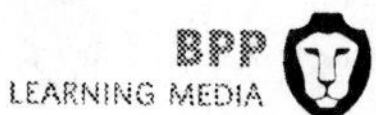

T Usually nil.

C Underlying scleral perforation.

Episcleritis

P Inflammation of episclera.

A Often idiopathic.

S Episcleral inflammation / engorged vessels, common in young adults.

Sx Painful red eye.

T Usually self limiting, mild topical steroids for comfort.

Scleritis

P Inflammation of sclera.

A Often associated with systemic connective tissue disease, rheumatoid arthritis.

S Scleral / episclearal / conjunctival inflammation, engorged vessels.

Sx Severe eye pain, red eye, may have reduced vision.

I If history suggests: bloods including FBC, U&E, ESR, CRP, RhF, ANA, ANCA, urine dip.

T Oral NSAIDs / steroids.

C Sight threatening.

Keratitis

P Corneal inflammation, infective and non infective.

A Viral (herpes virus), bacterial, acanthamoeba, fungal.

S Ulcer / epithelial defect (check for dendrite in herpes simplex virus infection), corneal opacity, discharge, hypopyon, conjunctival injection.

Sx Painful red eye, possible associated skin rash (herpes zoster).

I Avoid contact lens wear, corneal scrape.

T Dependent on cause, topical antibiotics / antifungals / antivirals.

C Sight threatening.

Acute anterior uveitis (acute iritis)

P Inflammation of uveal tract (iris, ciliary body, choroid).

A Often idiopathic, can be associated with systemic disease (eg HLA-B27 linked disease, sarcoid), can be associated with infection (eg syphilis) and trauma.

S Keratitic precipitates, cells in AC, vessels on iris dilated, conjunctival injection.

Sx Painful, red, photophobic eye.

I If bilateral, severe, or recurrent: CXR, HLA-B27, syphilis serology, serum ACE.

T Topical steroids and mydriatics.

C Recurrence, persistence.

Acute angle closure glaucoma

P Angle closure between iris and trabecular meshwork, impairs aqueous outflow.

A Often due to pupil block (apposed lens and iris with subsequent blockage of aqueous outflow), leads to rise in intraocular pressure.

S Raised IOP, closed angle, conjunctival injection, fixed mid dilated pupil, hazy cornea.

Sx Painful red eye, blurred vision, headache, nausea, vomiting.

I Check IOP, gonioscopy (closed angle).

T Urgent ophthalmology referral (topical and systemic treatment required), regular IOP monitoring, laser iridotomy.

C Sight threatening.

Loss of vision

Sudden painless loss of vision

Central retinal artery occlusion

P Occlusion of central retinal artery, causing hypoxia and ischaemia of retina.

A Commonly atherosclerotic, also consider embolic and inflammatory (giant cell arteritis).

S White, swollen retina, cherry red spot at macula, RAPD.

Sx Sudden unilateral, painless, visual loss.

I BP, blood glucose, FBC, lipids, carotids (check for bruit, arrange doppler). Rule out GCA (raised ESR, CRP).

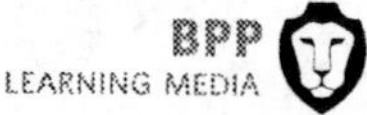

T Ocular massage, reduce IOP, PO / IV steroids if suspected GCA, treat underlying medical conditions.

C Sight threatening, neovascular glaucoma.

Central retinal vein occlusion

P Thrombosis of retinal vein.

A Diabetes, hypertension, hypercholesterolaemia, glaucoma.

S Retinal haemorrhages, tortuous veins, optics disc swelling, cotton wool spots, neovascularisation.

Sx Painless loss of vision in one eye.

I BP, bloods: lipids, glucose, FBC, ESR.

T Reduce IOP, photocoagulation if neovascularisation, treat underlying medical conditions.

Vitreous haemorrhage

P Bleed into vitreous.

A Diabetic retinopathy, posterior vitreous detachment, retinal tear / detachment, retinal vein occlusion, trauma, cancer.

S Blood within vitreous, obscured fundal view.

Sx Sudden, painless loss of vision.

I B scan if no retinal view.

T Treatment dependent on underlying pathology, may require surgical removal of blood (vitrectomy).

Giant cell arteritis

P Arterial inflammation, affects internal elastic lamina.

A Arterial inflammation and ischaemia of optic nerve head.

S RAPD, swollen pale disc, thick tender non pulsatile temporal artery.

Sx Sudden visual loss, scalp tenderness, jaw claudication, headache.

I ESR, CRP, FBC, consider temporal artery biospy.

T High dose steroids (PO/IV).

C Second eye involvement, visual loss.

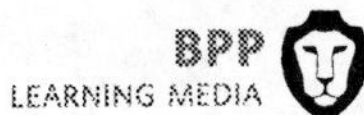

Trauma

Penetrating trauma / globe rupture

A Injury / foreign body to eye.

S Scleral / corneal laceration, severe subconjunctival haemorrhage, hyphema.

Sx Pain, reduced vision, fluid from eye.

I May require CT orbits / brain.

T Antibiotics, check tetanus status, arrange for surgical repair.

C Loss of eye / vision.

Surface foreign body

A Foreign body to conjunctiva / cornea.

S Foreign body seen, rust ring, conjunctival injection.

Sx Foreign body sensation, tearing.

T Topical anaesthetic, remove FB and rust ring, topical antibiotic.

C Corneal scarring.

Corneal abrasion

A Injury / foreign body.

S Epithelial defect, stains with fluorescein.

Sx Pain, photophobia, foreign body sensation, tearing.

T Topical antibiotic, cycloplegic if traumatic iritis.

C Corneal scarring.

Detachments

Posterior vitreous detachment

P Separation of vitreous and retina.

A Ageing process, may occur earlier in myopia, trauma, inflammation, connective tissue disease.

S Weiss ring, visible posterior hyaloid face.

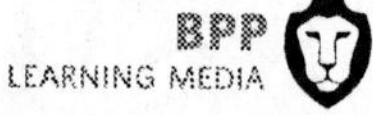

Sx Flashes of light, floaters.

T Monitor and give retinal detachment warning (if new flashes / floaters / black curtain in vision occur seek urgent ophthalmology review).

C Retinal tear / detachment.

Retinal detachment

P Separation of neuroretina from pigment epithelium.

A Retinal tears, traction, accumulated fluid in subretinal space.

S Elevation of retina from RPE, anterior pigmented cells, vitreous haemorrhage, tears in retina.

Sx Flashes of light, floaters, black curtain / shadow moving across vision, visual loss.

I B-scan.

T Surgical repair.

C Sight threatening.

Sub-acute loss of vision

Optic neuritis

P Inflammation of the optic nerve.

A Most common cause is demyelination.

S Reduced VA, reduced colour vision, RAPD.

Sx Reduced VA, field loss, retrobulbar pain.

I Consider MRI, LP.

T IV steroids.

C Visual loss, may develop MS.

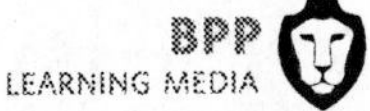

Gradual loss of vision

Cataract

- **P** Opacity of lens.
- **A** Age, sunlight, smoking, alcohol, dehydration, corticosteroid use, diabetes mellitus.
- **S** Opacity of lens.
- **Sx** Reduced vision, glare.
- **T** Surgical (phacoemulsification and intraocular lens insertion).

Chronic open-angle glaucoma

- **P** Optic neuropathy (disc cupping), visual field loss, raised intraocular pressure.
- **A** Primary, secondary (eg due to trauma / uveitus), congenital.
- **S** Disc cupping, raised IOP, visual field defect.
- **Sx** Usually asymptomatic, tunnel vision occurs late.
- **I** Visual field test.
- **T** Topical drops eg prostaglandin agonists, beta blockers.
- **C** Visual loss.

Age related macular degeneration

- **P** Non exudative (dry) or exudative (wet).
- **A** Ageing, smoking.
- **S** Drusen. Retinal fluid if wet.
- **Sx** Gradual loss of central vision.
- **I** Amsler grid, OCT, FFA.
- **T** Supportive if dry. Anti VEGF therapy if wet.
- **C** Visual loss.

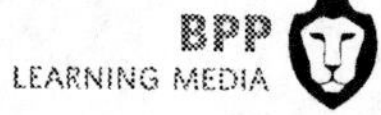

The eye in systemic disease

Hypertensive retinopathy

P Systemic hypertension affecting retinal vessels.

Arteriosclerosis and fibrosis occurs due to chronically raised pressure.

A Systemic hypertension.

S Arteriolar narrowing, arteriovenous narrowing at crossings, cotton wool spots, retinal haemorrhages, hard exudates, optic disc swelling.

Sx Usually asymptomatic, may have visual loss.

I Measure BP.

T Control of hypertension.

Grade 0: Normal
Grade 1: Minimal arteriolar narrowing
Grade 2: Widespread arteriolar narrowing, arteriovenous crossing narrowing
Grade 3: Retinal haemorrhages or exudates
Grade 4: Optic disc swelling

Box 22.2: Classification hypertensive retinopathy

Diabetic retinopathy

P Diabetes can lead to visual loss due to macular oedema, macular ischaemia, vitreous haemorrhage and tractional retinal detachment.

A Hyperglycaemia causing microvascular complications.

S Microaneurysm, haemorrhages, cotton wool spots, venous beading, neovascularisation.

Sx Reduced vision.

I BP, fasting glucose, FFA, OCT.

T Manage BP, BMs, may require laser.

C Visual loss.

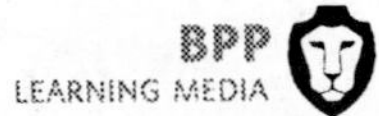

Background retinopathy '**HOME**'
- **H**aemorrhage
- **O**edema
- **M**icroaneurysms
- **E**xudates

Pre-proliferative retinopathy
- 'Cotton wool' spots: a focal infarct
- Venous looping and engorgement

Proliferative retinopathy
- New vessel growth from retina, optic disc and iris (rubeosis)

Advanced retinopathy
- Scarring (retinal gliosis)
- Vitreous haemorrhage
- Retinal detachment

Box 22.3: Classification of diabetic retinopathy

CMV retinitis

P Infection associated with HIV / immunosuppression (usually CD4<50).

A Cytomegalovirus.

S Retinal haemorrhage and whitish areas.

Sx Floaters, visual reduction.

I CD4 count.

T HAART, antivirals eg ganciclovir.

C Retinal detachment, retinal and optic nerve disease.

Papilloedema

P Optic disc swelling due to raised intracranial pressure.

A Intracranial mass (tumour, abscess, haemorrhage), idiopathic intracranial hypertension.

S Swollen optics disc / blurred / elevated disc margins.

Sx Reduced visual acuity, field defects, headache, nausea / vomiting.

I MRI, LP.

T Depends on underlying cause. Weight loss recommended in idiopathic intracranial hypertension, intracranial masses may require surgery.

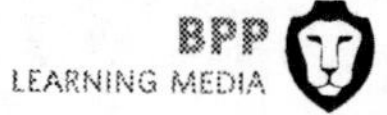

Practice Questions

Single Best Answers

1. Common topical drug used for pupil dilation

    A Tropicamide
    B Pilocarpine
    C Carbachol
    D Fluorometholone

2. When examining a corneal abrasion

    A Fluorexcein will not stain a corneal defect
    B Fluorescein will be excited by a blue light and shows green over the corneal defect
    C Fluorescein will be excited by a green light and shows blue over the corneal defect
    D Fluorescein will be excited by a white light

3. Key difference between orbital and preseptal cellulitis.

    A Erythema
    B Swelling
    C Restricted eye movements
    D Pain

4. Cause of dendritic ulcer.

    A Herpes simplex virus
    B Stap aureus
    C Streptococcus
    D CMV

5. Most likely diagnosis: patient with painful red eye with pupil fixed in mid dilation.

    A Conjunctivitis
    B Iritis (acute anterior uveitis)
    C Corneal ulcer
    D Acute angle closure glaucoma

6. Most likely diagnosis: patient with flashing lights, floaters, significant reduction in vision.

    A Retinal detachment
    B Glaucoma
    C Cataract
    D Conjunctivitis

7. Key blood tests for: patient with monocular loss of vision, scalp tenderness, jaw pain.

   A LFT, CRP
   B U&E, CRP
   C FBC, U&E
   D ESR, CRP

8. Common topical anaesthetic used when examining the eye.

   A Pilocarpine,
   B Fluorescein
   C Proxymetacaine
   D Carbachol

9. Presbyopia refers to

   A Improved visual acuity
   B Loss of accommodation with age
   C Loss of colour vision with age
   D Cataract

10. Most appropriate next step: 67-year-old presents to A&E with a painful red eye, cloudy cornea and vomiting.

   A Urgent ophthalmology referral
   B Arrange for outpatient ophthalmology assessment in one week
   C Start PO antibiotics
   D Discharge home

11. Herpes zoster ophthalmicus affects

   A Ophthalmic division of trigeminal nerve
   B Ophthalmic division of facial nerve
   C Optic nerve
   D Trochlear nerve

12. In myopia, the patient may have

   A A short eye
   B A long eye
   C Reduced refractive power
   D Good night vision

13. Cataract is

   A Vitreous opacity
   B Lens opacity
   C Corneal opacity
   D Treated with topical drops

14. CMV retinitis is associates with

   A Diabetes
   B Hypertension
   C MS
   D HIV

15. The most severe stage in diabetic retinopathy involves

    A Extensive haemorrhages
    B Cotton wool spots
    C Cotton wool spots plus haemorrhages
    D Neovasculaisation

Extended Matching Questions

Topical eye drops

A Tropicamide
B Chloramphenicol
C Fluorescein
D Pilocarpine
E Aciclovir

For each situation below, choose the **single** most likely answer from the above list of options.

1. Most useful for examining corneal defects

2. Most useful for examining the retina

3. Common topical antibiotic

4. Causes pupil constriction

5. Used when measuring intraocular pressure

Eye infections

A CMV
B Herpes simplex
C Herpes zoster ophthalmicus
D Acanthamoeba
E HIV

For each situation below, choose the **single** most likely answer from the above list of options.

6. Causes dentritic ulcers

7. Viral reactivation causes this

8. Is associated with the trigeminal nerve

9. Infection with this may occur after swimming with contact lens in situ

10. Check for Hutchinson's sign if this infection is suspected

Diabetic retinopathy

A Hard exudates
B Cotton wool spots
C Neovascularisation
D Maculopathy
E Cataract

For each situation below, choose the **single** most likely answer from the above list of options.

11. Common condition in elderly, but can affect patients with diabetes earlier

12. Signifies advanced disease

13. Fluffy white lesions due to infarcts

14. Release of VEGF results in this

15. Disease at the macula

Orbital trauma

A Globe rupture
B Surface foreign body
C Frontal bone
D Maxillary bone
E Chemical injury

For each situation below, choose the **single** most likely answer from the above list of options.

16. Requires immediate irrigation

17. Bone most commonly fractured in orbital injury

18. Requires urgent surgical repair

19. May involve lens subluxation

20. Bone least commonly fractured in orbital injury

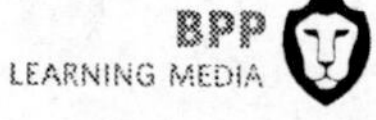

Emergencies

A Acute angle closure glaucoma
B Orbital cellulitis
C Globe rupture
D Retinal detachment
E Temporal arteritis

For each situation below, choose the **single** most likely answer from the above list of options.

21. Is most likely to present with flashing lights and floaters

22. Painful eye movements, diplopia, eyelid erythema / inflammation

23. Commoner in myopia

24. Painful eye, temporal headache and jaw pain with raised ESR

25. Artery biopsy may aid diagnosis for this condition

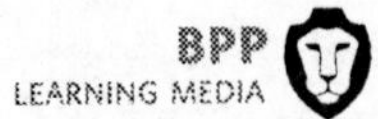

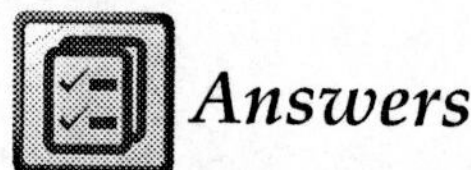

Answers

SBAs		EMQs	
1	A	1	C
2	B	2	A
3	C	3	B
4	A	4	D
5	D	5	C
6	A	6	B
7	D	7	C
8	C	8	C
9	B	9	D
10	A	10	C
11	A	11	E
12	B	12	C
13	B	13	B
14	D	14	C
15	D	15	D
		16	E
		17	D
		18	A
		19	A
		20	C
		21	D
		22	B
		23	D
		24	E
		25	E

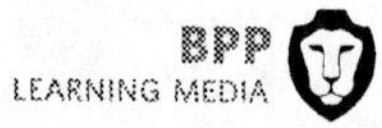

Chapter 23

Obstetrics and gynaecology

Dr William Dougal

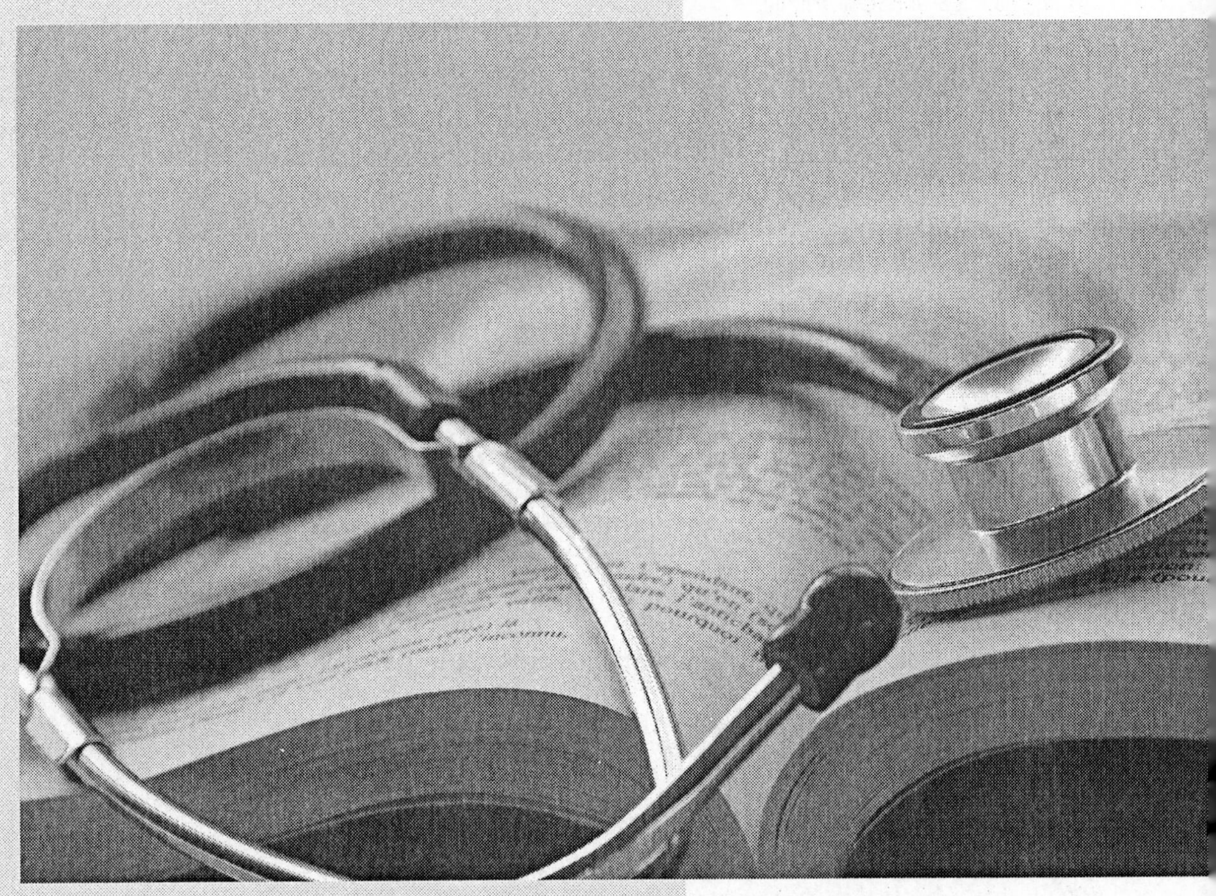

Obstetric emergencies

Pre-eclampsia / eclampsia

P Pre-eclampsia: hypertension (>140/90) plus proteinuria (>0.3 g/L).

Eclampsia: above plus tonic-clonic seizures.

A Pre-eclampsia affects 5–10% of pregnant women.

Sx Malaise, vomiting, headache.

S Hypertension and proteinuria, hyperreflexia, tonic-clonic seizures.

HELLP syndrome: Haemolysis, Elevated Liver enzymes, Low Platelets.

I BP, urinalysis, foetal USS, FBC, U&Es.

T Delivery is curative.

Antihypertensives, induction of labour magnesium sulphate for seizure prevention.

C See Box 23.1.

Mother	Foetus
• HELLP syndrome • Papilloedema • DIC • Cerebral haemorrhage • Renal failure • Liver failure • Death	• Intrauterine growth restriction • Death

Box 23.1: Complications of pre-eclampsia

Hyperemesis gravidarum

P Severe 'morning sickness' may be due to high levels of beta-HCG.

A 0.3–2% women affected.

Sx Nausea, vomiting, dehydration, loss of body weight, electrolyte imbalance, nutritional deficiencies, ketosis.

I Clinical diagnosis, FBC, U&E, LFT, pelvic USS, urine M,C&S.

T Supportive: fluids, antiemetics, nutritional and electrolyte replacement.

C Renal failure, nutritional and electrolyte imbalance.

Pr Usually improves as B-HCG levels fall.

Ectopic pregnancy

P Embryo implantation outside of the uterus. Rupture causes pain and bleeding into abdomen.

A 98% are in the fallopian tubes, also ovary, cervical and abdominal.

Often no cause identified. Risk factors include: PID, use of intrauterine device (IUD), tubal surgery, infertility, previous ectopic.

S Sx Abdo pain, pelvic pain, mild PV bleeding.

I B-HCG, FBC, transvaginal USS, diagnostic laparotomy.

T Medical: methotrexate.

Surgery: laparoscopic salpingectomy. Laparotomy if patient unstable.

C Rupture leading to hypovolaemic shock.

Pr Further ectopic pregnancy in 10–15%.

Miscarriage / spontaneous abortion

P Spontaneous end of pregnancy <20 weeks gestation.

A Commonest complication of early pregnancy, mostly in first trimester due to chromosomal abnormality.

- Threatened: bleeding and pain with a closed os and viable foetus on USS
- Inevitable: bleeding and pain with an open os
- Missed: death of foetus / embryo but no signs or symptoms of miscarriage
- Incomplete: death of foetus / embryo, open cervix but retained products of conception yet to be passed
- Complete: death of foetus, all products of conception passed

Box 23.2: Classification of Miscarriage

S Sx PV bleeding, abdo pain.

I Clinical with USS.

T No treatment: 'watchful waiting' for resolution.

Medical: misoprostol.

Surgery: vacuum aspiration / D&C.

Placental abruption

P Placental lining separates from uterine wall >20 weeks.

A Commonest cause of late partum bleeding.

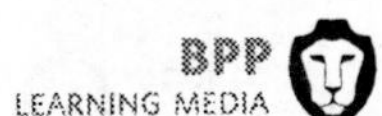

Trauma, hypertension and coagulopathy linked, also higher incidence in smokers and polyhydramnios.

S Sx Painful PV bleeding, enlarged, hard uterus, abdo tenderness, contractions.

I Clinical with USS.

T Dependent on volume of blood loss and foetal distress.

Immediate delivery may be required.

C Hypovolaemic shock, premature delivery, foetal death.

Pr 20–30% foetal mortality.

Placenta praevia

P Placenta is attached to the uterine wall close to or overlying the cervix.

A Leading cause of antepartum haemorrhage.

S Sx Asymptommatic or painless PV bleeding.

I USS.

T Caesarean section delivery.

C Increased risk of sepsis and postpartum haemorrhage.

Umbilical cord prolapse

P Umbilical cord descends through cervix ahead of the foetus.

The following foetus puts pressure on the cord, oxygen and blood supply to foetus obstructed.

A Rare, 0.1–0.6% of all births.

S Sx Palpable or visible cord outside of uterus.

I Clinical.

T Emergency C-section.

C Hypoxic encephalopathy, cerebral palsy, foetal death.

Post-partum haemorrhage

P Primary: >500ml blood loss < 24 hours of delivery.

Secondary: >500ml blood loss >24 hours after delivery.

A See Box 23.3.

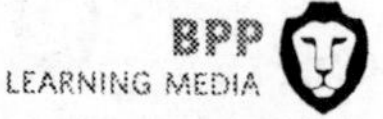

The 4 'Ts'

- Tissue: retained placental or foetal tissue
- Tone: uterine atony (inability of uterus to contract)
- Trauma: perineal, vagina, cervical, uterine tears
- Thrombin: coagulopathies

Box 23.3: Causes of PPH

S Sx PV bleeding, signs of hypovolaemic shock.

I FBC, INR, USS.

T IV oxytocin, transfusion, correct coagulopathy, uterine artery embolisation, laparotomy, hysterectomy.

C Hypovolaemic shock, death.

Rhesus disease

P Exposure of Rh –ve mother with Rh +ve foetus' blood causes production of maternal IgM antibodies against Rh antigen (these abs do not cross the placenta).

In future pregnancies IgG is produced, crosses the placenta and causes haemolytic anaemia in the foetus.

A Rh –ve mother and Rh +ve father.

S Sx Foetal distress, hyrops fetalis.

I USS, foetal blood sampling for foetal monitoring.

T All Rh –ve mothers given anti-D IgG throughout pregnancy.

C Haemolytic disease of the newborn, hydrops fetalis, stillbirth.

Pr Good due to anti-D.

Gynaecology

Pelvic inflammatory disease

P Inflammation of uterus, fallopian tubes or ovaries.

A Usually due to ascending bacterial infection.

Common organisms include neisseria gonorrhoea (40–60%) and chlamydia trachomatis (60%).

S Sx Lower abdo pain, vaginal discharge, pyrexia, PV bleeding, painful intercourse.

I FBC, CRP, B-HCG, urine MC&S, high vaginal swab, pelvic USS.

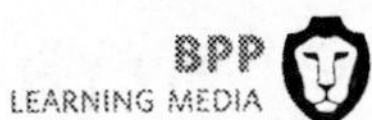

T Oral or IV antibiotics eg ceftriaxone and metronidazole.

C Scarring leading to ectopic pregnancy, infertility and chronic pain.

Endometriosis

P Presence of endometrial tissue outside of uterus producing an inflammatory reaction.

A Most often in ovaries, pelvis and abdomen.

S Sx Triad of: pelvic pain, pain during intercourse, history of difficulty conceiving. May be asymptomatic.

I Laparoscopy is gold standard, USS pelvis, MRI pelvis.

T Medial: oral contraceptive pill, GnRH analogues.

C Infertility, adhesions.

Pr Progressive in 30%.

Uterovaginal prolapse

P Weakness of muscles and ligaments supporting the uterus causing it to prolapse with gravity.

A Old age, child birth.

S Sx 'Feeling of a mass', associated urinary incontinence.

I Speculum examination.

T Conservative: pelvic floor exercises, ring / shelf pessary.

Surgical: hysterectomy, anterior / posterior vaginal wall repair.

Polycystic ovarian syndrome

P Criteria is two out of three **POS**:

- Polycystic ovaries on USS
- Oligo / anovulation
- Signs of androgen excess (hirsuitism)

A Genetic component, affects 5–10% women of reproductive age.

S Sx Oligo / amenorrhoea, infertility, hirsuitism, acne, obesity (due to insulin resistance).

I USS pelvis, glucose tolerance test, sex-hormone binding globulin.

T Aimed at lowering insulin levels, treating hirsuitism and restoring fertility, weight loss, OCP.

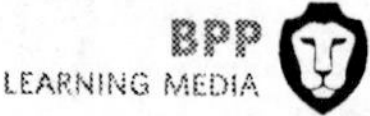

C Type II diabetes, endometrial hyperplasia, endometrial carcinoma.

Fibroids (Leiomyomas)

P Benign tumours originating from the uterine myometrium.

A 20% women, more common in Afro-Caribbean women.

S Sx Menorrhagia, dysmenorrhoea, abdo pain, red degeneration (capsular vessel thrombosis), mass on PV examination.

I FBC, B-HCG, USS pelvis.

T Conservative: analgesia and rest.

Surgery: myomectomy, hysterectomy, uterine artery embolisation.

Cervical inta-epitheleal neoplasm (CIN)

P Potentially pre-malignant transformation and dysplasia of squamous cells in the transformation zone of the cervix.

A Increased risk in HPV infection (particularly HPV 16 and 18), smoking, multiple sexual partners.

S Sx Usually asymptomatic due to cervical screening.

Age 25–6, cervical smear test every 3 years <50, every 5 years >50

- CIN I mild dysplasia: confined to basal 1/3 epithelium. 80% regress to normal, 20% progress to grade II
- CIN II moderate dysplasia: confined to basal 2/3 epithelium. 25% progress to grade III
- CIN III severe dysplasia / carcinoma in-situ (CIS) greater than 2/3 epithelium

Box 23.4: Cervical screening

I Cervical smear grades CIN on histology.

T CIN I: conservative management and regular smears.

CIN II + III: large loop excision of transformation zone (LLETX).

C Progression to cervical cancer.

Pr Regular smears.

Cervical cancer

P 80–90% are squamous cell carcinomas, 10–20% adenocarcinomas.

A HPV, smoking, HIV. 12th commonest female cancer.

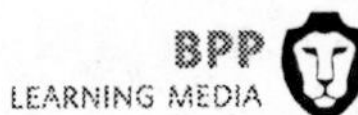

Sx Vaginal bleeding, hard, craggy, bleeding cervix on pelvic examination. May be asymptomatic.

I Cervical biopsy, CT/MRI pelvis.

T Hysterectomy +/– lymphadenectomy with chemo and radiotherapy.

Pr Overall five-year survival 92%. Related to stage of carcinoma spread.

Stage	Features	Five-year survival
1	Confined to cervix	80–90%
2	Extends into parametrium	50–60%
3	Extends into pelvic wall	30–40%
4	Extended beyond the pelvis	15%

Box 23.5: Cervical cancer staging and prognosis

Endometrial cancer

P 95% adenocarcinoma.

A Obesity, HRT, early menarche, late menopause, oestrogen-secreting tumour, Tamoxifen.

Usually presents in first few decades after menopause.

S Sx Post-menopausal vaginal bleeding, anaemia, bleeding between normal periods.

I Transvaginal USS, endometrial biopsy, CT/MRI pelvis.

T Hysteretomy +/– bilateral salpingo-oopherectomy with radiotherapy.

Pr Five-year survival 75–90% for carcinoma confined to uterus, 10% in metastatic disease.

Ovarian cancer

P 90% epithelial cell adenocarcinoma.

A Genetic (BRCA1 and 2 genes), infertile women, endometriosis, HRT, nulliparity.

S Sx Asymptomatic or abdo pain, bloating, vaginal bleeding, weight loss, increased urinary symptoms.

I USS pelvis, CA125 tumour marker, CT/MRI pelvis.

T Hysterectomy and bilateral salpingo-oopherectomy +/– lymphadenectomy with radiotherapy.

Pr Poorest overall survival compared to other gynaecological malignancies.

Five-year survival 80% if limited to ovaries, 18% with mets.

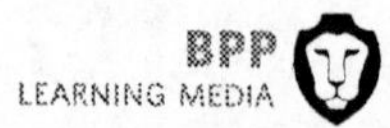

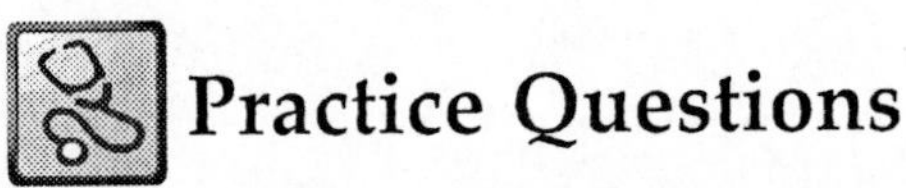

Practice Questions

Single Best Answers

1. HELLP syndrome is associated with

   A Pre-eclampsia
   B Polycystic ovarian syndrome
   C Endometriosis
   D Rheusus disease

2. Rhesus disease will occur with

   A Rh +ve mother and Rh +ve foetus
   B Rh –ve mother and Rh +ve foetus
   C Rh +ve mother and Rh –ve foetus
   D Rh –ve mother and Rh –ve foetus

3. Endometrial cancer is mainly due to

   A Squamous cell carcinoma
   B Adenocarcinoma
   C Sarcoma
   D Adenoma

4. The following is true of fibroids.

   A Are malignant
   B Are derived from ovarian tissue
   C Cause 'chocolate cysts'
   D Are more common in Afro-Caribbean women

5. Cervical cancer is associated with

   A HSV
   B EBV
   C HPV
   D VZV

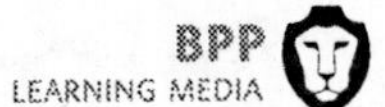

Extended Matching Questions

Match the following definitions and diseases.

A Primary PPH
B Secondary PPH
C Placental abruption
D Placenta praevia
E Hyperemesis gravidarum

1. Premature separation of placenta from uterine wall

2. > 500ml blood loss in first 24 hours after birth

3. Placenta covers cervical os

4. >500ml blood loss >24 hours after birth

5. Severe nausea and vomiting in pregnancy

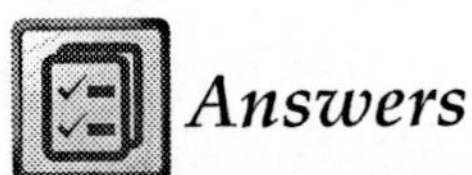

Answers

SBAs		EMQs	
1	A	1	C
2	B	2	A
3	B	3	D
4	D	4	B
5	C	5	E

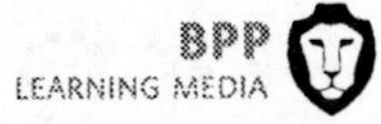

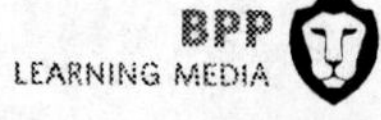

Chapter 24

Paediatrics

Dr Sarah Blackstock and
Dr Sarah Bird

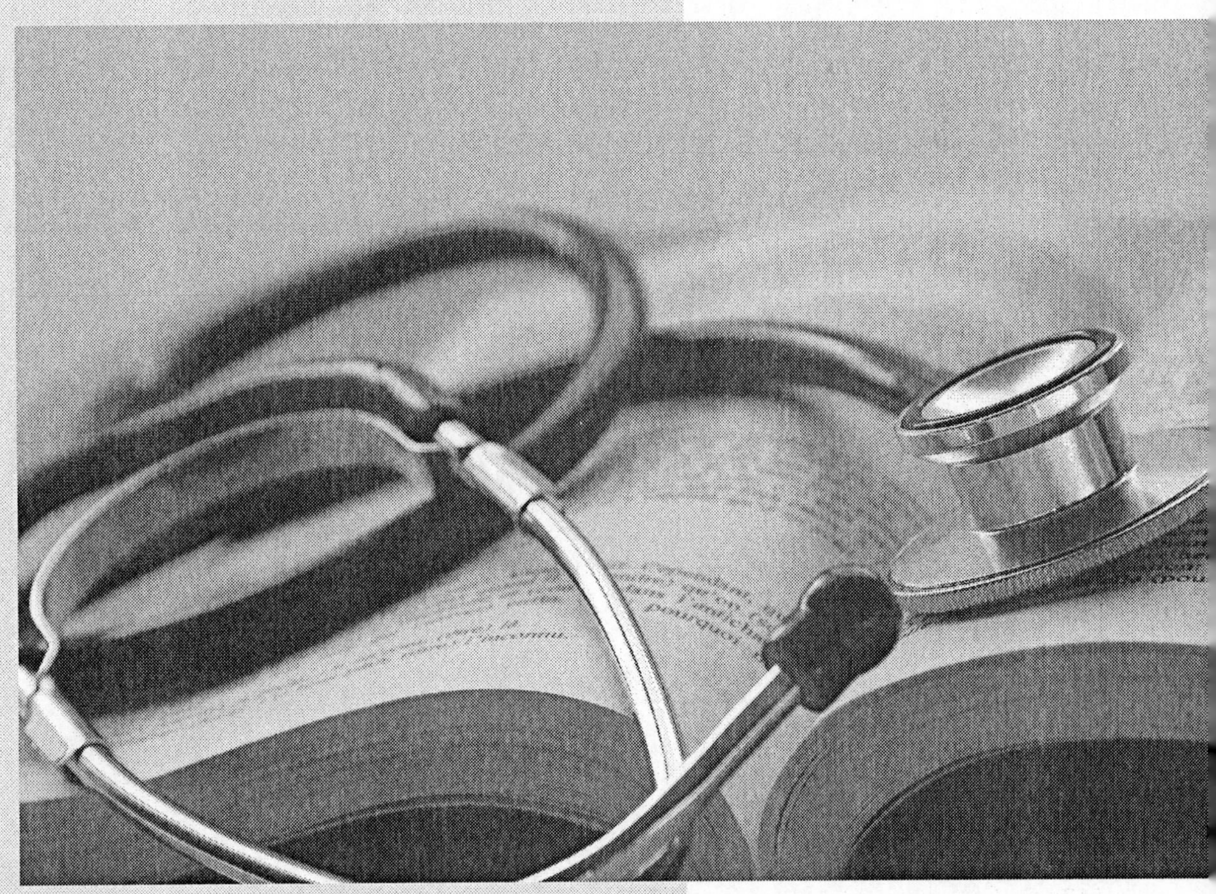

Paediatric values

Age	Heart rate	Respiratory rate
<1 Infant	100–160	30–60
1–2	90–150	24–40
2–5 Younger children	80–140	22–34
6–12	70–120	18–30
>12 Older children	60–100	12–16

Table 24.1: Normal vital sign values

Age	mL/kg/day
1st day	60
2nd day of life	90
Up to 9 months	120–140

Table 24.2: Fluid requirements

Weight	Fluid requirement per 24 hours
First 10kg = 100ml/kg	1,000ml
Second 10kg = 50ml/kg	500ml
Subsequent kgs = 20ml/kg	

Table 24.3: Maintenance IV fluid requirements

Example:

26kg child maintenance fluid for 24 hours = 1,000 + 500 + 120 = 1,620

1,620 ÷ 24 = 67.5 ml/hr

Deficit is based on the degree of acute weight loss from dehydration.

Deficit calculated as weight × % dehydration (e g 5%) × 10

The neonate

Neonate: less than/equal to 28 days.

APGAR scores are used to describe a newborn's condition 0, 5, and every 5 minutes after this if scores remain poor.

	APGAR score		
	0	1	2
Heart rate	Absent	< 100 beats/min	>100 beats/min
Respiratory effort	Absent	Gasping or irregular	Regular, strong cry
Muscle tone	Flaccid	Some flexion of limbs	Well, flexed, active
Reflex Irritability	None	Grimace	Cry, cough
Colour	Pale / blue	Body pink, extremities blue	Pink

Table 24.4: APGAR score

Brachial plexus injuries

A Birth injury, commonly breech delivery / large baby / shoulder dystocia / narrow canal, malpresentation e e breech.

Often subtle, may be picked up by asymmetrical Morro's reflex alone.

Erb's palsy

P Damage to C5 and C6.

S Upper arm adducted with elbow held in extension, forearm pronated, wrist flexed and fingers extended, 'waiter's tip' sign.

Klumpke's palsy

P Rare, damage to C7 and C8 and T1.

S Affects intrinsic hand muscles: flexion of wrist and fingers. Ipsilateral Horner's syndrome.

See also *Trauma and Orthopaedic Surgery* chapter.

T Occasionally in severe injury paralysis permanent. Physiotherapy to prevent contractures.

Surgical reconstruction occasionally attempted.

Pr Usually improves over a few weeks.

Hypoxic-ischaemic encephalopathy (HIE)

P The clinical manifestation of birth asphyxia.

A Hypoxic ischaemia resulting in depletion of brain phosphocreatine and ATP and rise in lactate.

Stage 1	Hyper-alert, tremulous, poor feeding, rarely seizures
Stage 2	Hypotonic, lethargic, obtunded, seizures may occur
Stage 3	Comatose, seizures within 12–24 hours

Box 24.1: Stages of HIE

Outcomes according to severity of HIE:

Stage 1	Largely normal
Stage 2	5% die, 25% suffer neurological injury
Stage 3	80% die, 20% suffer neurological injury

Box 24.2: Outcomes of HIE

I

Intrauterine distress noted by abnormal CTG, cord gases or foetal blood sampling revealing metabolic acidosis.

CTG is a poor assessor of severity of ischaemmia but a normal CTG is highly predictive of an absence of problems.

Persistently low APGAR scores can also be an indicator.

Neonatal sepsis

P

Bacterial, viral, fungal.

Early onset: often maternally acquired, up to 48 hours after birth. Commonest causes:

- Group B streptococcus (GBS). (Up to 20% of pregnant women have genital tract colonisation but this is not routinely screened for.)
- E. coli or other gram negative bacilli.
- Listeria monocytogenes (outbreaks in dairy products, patés and uncooked meats).

Late onset: usually acquired in hospital eg coagulase negative staphylococcus, s. aureus, e. coli, klebsiella, pseudomonas, candida.

S

Signs none specific. Early onset more likely to be associated with respiratory distress, shock, mortality higher. Late onset signs are more insidious.

- Respiratory distress / apnoeas
- Lethargy / irritability
- Seizures
- Poor feeding / vomiting
- Fever / hypothermia

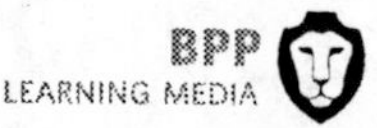

- Pre-term rupture of membranes (<37 weeks)
- Prolonged rupture of membranes (PROM)
- Maternal fever
- Maternal colonisation with GBS
- Foetal tachycardia
- Lack of intrapartum antibiotics with above risk factors

Foul smelling / stained amniotic fluid. Listeria causes green coloured liquor which can be mistaken for meconium.

Box 24.3: Risk factors neonatal sepsis

I Bloods and blood film, blood culture.

CXR: pneumonia may cause diffuse reticular nodular shadowing indistinguishable from hyaline membrane disease.

Urine culture, lumbar puncture.

T Empirical IV antibiotics pending culture results.

Usually a combination of a penicillin and gentamicin. Ampicillin would be used to cover listeria.

Treatment often commenced if there are a couple of risk factors for sepsis even if no symptoms.

Pr Good if commenced early.

TORCH infections

P Intrauterine infection with **T**oxoplasmosis, **O**ther (eg parvovirus), **R**ubella, **C**ytomegalovirus, **H**erpes simplex virus.

S Microcephaly, deafness, cataracts, deafness, congenital heart disease, IUGR.

I Viral PCR, serology, urine, throat swabs.

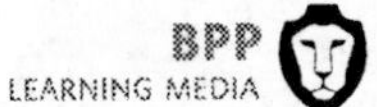

Neonatal jaundice

Jaundice < 24 hours	• Haemolytic disorders – Rhesus haemolytic disesase (mother RhD negative, baby Rh D positive, sensitisation from previous pregnancy / antepartum haemorrhage) – ABO compatibility (commonly group O mother, group A infant, occasionaly group B infants) – G6PD (Mediterranean / middle eastern variants) – Spherocytosis • Congenital infection
24 hours – 2 weeks	• Physiological jaundice (clinically well baby) • Breast milk jaundice (may also be assoc with poor feeding) • Polycythaemia (assoc with dehydration, IUGR, maternal diabetes, delayed cord clamping, twin-twin transfusion) • Infection eg UTI • Crigler-Najjar syndrome • Also Haemolytic causes
At > 2 weeks	• **Conjugated:** (pale stool, dark urine) – Bile duct obstruction – Biliary atresia – Progressive obliteration of extrahepatic ducts or intrahepatic eg Alagilles syndrome – Neonatal heptatitis (eg CMV, hep B) – Metabolic causes eg galactosaemia (assoc with cataracts) • **Unconjugated:** – Hypothyroidism – Physiological and breast milk – Infection

Box 24.4: Causes of neonatal jaundice by timing of onset

S Jaundice +/- lethargy, poor feeding, hepatosplenomegaly.

If haemolysis: bruising.

Severe unconjugated hyperbilirubinaemia: back arching.

Conjugated hyperbilirubinaemia: pale stools, dark urine.

I Exclude other causes before diagnosing physiological / breast milk jaundice.

FBC, total and direct bilirubin, total protein, blood group and film, (may see spherocytosis on film) direct Coombs' test CRP, blood culture.

Prolonged jaundice: neonatal screen, TFTs, urine reducing substances, urine culture, plasma cortisol.

Imaging: ultrasound, and radionuclide scan, for unconjugated hyperbilirubinaemia.

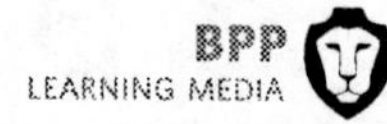

T Breast milk / physiological, no treatment required, continue to breast feed.

Phototherapy: for moderate-severe unconjugated hyper bilirubinaemia.

Exchange transfusion for severe unconjugated jaundice associated with anaemia.

Biliary atresia: surgery required. Kesai procedure.

C Very high levels of unconjugated bilirubin can cause kernicterus and resultant neurological damage eg choreoathetoid cerebal palsy.

Neonatal respiratory distress

S Tachypnoea (>60/min) nasal flaring, intercostal recession, grunting, cyanosis, poor feeding, tachycardia.

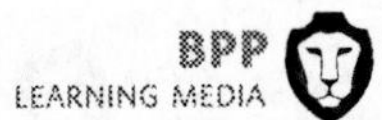

Common	**Transient tachypnoea of newborn:** (TTT) due to delay in reabsorption of lung fluid, more common post C-section therefore also macrosomic babies of diabetic mothers. CXR: fluid in horizontal fissure, resolves over 24 hours.
Less common	**Meconium aspiration syndrome**: meconium passed before birth causing chemical pneumonitis, classically associated with mature or post mature baby or intrapartum asphyxia. CXR: overinflated lungs, patches of collapse / consolidation. Requires suction if meconium below vocal cords, may require intubation, surfactant, ECMO. **Respiratory distress syndrome**: also known as hyaline membrane disease. Caused by surfactant deficiency, most commonly due to prematurity. Usually presents within four hours of birth. Can be prevented by giving mothers in premature labour glucocorticoids, ideally 24 hours before delivery. CXR: hypoinflated lungs, atelectasis, ground glass appearance, air bronchograms **Pneumonia / Sepsis** **Pneumothorax:** hyperresonant hyperexpanded assymetrical chest, history of traumatic delivery / ventilation. **Persistent pulmonary hypertension:** due to high pulmonary vascular resistance causing right to left shunting. Associated with birth asphyxia, meconium aspiration, RDS, sepsis. Urgent ECHO required. Treated with inhaled nitric oxide and ventilation. **Milk aspiration:** in babies with gastro-oesphageal reflux, also children with cleft palate.
Rare	**Congenital diaphraphmatic hernia**: caused by failure in closure of foramen of Bochdalek of the diaphragm resulting in abdominal contents herniating into chest causing hypolastic lungs. Signs include scaphoid abdomen, reduced breath sounds / bowel sounds in chest. Baby should ideally be intubated before any respiratory effort. When stable requires surgical repair. **Congenital heart disease:** usually presents after the first 24 hours. Signs include cyanosis, large liver, murmurs, absent pulses. May be history of maternal illness in pregnancy (rash / fever) or maternal drug ingestion. **Metabolic acidosis** eg due to sepsis or metabolic disorders. **Tracheo-oesphageal fistula:** (TOF) communication between oesophagus and trachea, usually associated with oesophageal atresia. Other signs include drooling and cyanosis. Diagnosed by failure of passage of size 10 catheter into stomach as coils in atretic pouch. CXR confirms this and also air in the stomach. Associated with polyhydramnios in pregnancy. Nearly half have other congenital malformations eg as part of VACTERL association (Vertebral, Anorectal, Cardiac, Trans-oesphageal, Renal and radial Limb anomalies.

Box 24.5: Causes of neonatal respiratory distress syndrome

Exomphalos

P Abdominal contents protrude through umbilical ring.

Defect covered by peritoneum. Approximately 70% have other congenital anomalies eg trisomies / congenital heart disease.

I Antenatal karyotype and a more detailed anomaly scan are recommended.

Postnatal CXR, ECHO, renal ultrasound blood glucose monitoring.

T Cover with cling film. Primary or staged closure is required. NGT decompression. IV fluids.

Pr 35% mortality – three times greater than gastroschisis.

Associated defects are the major influence on mortality.

Gastroschisis

P Herniation of bowel without covering sac.

Defect usually lateral to umbilical cord.

Rarer than exomphalos. Typically premature, SGA, oligohydramnios, associated with antenatal ingestion of aspirin, alcohol, illegal drugs.

Much greater risk of dehydration and protein loss.

T Wrap in cling film to minimise fluid and heat loss. Pass NG tube. IV infusion dextrose. TPN, electrolyte replacement.

Primary or staged closure.

Pr Usually good. 10% necrotising entercolitis.

Rarely associated with lethal chromosomal abnormalities.

Necrotising enterocolitis (NEC)

P Ischaemia of bowel wall, accelerated by feeding with milk. Occurs in 10% of VLBW infants.

Small amounts of early breast milk may be beneficial.

A Prematurity, APH, perinatal haemorrhage, polycythaemia, formula feeding.

Sx Vomiting, may be bile stained. Abdominal distension, stool containing fresh blood, infant rapidly shocked, apnoeas, respiratory failure.

I AXR: distended loops of bowel, thickening of bowel wall with intramural gas and air in portal tract.

Translumination of abdomen.

T Stop oral feeds, IV antibiotics.

Surgery performed for bowel perforation.

C Perforation occurs in 20–30% of confirmed cases. Overwhelming sepsis. DIC, strictures, recurrent NEC, short bowel syndrome, lactose intolerance.

Pr Morbidity and mortality of 20%.

Common presentations

Cardiology

Also see *Cardiology*, Chapter 1.

Hypoplastic left heart syndrome

P Underdevelopment of the left side of the heart (small mitral valve, left ventricle and aortic valve / aorta). Causes the left side of the heart to be unable to maintain effective cardiac output, therefore it is a duct-dependant syndrome.

S Neonates present with circulatory collapse (as the duct closes following birth the heart is unable to maintain cardiac output). Peripheral pulses are absent or weak. The neonate will be breathless and severely acidotic.

I ECG: absent / minimal left ventricular forces.

ECHO required to confirm diagnosis.

T Initial management is with resuscitation and prostaglandins to keep the duct patent.

Surgery is required following stabilisation three to five days later (Norwood's procedure) or heart transplant.

Pr Five-year survival 70–80% following Norwood's procedure.

Respiratory

Also see *Respiratory*, Chapter 2.

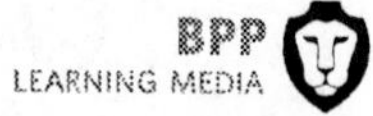

Wheeze

Bronchiolitis

P Commonest cause respiratory syncytial virus (RSV) in 90% cases. Other viruses include parainfluenza, adenovirus. Commonest in winter.

S Respiratory distress, coryza, hyperinflation, apnoea, crackles throughout lung fields +/- wheeze. Lasts five to seven days, may get worse day three to four. Most common in first year of life. In older children consider viral induced wheeze.

I NPA (nasopharyngeal aspirate) only for those admitted to hospital for cohorting patients.

CXR only if doubt of diagnosis eg asymmetrical wheeze.

Differential diagnosis: pneumonia, cardiac failure, CF, immunodeficiency.

T Largely supportive. Moderate / severe bronchiolitis may require admission to hospital if requiring oxygen support or poor feeding. Ensure adequate hydration. NG or IV fluids if significant work of breathing to decrease risk of aspiration.

Saline nebulisers and bronchodilators may be trialled, however evidence is not strong.

If severe respiratory distress CPAP or ventilator support may be required. For those at high risk (eg ex-premature babies) immunise with anti-RSV antibody eg palvizumab.

C Groups at risk of severe disease: congenital heart disease, chronic lung disease, immunosuppressed.

Asthma: See *Respiratory* Chapter 2

Cystic fibrosis: See Chapter 2

Cardiac failure: features include: shortness of breath, wheeze, hepatomegaly poor feeding +/- murmur, cyanosis, persistent tachycardia, decreased pulses, failure to thrive, phenotypic abnormality, FH of structural cardiac disease.

Box 24.6: Differential diagnosis of wheeze

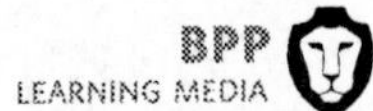

Acute stridor

Common	
Croup (acute laryngotracheobronchitis)	
A	Parainfluenza virus is the commonest cause. Also influenza virus, RSV, rhinovirus, age 1–4 years, boys > girls.
S	Stridor, coryza onset over a couple of days. Mild fever not usually toxic. Hoarse voice, barking cough, worse at night.
T	Steam mist vaporiser, monitor fluid intake, oral dexamethasone, steroid nebuliser, adrenaline nebuliser, intubation in 1% of cases.
Rare	
Bacterial tracheitis (pseudomembranous croup)	
A	Staphylococcus aureus or haemophilus influenza.
S	May follow on from croup-like illness. Similar symptoms but more severe. Child more toxic with rapidly progressive airway obstruction.
T	Treat as for epiglottis. Do not upset child as cannot completely exclude epiglottis.
Diphtheria	
P	Corynebacterium diphtheria. Release of toxin results in carditis week 2, with tachycardia and heart failure.
S	Coryzal symptoms and sore throat, followed by rapid development of pseudomembrane (grey / white) which causes airway obstruction.
T	Erythromycin or penicillin plus antitoxin, management of airway obstruction.
Very rare	
Acute epiglottitis	
A	Haemophilus influenza type b, rare since induction of HIB vaccine. Aged 2–6 years.
S	Acute onset stridor: within hours, toxic, high fever, drooling, anxiety no preceding coryza, no cough, reluctant to speak.
T	Urgent general anaesthesic and ENT review for visualisation of airway and intubation, bacterial swabs at intubation. IV 3rd generation cephalosporin. Do not examine throat / X-ray / take bloods / upset child.

Box 24.7: Differential diagnosis of acute stridor

Chronic stridor

Laryngomalacia

A Small larynx with floppy aryepiglottic folds. Common.

S Starts in first month of life.

Stridor mainly inspiratory and worse when child supine or after URTI.

Child well, growing and developing normally.

T None required. Endoscopy if faltered growth, respiratory distress.

Pr Resolves by 1–3 years life.

Subglottic stenosis

A Congenital or acquired. Common.

Stenosis just below level of vocal cords.

Risk factors include prematurity, recurrent, prolonged or traumatic intubation.

S Stridor.

T Systemic steroids may facilitate extubation in mild to moderate cases.

Laser or cryotherapy may be beneficial. Severe cases may require surgery eg cricoid split or tracheostomy.

Pr As child grows stenosis becomes less severe.

Compression leading to obstruction:

Intraluminal, luminal or extraluminal eg subglottic haemoangioma, vascular rings, laryngeal web, neoplasia.

Box 24.8: Differential diagnosis of chronic stridor

Whooping cough / pertussis

A Bordetella pertussis.

S Two to three days coryza then characteristic paroxysmal or spasmodic cough followed by an inspiratory whoop. Spasms worse at night and may culminate in vomiting. Subconjunctival haemorrhages and epistaxis can occur.

I Culture per nasal swab. There is also marked lymphocytosis.

T Erythromycin. Immunisation (it is in the UK routine immunisation programme) reduces risk by 80–90%.

Often prolonged cough '100 day cough'.

C Pneumonia, convulsions, bronchiectasis, apnoeas, sudden death.

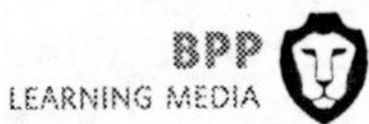

Gastrointestinal

Also see *Gastroenterology,* Chapter 3 for coeliac disease, inflammatory bowel disease and *General Surgery,* Chapter 12 for pyloric stenosis, Meckel's diverticulum and intussusception.

Gastroesophageal reflux

P Functional immaturity of the lower oesophageal sphincter.

High risk groups include those with neurodisability eg cerebral palsy, as they have poor bulbar tone.

S Vomiting, regurgitation, arching / irritability with feeds, weight loss, excessive hiccups, anaemia, aspiration pneumonia.

Atypical: wheeze / intractable asthma.

I No investigation for mild.

If severe / features of oesophagitis consider barium radiology / pH study (gold standard) / nuclear medicine 'milk scan'.

T Positioning, diet change, antacids, thickeners, PPIs, surgery.

C Oesophagitis, aspiration pneumonia.

Pr Good. Very common, most resolved by 12 months once children are sitting / eating solids.

Malrotation

P Occurs as a result of incomplete rotation of the gut in foetal life. There is intermittent and incomplete obstruction by Ladd's bands. Associated with diaphragramatic hernia and atresias.

Usually presents within the first four weeks of life, but can present at any age.

S Bilious vomiting, abdominal distension. Anyone with bilious vomiting has a malrotation and possible volvulus until proven otherwise.

I Upper gastrointestinal contrast studies show the duodenal-jejunal flexure on the right abdomen with a high caecum.

T Surgery.

Hirshsprung's disease

P Absence of ganglion cells from the myenteric and submucosal plexuses in the bowel. Rectum and sigmoid are most often affected.

S Delayed passage of meconium (> 24 hours), bowel obstruction, enterocolitis or later constipation.

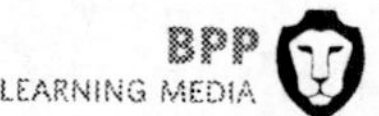

I Rectal biopsy.

T Regular rectal washouts. Temporary colostomy (usually reversed at 6 months).

Neurology

Also see *Neurology*, Chapter 6.

Febrile convulsions

P Usually caused by a viral infection. Seizures are usually generalised tonic-clonic and brief lasting one to two minutes.

A Commonest from 6 months to 6 years. Occurs in 3% of children and in 15% seizures reoccur.

Genetic predisposition (10–20% relatives).

Need to be differentiated from rigors, reflex anoxic seizures and sepsis / meningitis.

S Seizure, temperature, viral symptoms.

I Essential to establish child does not have meningitis or other serious bacterial infection that requires treatment. Therefore child may need infection screen including LP and urine culture depending on clinical findings.

T Anti-pyretics, tepid sponging.

Pr Good. 1% develop epilepsy (usual population risk).

Cerebral palsy

P Disorder of movement and posture due to a non-progressive lesion of the developing nervous system.

The clinical manifestations evolve with the developing brain.

- *Prenatal (80% of causes)*: intrauterine hypoxic-ischaemic injury, congenital infection, chromosomal disorders, toxins, cerebral malformation / dysgenesis.
- *Intrapartum (10%)*: hypoxic ischaemic injury (asphyxia), intracranial haemorrhage.
- *Postnatal (10%)*: trauma, meningitis / encephalitis, bilirubin encephalopathy, hydrocephalus.

S Developmental delay, joint contracture, epilepsy, perceptual difficulties, visual and hearing impairment, poor growth, feeding difficulties.

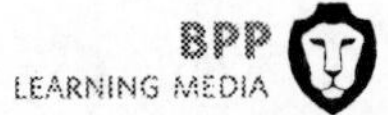

Classification

- *Spastic*: increase in muscle tone hemiplegia / diplegia / quadraplegia. Commonly seen due to periventricular leukomalacia in pre-term infants.
- *Athetoid*: writhing, involuntary pronation / flexion of distal extremity. Choreform 'dancing' movements.
  Commonly seen after bilirubin encephalopathy.
- *Ataxic*: mixed.

T Multidisciplinary team approach, physiotherapy.

C Aspiration pneumonia, contractures.

Neural tube defects

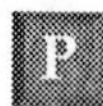

- *Anencephaly*: failure of closure of the rostral aspect of the neural tube.
  75% of affected infants are stillborn the rest die shortly after birth.
- *Encephalocoele*: protrusion of cerebral tissue through midline cranial defect in the frontal or occipital regions.
- *Myelomeningocoele*: herniation of meninges, nerve roots and spinal cord through dorsal vertebral defect.
  Results in sensory and motor defects below lesion including sphincter disturbance.
  Associated with Arnold Chiari malformation. Hydrocephalus may coexist.
- *Meningocoele*: cyst formation by herniation of meninges, usually over dorsum of spine.
  Neurological disability minimal, risk of bacterial meningitis.
- *Spina Bifida Occulta*: asymptomatic consition characterised by failure of closure of vertebral arch.
  Occurs in 5% of population.

I Antenatal scanning.

T Surgical repair of meningocoele, encephaloele, and myelomeningocoele.

Close observation for hydrocephalus and shunt insertion if required.

Orthopaedic management of limb deformities, management of bladder and bowels, eg intermittent bladder drainage.

Treatment of seizures, physiotherapy.

Duchenne muscular dystrophy

P Commonest neuromuscular condition.

Caused by mutation in the dystrophin gene. X-linked recessive inheritance. One-third are new mutations. Females are asymptomatic carriers.

Incidence is 1 in 3,500 male births.

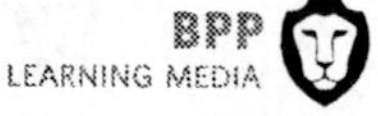

S Onset in early years (but average age of diagnosis 5.5 years). Delay in motor milestones, clumsy, waddling gait, proximal muscle weakness. Typically patients lose ability to walk by 8–12 years. Pseudohypertrophy of calves, scoliosis. Gowers sign positive (using hands and arms to 'walk up' own body from squatting position due to lack of hip and thigh strength).

I High plasma creatine kinase (> 5000 iu/L), mutations in dystrophin gene, muscle biopsy (dystrophic picture with absent dystrophin).

T No curative treatment. Physiotherapy for contractures. Non-invasive respiratory support may be used to improve quality of life.

Corticosteroids improve muscle power. Self help groups.

Pr Poor. Death late teens from respiratory failure or associated cardiomyopathy.

Renal

Also see *Renal*, Chapter 4.

Urinary tract infection / Vesico ureteric reflux

A 1% boys versus 3% girls. More than 90% of UTIs are caused by E. coli.

Risk factors for urinary tract infections include: vesicouretic reflux (this tends to be of familial inheritance), incomplete bladder emptying, catheterisation / instrumentation, renal stones.

Sx In babies / infants the presentation is non-specific with pyrexia, vomiting and unsettled they may present with features of sepsis. In older children, they may present with dysuria, frequency and loin pain.

Atypical UTI	Recurrent UTI
• Severely unwell at presentation • Poor urinary flow • Abdominal mass • Raised creatinine • Septicaemia • Failure to respond to antibiotics within 48 hours • Infection with non E. coli organisms	• Two or more episodes of acute UTI with pyelonephritis / upper urinary tract infection. • One episode of acute UTI with pyelonephritis / upper urinary tract infection **plus** one or more episodes of cystitis / lower urinary tract infection. • Three or more episodes of cystitis / lower urinary tract infections.

Box 24.9: Symptoms of atypical and recurrent UTIs

I Collection of a sterile urine sample for M,C &S.

Imaging aims to identify structural abnormalities (eg VUR) or identify renal scarring as a result of infection.

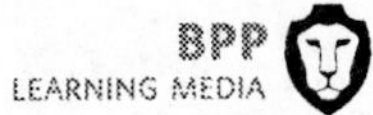

	Responds within 48 hours to abx	Atypical UTI	Recurrent UTI
Under 6 months	USS in 6 weeks	USS during illness MCUG DMSA in 6 months	USS during illness MCUG DMSA in 6 months
6 months – 3 years	Nil	USS during illness DMSA in 6 months	USS in 6 weeks DMSA in 6 months
Over 3 years	Nil	USS during illness	USS in 6 weeks DMSA in 6 months

Table 24.5: Investigations required in each age group

T Oral antibiotics, IV antibiotics in pyelonephritis or sepsis.

Treatment of VUR: low dose prophylactic antibiotics (eg trimethoprim). Surgery may be required if there are frequent UTIs despite prophylactic antibiotics.

C Renal scarring following a UTI carries a 15–20% risk of hypertension. Reflux nephropathy carries a 15–20% risk of renal failure.

Undescended testes (Cryptorchidism)

P The testes descend through the inguinal canal during foetal life. 50% of undescended testes descend spontaneously by 6 months of age, and are unlikely to occur after this.

A 3% of term babies, 30% of premature babies.

S Sx See Box 24.10.

T See Box 24.10.

- *Palpable undescended testes (80%):* testes are palpable usually at the inguinal canal but cannot be manipulated into the scrotum.
  - These are usually brought down into the scrotum with an orchidopexy.
- *Impalpable testes (20%):* the testes are impalpable in the scrotum or inguinal ring. They may be intra-abdominal, within the inguinal canal or absent.
  - Laparoscopy is required to locate the testes and either surgically remove or bring down the testes via orchidopexy.
- *Retractile testes:* these are not true undescended testes. The testes may be manipulated into the scrotum but then self-retract into the inguinal region due to overactive cremasteric muscle.
  - Follow-up is required, but surgery is rarely required.

Box 24.10: Classification and treatment of undescended testes

C Boys requiring bilateral orchidopexy are at risk of being sterile.

Fertility for unilateral orchidopexy is close to normal.

Undescended testes produce an increased risk of malignancy, with the greatest risk for intra-abdominal testes.

Early orchidopexy (usually in the second year of life) can reduce this risk.

Hypospadias

P An abnormality of the urethral meatus, with a position more proximal to the tip of the penis.

A Unknown in most cases, 1 in 300 live births.

S Abnormal position of the urethral meatus on the ventral surface of the penis, may be associated with a ventral curvature of the penis (chordee) or a hooded foreskin (due to ventral deficiency of the foreskin).

Sx Difficulty urinating while standing. Sexual dysfunction is not present unless there is also a severe chordee, which may cause painful erections.

T Surgical correction is often required before 2 years of age.

Growth

Age	Gross motor	Fine motor and vision	Language	Social
6 weeks	Good head control. No head lag	Able to fix and follow through 90°	Makes throaty noises	Smiles responsively
3 months	Raise head and chest on forearms	Fix and follow through 180°	Begins to vocalise, coos and laughs	Aware smile attracts attention
6 months	Sits supported	Palmar grasp, transfers objects	Babbles, turns to name	Plays with feet, holds bottle
9 months	Sits unsupported, crawling	Looks for hidden objects	Two-syllable babble	Finger feeds
12 months	Cruising round furniture	Pincer grasp, bangs blocks together	Two words with meaning	Waves bye-bye, plays peek a boo
15 months	Walking steadily	Scribbles	Several words	Able to drink from a cup
18 months	Stoops to carry objects	Delicate pincer grasp	Up to 25 words, points to body parts	Holds a spoon and feeds self
2 years	Climbs one stair at a time	Tower of eight bricks, draws a line	Simple phrase of two to three words	Dry by day, plays alone
3 years	Rides tricycle	Copies circle	Three- to four-word sentences	Interactive play
4 years	Hops	Copies cross and square	Counts to ten	Dry by night, brushes teeth
5 years	Walks down stairs one foot at a time	Copies triangle	Develops comprehension	Acts out role play

Table 24.6: Developmental milestones

Failure to thrive

P Failure to gain weight / grow at an appropriate / expected rate. This is measured by using centile charts.

Mild failure to thrive: a fall across two centiles.

Severe failure to thrive: a fall across three or more centiles.

A Separated into organic and non-organic causes.

Organic causes	Non-organic causes
• Gastro-oesophageal reflux • Coeliac disease • Cow's milk protein intolerance • Cystic fibrosis • Congenital heart disease • Malignancy • Hypothyroidism • Cerebral palsy • Infection / immunodeficiency (eg HIV) • Malignancy • Chromosomal / genetic disorders	• Insufficient breast milk • Poor feeding technique • Inadequate maternal food intake • Maternal depression • Munchausens syndrome by proxy • Lack of awareness of required intake • Child neglect • Financial difficulties

Box 24.11: Causes of failure to thrive

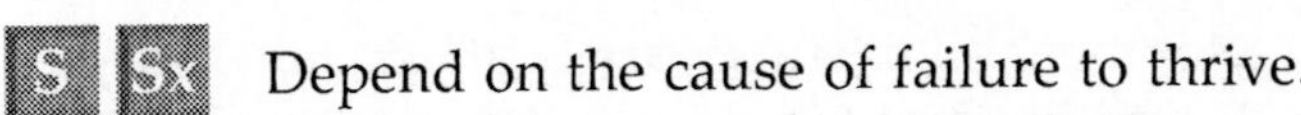

S Sx Depend on the cause of failure to thrive.

I A thorough history and examination in combination with a growth chart are essential in investigating failure to thrive.

Other investigations may include:

Investigation	Cause
Bloods: FBC, U&Es, LFTs, TFTs	Anaemia, immunodeficiency, infection, renal insufficiency, malabsorption, hypothyroidism
Ferritin	Iron deficiency anaemia
Anti-endomysial / anti-gliadin antibodies	Coeliac disease
Urine / stool MC&S	Urine infection, intestinal parasites
Genetic testing	Eg Turner's syndrome
Sweat test	Cystic fibrosis

Table 24.7: Other investigations for failure to thrive

T The management of failure to thrive is often multidisciplinary depending on the cause.

Precocious puberty

P Early puberty which is younger than 8 years in females and younger than 9 years in males.

A Causes can be divided into central (true or gonadotrophin-dependant) or peripheral (gonadotrophin-independent) precocious puberty.

Central precocious puberty is usually due to premature activation of gonadotrophin releasing hormone (GnRH). Peripheral causes depend on the location (Table 24.12).

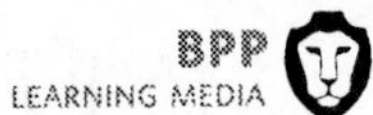

Location	Causes
Adrenal	• Congenital adrenal hyperplasia • Adrenal tumour
Gonadal	• Testicular / ovarian tumour • McCune-Albright syndrome
Iatrogenic	• Exogenous sex-steroid administration

Table 24.8: Peripheral causes of precocious puberty

S Precocious puberty is the early development of sexual characteristics accompanied by a growth spurt.

This must be differentiated from the following terms:

- *Thelarche:* premature breast development alone, this usually affects females aged 6 months to 2 years, usually self-limiting and requires no further investigation
- *Adrenarche:* premature pubic hair development alone, more common in Asian / Afro-caribbean children, usually self-limiting

I Oestradiol / testosterone levels, adrenal androgens, bone age, pelvic ultrasound, MRI and CT.

T Gonadotrophin-releasing hormone analogues in gonadotrophin-dependant causes of precocious puberty.

In gonadotrophin independent causes, the source of excess sex steroids must be identified and inhibitors of androgens / oestrogens (eg cyproterone acetate) used.

Pr An early growth spurt may result in premature closure of the epiphyses and thus result in small adult height.

Delayed puberty

P Delayed puberty is the absence of secondary sexual characteristics by 14 years in females and 15 years in males.

A In contrast to precocious puberty, it is normally idiopathic (constitutional delay) in boys, however in girls further investigation is required to identify a cause.

- Constitutional delay
- Hypogonadotrophic hypogonadism
- Intracranial tumours
- Anorexia nervosa
- Systemic disease (eg CF, Crohns)
- Kallmans syndrome (LHRH deficiency + anosmia)
- Chromosomal (Turner's / Klinefelter's syndrome)
- Hypothyroidism
- Panhypopituitarism

Box 24.12: Causes of delayed puberty

I In males, as delayed puberty is often due to constitutional delay, further investigations are not usually required.

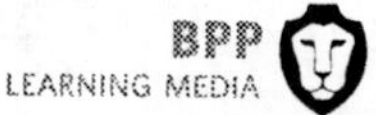

In females delayed puberty must be investigated with the following: karyotyping, LH / FSH / oestrogen levels, pelvic ultrasound, thyroid hormone levels.

T Constitutional delay often only requires reassurance. Androgens may also be used in some cases (oxandrolone).

Genetic disorders

Down's syndrome

P Trisomy 21, typically due to non-disjunction during maternal oogenesis. 2% are due to Robertsonian translocation and 2% are mosaic.

A 1 in 700 live births (incidence rises with maternal age).

S Sx See Box 24.13.

Typical facial features:	Other common features:	Increased incidence of:
• Brachycephaly (flat occiput) • Epicanthic folds • Protruding tongue • Small ears • Upslanting palpebral fissures • Brushfield spots on iris	• Single palmar crease • Wide sandal gap • Hypotonia • Fifth finger clinodactyly • Small stature	• Heart defects – AVSD • Duodenal atresia • Hypothyroidism • Cataracts • Learning difficulties • Leukaemia

Box 24.13: Clinical features of Down's syndrome

I Screening for Down's syndrome is undertaken in all women despite maternal age.

Screening consists of nuchal translucency measurements combined with a maternal blood test. Confirmation of the screen is via either amniocentesis or chorionic villus sampling to sample the foetal tissue.

T Initial management necessitates a thorough examination of the newborn to check for common complications (eg congenital heart disease that may require surgery, cataracts).

Pr There is a shorter life expectancy, with an average lifespan of 49 years. Life expectancy has increased in recent years and people with Down's syndrome are now beginning to suffer with Alzheimer's disease / dementia.

Turner's syndrome (45, X)

P Monosomy X, the normal karyotype, has 46 chormosomes with two being the sex chromosomes (XX in females). Turner's is a chromosomal abnormality in which the second X chromosome is absent or partly missing (mosaicism).

A 1 in 2,500 liveborn females (NB: >95% result in early miscarriage).

S Sx See Box 24.14.

Typical features	Increased incidence of
• Short stature • Webbed neck • Widely spaced nipples • Wide carrying angle • Lymphoedema of hands / feet • Normal intellectual development	• Reproductive sterility • Amenorrhoea • Coarctation of aorta • Bicuspid aortic valve • Horseshoe kidney

Box 24.14: Clinical features of Turner's syndrome

I Diagnosis can be made by amniocentesis during pregnancy. Karyotyping (chromosomal analysis) is the test of choice to diagnose Turner's syndrome.

T Initial management necessitates a thorough examination of the newborn to check for common complications (eg congenital heart disease that may require surgery, renal abnormalities).

Secondary sexual characteristics can be induced with oestrogen therapy.

Final height can be increased with growth hormone therapy.

Pr Physical findings do not affect prognosis, however the accompanying medical problems as listed above may cause significant morbidity.

Kleinfelter's syndrome (47, XXY)

P Klinefelter's syndrome is a chromosomal abnormality in which there is an extra X chromosome in the male karyotype, due to non-disjunction during meiosis.

A 1 in 600 liveborn males.

S Sx See Box 24.15.

Typical features	Increased incidence of
• Tall stature • Gynaecomastia • Hypogonadism • Poor growth of facial / body hair	• Infertility • Mild learning difficulties • Germ cell tumours • Osteoporosis

Box 24.15: Clinical features of Kleinfelter's syndrome

I The diagnosis can be made antenatally via amniocentesis or chorionic villus sampling. Karyotyping is necessary to confirm the diagnosis.

T Testosterone treatment is optional to achieve a masculine appearance.

Pr Normal life expectancy.

Fragile X

P X-linked recessive inheritance. Complex inheritance pattern based on the fragile site in the long arm of the X chromosome (CGG trinucleotide repeat expansion).

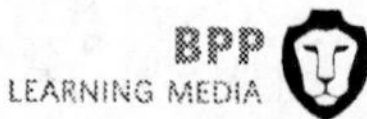

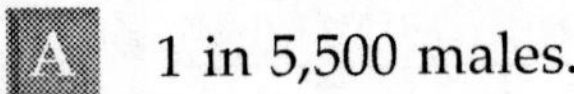

A 1 in 5,500 males.

S Sx See Box 24.16.

Typical features:	Increased incidence of:
Large everted ears Prominent mandible Large forehead Macro-orchidism Macroencephaly	Learning difficulties Seizures Autistic spectrum disorder Hyperactivity/repetitive behaviour

Box 24.16: Clinical features of fragile X

I None.

T Behavioural therapy and special education are often required.

Pr No effect on life expectancy.

Paediatric tumours

CNS tumours

P Brain tumours in children are mostly primary tumours. They rarely metastasise outside of the CNS.

S Sx Due to raised intracranial pressure: headache (worse in the morning), vomiting (worse in the morning), papilloedema, changes to personality / behaviour, squint (with VIth nerve plasy), nystagmus, ataxia, seizures, disturbance of speech.

I A CT or MRI scan is required to diagnose an intracranial tumour.

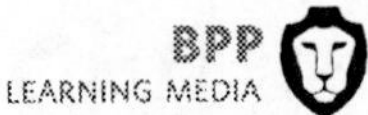

Type of CNS tumour	Details
Astrocytoma	Most common brain tumour in children (>40%). Range from low-grade, benign tumours (cerebellar) to high-grade malignant tumours (supratentorial/brainstem). Require surgical resection plus radiotherapy.
Medulloblastoma	20% of childhood brain tumours. Arise in the midline of the posterior fossa (causes ataxia). High-grade tumour. 20% have spinal metastases at diagnosis. Can metastasis outside the CNS. Require surgical resection, radiotherapy +/- chemotherapy. 50% five-year survival.
Brain stem glioma	20% of childhood brain tumours. Presents with cranial nerve palsies, ataxia and pyramidal tract sign (rarely presents with raised intracranial pressure). Radiotherapy is often palliative. Poor prognosis (<10% survival rate).
Craniopharyngioma	8% of childhood brain tumours. Located in suprasellar region / remnant of Rathke's pouch. Not truly malignant. Presents with raised ICP, visual field loss, pituitary dysfunction. Surgical excision +/- radiotherapy.

Table 24.9: Common types of intracranial tumours

Neuroblastoma

P Arises from the neural crest tissue and sympathetic nervous system.

S Most present with an abdominal mass of adrenal origin (but can lie anywhere along the sympathetic tract from the neck to the pelvis). Often a large mass, which crosses the midline.

Sx Bone pain (from metastases), weight loss and malaise.

I Urine reveals raised urinary catecholamine levels; biopsy.

T Surgical resection.

Chemotherapy and radiotherapy may be required for tumours that cannot be completely removed.

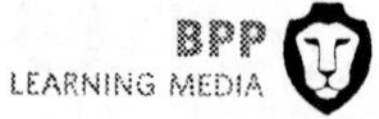

C Paravertebral tumours may cause spinal cord compression.

Pr Age and stage of disease at diagnosis are important prognostic factors. Presenting over 1 year of age is a poor prognostic factor.

Wilms' tumour

P Wilms' tumour (nephroblastoma) is a form of renal cancer which originates from the embryological renal tissue.

Most are unilateral (5% bilateral) and do not cross the midline of the abdomen as they are encapsulated.

A Most cases are sporadic. A Wilms' susceptibility gene has been identified which is associated with loss of genetic material from chromosome 11.

Sx Often asymptomatic, but may present with abdominal pain (from haemorrhage into the mass) or nausea / vomiting.

I USS and CT: identify a mass (claw sign).

Staging is also required to detect the presence of metastases (commonly to the lung).

T Nephrectomy is required, however for large masses, chemotherapy is initially required to reduce the size prior to surgery.

C Haemorrhage into the tumour may present as acute abdominal pain.

80% of cases are cured and there is a 90% five-year survival.

Pr Relapse is associated with a poor prognosis.

Rhabdomyosarcoma

P Rhabdomyosarcoma is a soft-tissue sarcoma arising from striated muscle cells.

A It is the most common soft tissue malignancy of childhood.

They can occur anywhere in the body, common sites are shown below (see Table 24.10).

S Sx Depend on the location of the tumour.

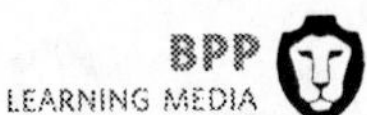

Location	Signs / symptoms
Head and neck	Proptosis Nasal obstruction Blood stained nasal discharge
Genitourinary	Dysuria Urinary outflow obstruction Bloodstained vaginal discharge
Metastatic disease	Dependent on site metastatic spread

Table 24.10: Location and signs / symptoms of rhabdomyosarcoma

T Initial treatment with six to nine courses of chemotherapy.

Surgery in cases where the tumour is excisable (usually following chemotherapy).

Radiotherapy may be required following surgery.

Pr Dependant on the extent of the disease, 70% in those with excisable tumours compared to <10% with bony metastases.

Retinoblastoma

P Retinoblastoma is a malignancy of the retinal cells of the eye.

A Retinoblastoma can be either hereditary or sporadic.

The hereditable form is due to the deletion of a tumour suppressor gene on chromosome 13.

S The two most common presentations of retinoblastoma are either a white papillary reflex (lack of the red reflex) or a squint.

Sx Retinoblastoma may be asymptomatic. In some cases there may be visual impairment.

I If a retinoblastoma is suspected, further imaging studies may include CT, MRI and ultrasound.

T Treatment options include surgery (enulceation of the eyeball), chemotherapy (via vessels in the groin through to the optic vessels), laser therapy or radiotherapy.

C Hereditary retinoblastoma carries a risk of a second primary malignancy (osteosarcoma being the most common).

Pr Most cases are cured with a 90% five-year survival.

Practice Questions

Single Best Answers

1. Which one of the following conditions presents with cyanosis?

   A Atrial septal defect
   B Ventricular septal defect
   C Patent ductus arteriosus
   D Tetralogy of Fallot

2. A 6-week-old infant presents with projectile vomiting after feeds. He is hungry after feeds. A gas shows a hypochloraemic hypokalaemic alkalosis. What is the likely cause?

   A Gastroenteritis
   B Gastroesophageal reflux
   C Pyloric stenosis
   D Cow's milk protein allergy

3. Which of the following is *not* a feature of Down's syndrome?

   A Hypotonia
   B Single palmar crease
   C Coarctation of the aorta
   D Low set ears

4. Which of the following is correct regarding undescended testes?

   A Are associated with a reduced risk of testicular malignancy
   B 20% descend in first year of life
   C Surgery is contraindicated in the neonatal period
   D 30% occur in premature babies

5. Concerning cerebral palsy

   A Aspiration pneumonia is a complication
   B All have learning difficulties
   C Birth asphyxia is the commonest cause
   D The athetoid form is the commonest form

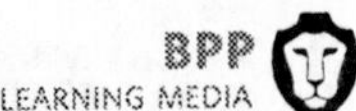

Extended Matching Questions

Developmental milestones in children

A 6 weeks
B 6 months
C 9 months
D 1 year
E 15 months
F 2 years
G 3 years
H 4 years

From the list above, select the age at which a normal child would be expected to do the following:

1. Walk steadily

2. Two syllable babble

3. Palmar grasp

4. Copy a circle

5. Sit unsupported

Neonatal jaundice

A Breast milk jaundice
B Biliary atresia
C ABO incompatibility
D Gilbert's syndrome
E Hereditary spherocytosis
F Congenital infection

From the list above, select the correct cause of neonatal jaundice in the following scenarios:

6. A 7-day-old baby was born at term by normal vaginal delivery. During a home visit the midwife notices that he appears jaundiced. He is a well baby and breastfeeding well.

7. A newborn baby was born at 39 weeks by normal vaginal delivery. At 12 hours of life the midwife notices she appears jaundiced. A blood gas shows a severe metabolic acidosis.

8. A 14-day-old baby has ongoing jaundice. Bloods show a conjugated hyperbilirubinaemia.

9. A 2-day-old baby attends A&E with a temperature of 38 degrees, not waking for feeds and jaundice.

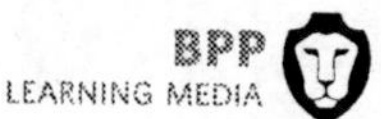

Respiratory conditions

A Croup
B Bronchiolitis
C Cystic fibrosis
D Epiglottitis
E Pertussis
F Foreign body
G Asthma

From the list above, select the cause of the following presentations:

10. A 6-month-old baby with coryzal symptoms for two days. She has difficulty in breathing and reduced feeding. On auscultation there are bilateral crackles heard.

11. A 2-year-old girl has a 12-hour history of coryzal symptoms, fever and a barking cough which is worse at night. She has an audible inspiratory stridor.

12. A 4-year-boy presents to A&E with a temperature, sore throat and difficulty in breathing. He is sat upright and noted to be drooling and unable to swallow his secretions.

13. A 1-year-old girl has a sudden onset of inspiratory stridor and difficulty in breathing. She has been otherwise well.

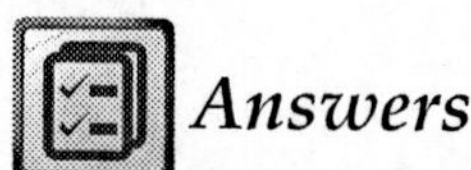

Answers

SBAs		EMQs	
1	D	1	E
2	C	2	C
3	C	3	B
4	D	4	G
5	A	5	B
		6	A
		7	C
		8	B
		9	F
		10	B
		11	A
		12	D
		13	F

Chapter 25

Psychiatry

Dr Philip Brooks

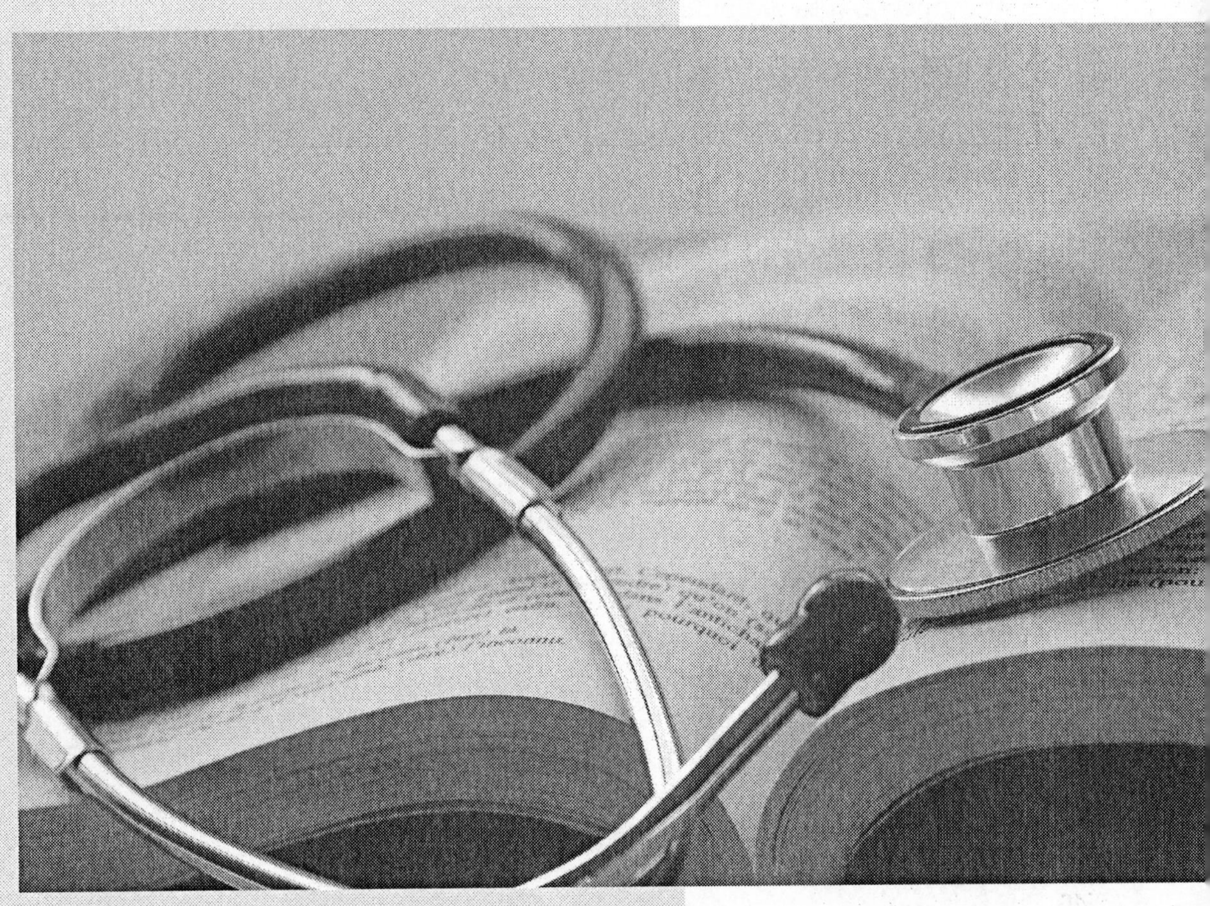

Mood disorders

Depression

P Two core symptoms for >2 weeks: low mood, anhedonia, loss of energy plus one other symptom.

A Lifetime prevalence 4.4%. M:F 1:2, high prevalence in low income groups.

Primary: genetic / environmental interplay or secondary.

- **Drugs**:
  - Anti-HTN: methyl-dopa, reserpine, propranolol, clonidine
  - Corticosteroids
  - Anti-malaria: chloroquine
  - ETOH
- **Endocrine**: hypothyroidism, Sheehan's syndrome
- **Neurological:** Parkinson's, post-stroke depression
- **Post-natal depression:** 25% of women after birth
- **Chronic diseases**: CRF, malignancies
- **Adverse life events**: bereavement, abuse, unemployment

Box 25.1: Secondary causes of depression

Sx *Cognitive:* anhedonia (core), guilt, reduced concentration, hopelessness, reduced self-esteem.

Biological: low mood (core), loss of energy (core), early morning waking, loss of appetite, loss of libido, reduced concentration.

I Depression score, FBC, TFTs.

T Lifestyle advice, CBT, anti-depressants (see below), ECT, suicide risk assessment.

C Major cause of low quality of life, DSH, suicide.

Mania

P State of abnormally elevated mood.

A Organic causes: infections, hyperthyroidism, SLE, thrombotic thromocytopenic purpura, stroke, ECT, drugs.

Part of bipolar disorder (see below).

Sx *Mood symptoms:* irritability, euphoria, lability.

Cognitive symptoms: grandiosity, flight of ideas, racing thoughts, distractibility, poor concentration, confusion.

Behavioural symptoms: hyperactivity, decreased sleep, rapid speech, hypersexuality, extravagance.

Psychotic symptoms: delusions, hallucinations.

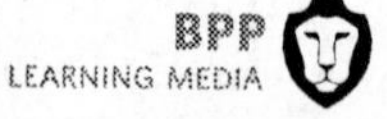

I Exclude organic symptoms.

T *Acute:* olanzapine, benzodiazepines.

Prophylaxis: mood stabiliser eg lithium.

C Hypomania: mildly elevated mood that does not interfere with ADLs.

90% of single manic episodes go on to develop bipolar disorder.

Bipolar disorder

P Repeated episodes of mania and depression with recovery in between.

A Risk to 1st degree relative 12%.

Sx Manic episodes last around three weeks, depressive episodes three to six months.

I Exclude organic cause.

T Mood stabiliser: lithium.

Neuroses

Anxiety disorders

P Abnormal psychiatric features without an organic psychiatric disorder.

Anxiety disorders are usually precipitated by stress.

A Genetic predisposition, stress, life events.

- Generalised anxiety disorder (GAD)
- Post-traumatic stress disorder
- Obsessive compulsive disorder (OCD)
- Panic disorder
- Agoraphobia
- Simple phobia
- Social phobia

Box 25.2: Types of anxiety disorders

Sx Tension, agitation, feelings of impending doom, insomnia, poor concentration, hyperventilation, headaches, sweating, palpitations, poor appetite, lump in the throat (globus hystericus), repetitive thoughts and activities.

I Clinical.

T CBT, graded exposure to anxiety provoking stimuli.

Anxiolytics eg diazepam, SSRI eg paroxetine.

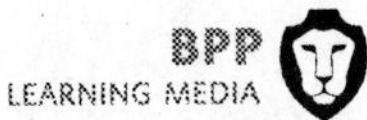

C Poor daily functioning.

Eating disorders

Anorexia

P Weight <85% of predicted by starvation, increased exercise or diet pills.

A Young females (10% male).

Sx Amenorrhoea, <85% body weight, fear of weight gain.

I FBC, U&Es, ECG.

T CBT, BMI <15kg/m^2 requires admission for re-feeding.

C Cardiac arrhythmias, nutritional deficiencies, re-feeding syndrome.

Pr 40% recover completely, 5% mortality.

Bulimia nervosa

P Recurrent episodes of binge eating characterised by uncontrolled overeating.

A Young females, higher prevalence in developed countries.

Sx Irregular menstruation, metabolic alkalosis, eroded dental enamel.

I FBC, U&Es, ECG.

T CBT, anti-depressants.

C Dental erosion, cardiac arrhythmias.

Pr 50% improve in ten years.

Psychoses

Schizophrenia

P Acute psychosis with hallucinations and thought disorder.

A Presents in early adult life, male = female, one-third single episode, one-third relapsing illness, one-third have progressive deterioration.

Sx *1st Rank symptoms*: Auditory hallucinations (3rd person), Broadcasting of thought, Controlled thoughts, Delusions.

Positive symptoms	Negative symptoms
• Hallucinations – auditory, visual • Delusions – paranoia, controlling, grandiose • Thought disorders – insertion, withdrawl, broadcasting, blocking, – 'Knight's-move thinking'	• Reduced speech • Flattened affect • Reduced energy • Low energy

Table 25.1: Schizophrenia symptoms

I Exclude organic cause.

T Atypical anti-psychotics: risperidone, olanzapine, clozapine lorazepam or haloperidol for sedation.

C Neuroleptic malignant syndrome.

	Typical (1st generation)	Atypical (2nd generation)
Drug	• Phenothiazines • Haloperidol	• Risperidone • Olanzapine • Clozapine • Quetiapine
Side effects	• Extrapyramidal • Neuroleptic malignant syndrome • Tachyarrhythmias	• Fewer SEs than typical. • Weight gain

Table 25.2: Anti-psychotics

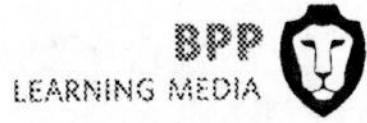

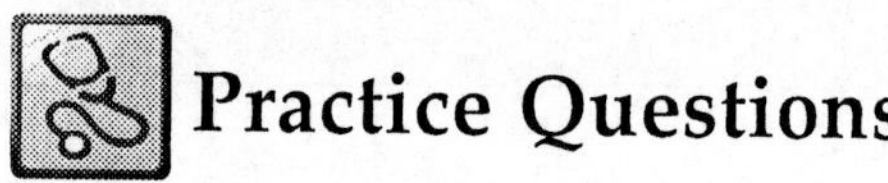

Practice Questions

Single Best Answers

1. Which of the following thoughts suggests depression?

   A 'Aliens are putting thoughts in my head'
   B 'TV sending me messages'
   C 'I'm dead inside'
   D 'I can save the world'

2. Which of the following is **not** an organic cause of depression?

   A Parkinson's disease
   B Hyperthyroid
   C Hypopituitary
   D Cushing's syndrome

3. Which of the following is true regarding anorexia nervosa?

   A It is typically associated with binge eating
   B It is associated with hyperalbuminaemia
   C It is always secondary to malignancy
   D It is associated with lethal cardiac complications

4. Select the most appropriate treatment for the corresponding overdose.

   A IV n-acetylcysteine (Parvolex) for paractemol
   B Disulfiram (Antabuse) for alcohol intoxication
   C Naloxone for benzodiazepine overdose
   D Gastric lavage for aspirin overdose

5. Deliberate self harm (DSH) is:

   A More common in young boys than girls
   B Includes attempted suicides
   C Reduces the risk of suicide
   D Usually requires admission

Extended Matching Questions

Symptoms and disease

A Mania
B Depression
C Schizophrenia
D Anxiety
E Bulimia nervosa

For each of the following situations choose the **single** most likely answer from the above list of options. Each option may be used once, more than once or not at all.

1. Overeating
2. 'Lump in throat'
3. Flight of ideas
4. Knight's move thinking
5. Loss of libido

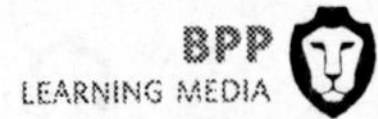

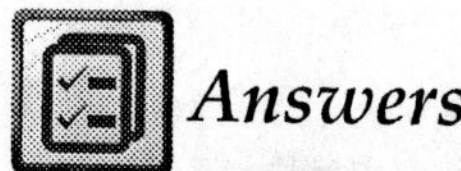

Answers

SBAs		EMQs	
1	C	1	E
2	B	2	D
3	D	3	A
4	A	4	C
5	B	5	B

Chapter 26

Statistics and epidemiology

Mr Alexander Young

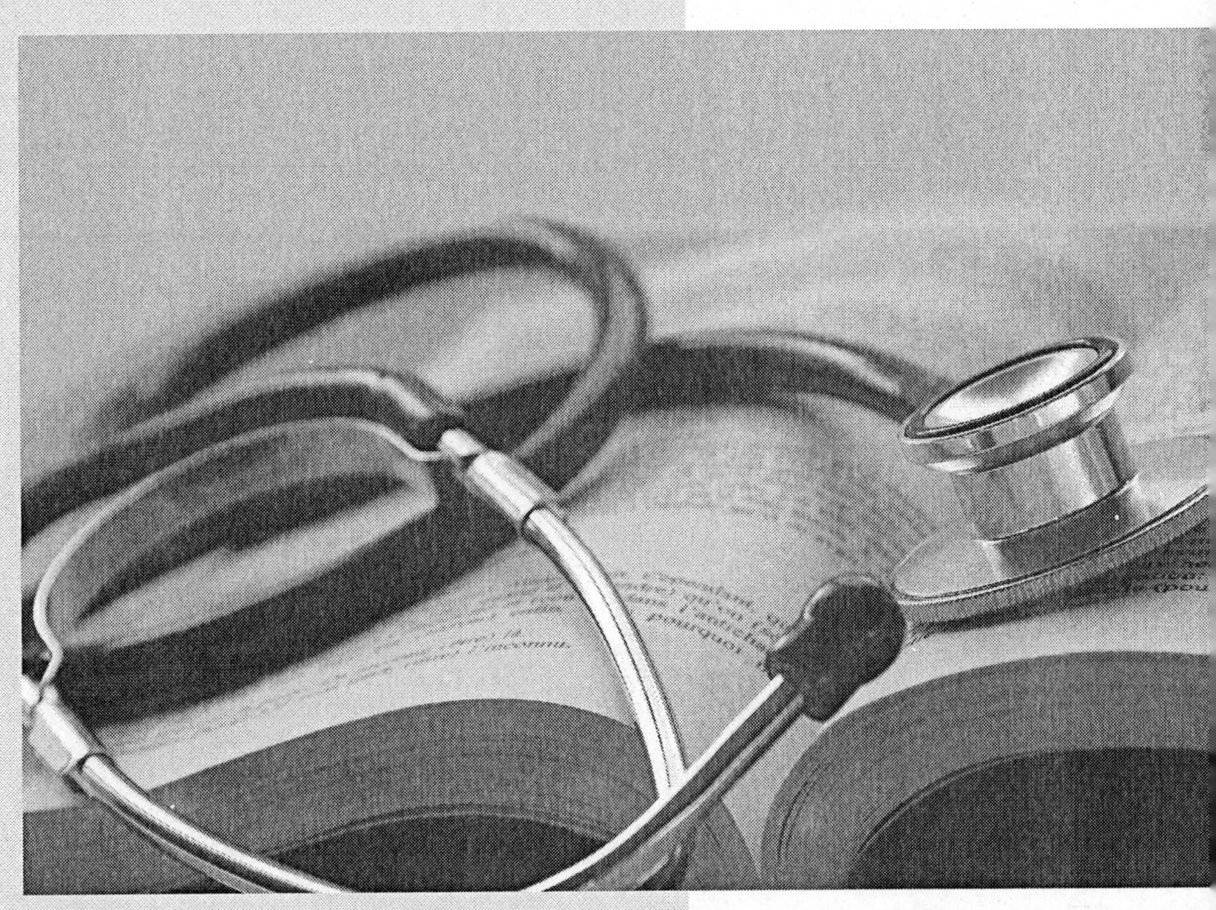

Terminology

- **Bias**: systematic flaw in data collection or interpretation resulting in erroneous results
  - *Selection bias:* study subjects selected do not accurately reflect the population at large
  - *Randomisation bias:* subjects are not truly randomised to intervention arms
  - *Funding bias*: data collection is influenced by funding received
  - *Lead time bias*: diagnosis of a condition earlier results in an apparent longer survival time
  - *Follow-up bias:* patients lost to follow up may reduce data reliability
  - *Interviewer bias:* an interviewer may ask different questions to different patients
  - *Interpretation bias:* researchers may analyse data to report a desired result
  - *Publication bias:* studies with a positive outcome are more likely to be published
- **Incidence**: number of new cases of a disease in a specified time period
- **Interquartile range**: the distribution between first and third quartile
- **Mean**: the average ie the sum of variable divided by the number
  - *Formula:* $(n_1 + n_2 + n_3 + n_{4...}) / n_{total}$
- **Median**: the mid point with 50% of variables above and 50% of variables below
  - *Formula:* $(n_{total} + 1) / 2$
- **Mode**: the most common variable
- **Number needed to treat**: number of people needing to receive a treatment for one person to benefit
- **Prevalence**: proportion of a population with a disease at a specific time
- **Range:** the distribution between maximum and minimum value
- **Relative risk**: risk of developing a disease in a population with an exposure compared to a population without an exposure
- **Standard deviation**: the distribution around the mean in a 'normally' distributed population

Tests

- **Sensitivity**: the percentage of people in a group with disease that will test positive
- **Specificity**: the percentage of people in a group without disease that will test negative
- **Positive Predictive Value (PPV)**: in a subject with a positive test the chance that they will actually have the disease
- **Negative Predictive Value (NPV)**: in a subject with a negative test the chance that they will not have the disease

	Condition positive	Condition negative	
Test positive	True positive (A)	False positive (C)	**PPV =** True positive (A) ÷ Test positive (A + C)
Test negative	False negative (B)	True negative (D)	**NPV =** True negative (D) ÷ Test negative (B + D)
	Sensitivity = True positive (A) ÷ Condition positive (A + B)	**Specificity =** True negative (D) ÷ Condition negative (C + D)	

Figure 26.1: Summary of tests

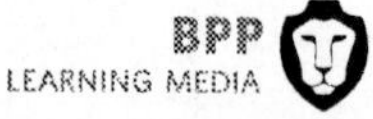

Hierarchy of evidence

The strength of a study depends on its design.

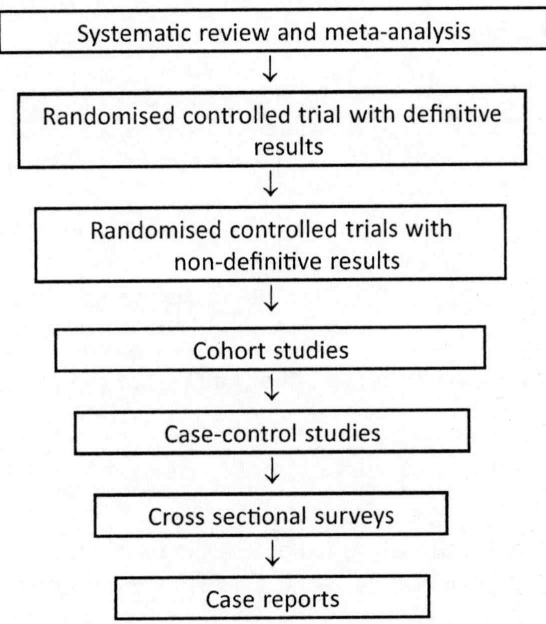

Figure 26.2: Hierarchy of evidence (decreasing in strength)

Randomised controlled trial (RCT)

- In RCT participants are randomly allocated to one intervention or another.
- Both groups are followed up for a specified period.
- Groups are analysed in terms of outcome defined at the outset.
- If groups are similar at outset any difference should be due to intervention.

Advantages of RCTs	Disadvantages of RCTs
Allows evaluation of a single variable in a defined patient group Potentially eradicates bias by comparing identical groups Allows for meta-analysis	Expensive and time-consuming Too few patients or too short a follow-up period Artificial endpoints may be used in preference to clinical outcome measures Randomisation bias

Table 26.1: Advantages and disadvantages of RCTs

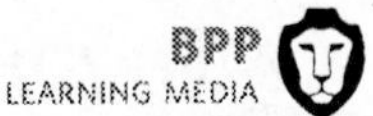

Cohort study

- Compares groups exposed to different factors
- Usually used to study disease aetiology or assess disease prognosis
- Followed up to see whether there is a difference in outcome

Advantages of cohort studies	Disadvantages of cohort studies
Allows direct incidence calculation	Inefficient for evaluating rare disease
Can reveal temporal relationship between exposure and disease	Losses to follow up can greatly impact results
Useful in rare exposures	Retrospective or prospective studies, dependent on notes and time respectively

Table 26.2: Advantages and disadvantages of control studies

Case-control study

- Case-control studies match patients with a disease to controls.
- Data is then collected retrospectively to find a difference between the groups.

Advantages of case-control studies	Disadvantages of case-control studies
Quick and inexpensive	Inefficient for evaluating rare exposures
Useful in rare disease	Inefficient in identifying temporal relationships
Can analyse multiple factors for a single disease	Unable to derive incidence
Useful over long time periods	

Table 26.3: Advantages and disadvantages of case-control studies

Index

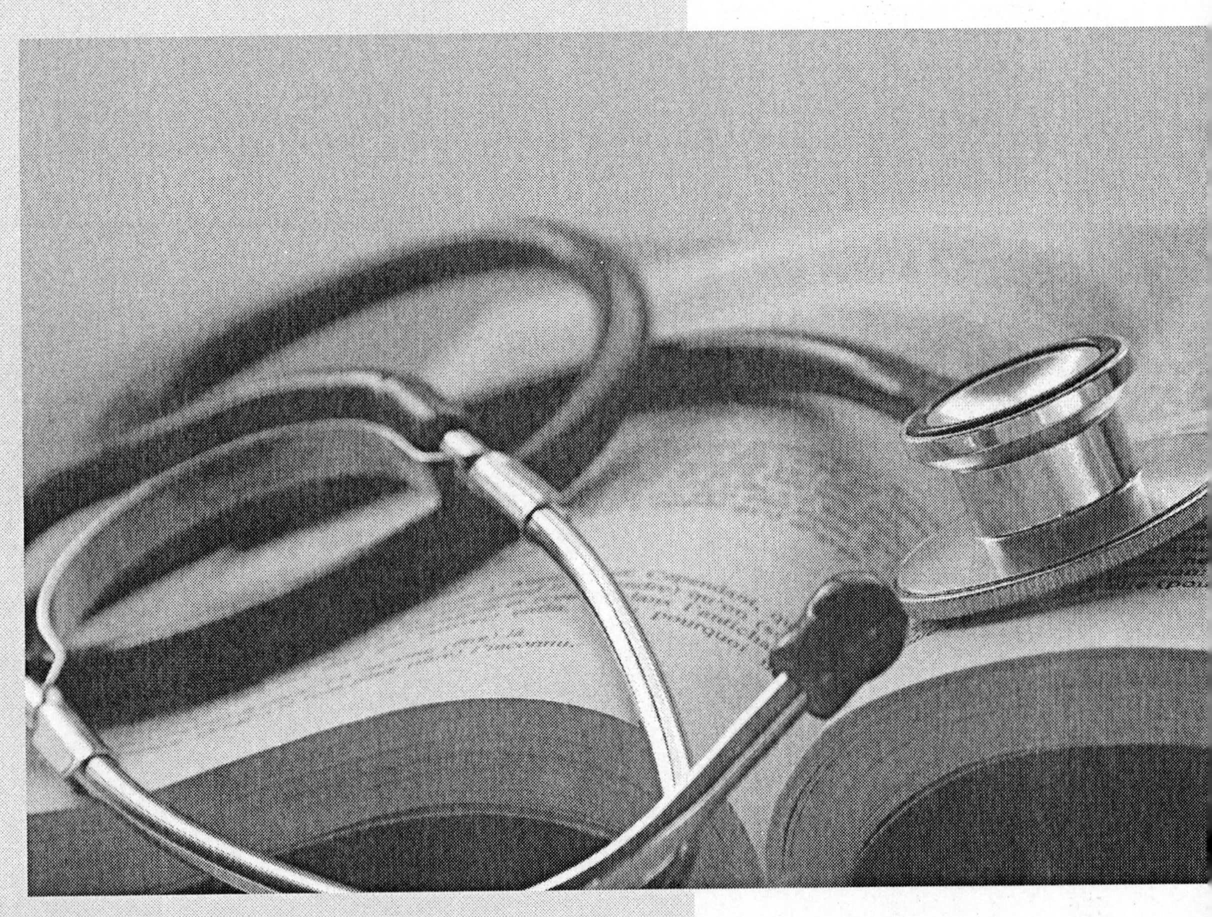

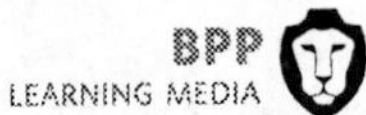
BPP
LEARNING MEDIA

B

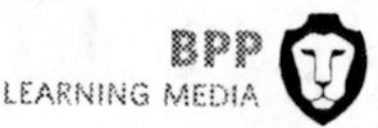

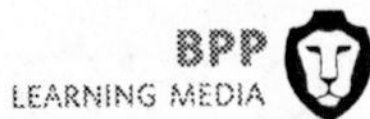
BPP
LEARNING MEDIA

D

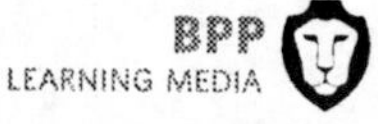

E

F

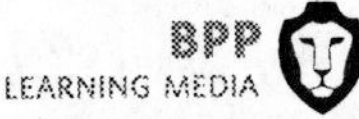

G

H

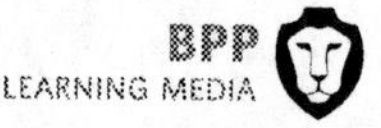

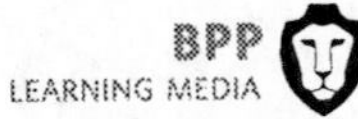
BPP
LEARNING MEDIA

N

O

P

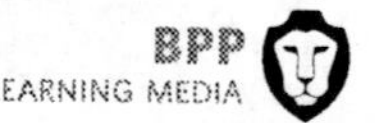

Q

R

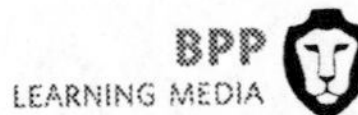

S

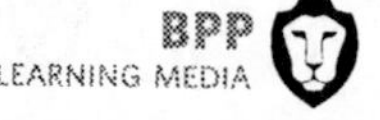

T

U

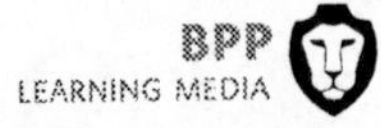

V

W

X

Z